www.bma.org.uk

OXFORD MEDICAL PUBLICATIONS

Oxford Handbook of Pre-Hospital Care

Published and forthcoming Oxford Handbooks

Oxford Handbook of Clinical Medicine 7/e
Oxford Handbook of Clinical Specialties 7/e
Oxford Handbook of Acute Medicine 2/e
Oxford Handbook of Anaesthesia 2/e
Oxford Handbook of Applied Dental Sciences
Oxford Handbook of Cardiology
Oxford Handbook of Clinical Dentistry 4/e
Oxford Handbook of Clinical and Laboratory Investigation 2/e
Oxford Handbook of Clinical Diagnosis
Oxford Handbook of Clinical Haematology 2/e
Oxford Handbook of Clinical Immunology and Allergy 2/e
Oxford Handbook of Clinical Pharmacy
Oxford Handbook of Clinical Surgery 2/e
Oxford Handbook of Critical Care 2/e
Oxford Handbook of Dental Patient Care 2/e
Oxford Handbook of Dialysis 2/e
Oxford Handbook of Emergency Medicine 3/e
Oxford Handbook of Endocrinology and Diabetes
Oxford Handbook of ENT and Head and Neck Surgery
Oxford Handbook for the Foundation Programme
Oxford Handbook of Gastroenterology and Hepatology
Oxford Handbook of General Practice 2/e
Oxford Handbook of Genitourinary Medicine, HIV and AIDS
Oxford Handbook of Geriatric Medicine
Oxford Handbook of Medical Sciences
Oxford Handbook of Nutrition and Dietetics
Oxford Handbook of Neurology
Oxford Handbook of Obstetrics and Gynaecology
Oxford Handbook of Oncology 2/e
Oxford Handbook of Ophthalmology
Oxford Handbook of Palliative Care
Oxford Handbook of Practical Drug Therapy
Oxford Handbook of Psychiatry
Oxford Handbook of Public Health Practice 2/e
Oxford Handbook of Rehabilitation Medicine
Oxford Handbook of Respiratory Medicine
Oxford Handbook of Rheumatology 2/e
Oxford Handbook of Tropical Medicine 2/e
Oxford Handbook of Urology

Oxford Handbook of Pre-Hospital Care

Ian Greaves
Visiting Professor of Emergency Medicine
University of Teesside, UK;
Consultant in Emergency Medicine
British Army

and

Keith Porter
Professor of Clinical Traumatology
University Hospital
Birmingham, UK

OXFORD
UNIVERSITY PRESS

OXFORD
UNIVERSITY PRESS
Great Clarendon Street, Oxford OX2 6DP

Oxford University Press is a department of the University of Oxford.
It furthers the University's objective of excellence in research, scholarship, and education by publishing worldwide in

Oxford New York

Auckland Cape Town Dar es Salaam Hong Kong Karachi
Kuala Lumpur Madrid Melbourne Mexico City Nairobi
New Delhi Shanghai Taipei Toronto

With offices in

Argentina Austria Brazil Chile Czech Republic France Greece
Guatemala Hungary Italy Japan Poland Portugal Singapore
South Korea Switzerland Thailand Turkey Ukraine Vietnam

Published in the United States
by Oxford University Press, Inc., New York

First published 2007
Reprinted in 2009, 2011 (with corrections), 2012

British Library Cataloguing in Publication Data
Data available

Library of Congress Cataloging in Publication Data
Data available

Typeset by Newgen Imaging Systems (P) Ltd., Chennai, India
Printed in China
on acid-free paper through
Asia Pacific Offset

ISBN 978–0–19–851584–5 (flexicover: alk. paper)

10 9 8 7 6

Foreword

By Rudy Crawford

There have been many changes in clinical medicine and in the UK National Health Service since the publication of *Pre-Hospital Medicine: The Principles and Practice of Immediate Care*, in 1999.[1] Advances in the treatment of cardiac emergencies have moved time critical interventions such as thrombolysis for acute myocardial infarction to the prehospital arena, while in-hospital primary percutaneous coronary intervention is increasingly the treatment of choice in hospitals for patients with acute coronary syndromes. The introduction of thrombolysis for acute ischaemic stroke (brain attack) is a time critical treatment that places further pressure on pre-hospital practitioners involved in the care of patients with acute cerebrovascular emergencies. These developments have increasing implications for those involved in pre-hospital care, which is the first step in the process of care for the acutely ill and injured. In addition, changes in primary care have resulted in many general practitioners no longer providing 24-hour care. This has left a gap in health-care provision, which is driving the development of the role of existing pre-hospital care providers to include activities previously undertaken by medical practitioners only, and is introducing new roles, such as the emergency care practitioner, to fill the unmet need for out-of-hours care.

The rapidity of National Health Service reform means that most of these changes are being introduced without any clinical evidence base to support their effectiveness or appropriateness. There has been very little research done to demonstrate the value of advanced pre-hospital care, although there is some evidence in the area of basic life support and defibrillation. Consequently, defibrillation has moved from being an advanced life support technique to a basic one and volunteer first aiders and other lay people have been trained in its use with additional lives being saved. In the past ten years, the Faculty of Pre-hospital Care has become firmly established as the authoritative body in the field of pre-hospital care, both setting and raising standards and supporting research to provide a firm evidence base for what we do.

Pre-hospital care is becoming increasingly specialized and may eventually be recognized as a separate subspecialty within Emergency Medicine. Nowadays, practitioners who are committed to pre-hospital care not only have to be competent in dealing with individual casualties in an environment that brings unique challenges, but also increasingly have to be able to respond effectively to civil emergencies involving mass casualties or terrorist threats which include bomb, chemical, biological, radiological, or nuclear threats. The Faculty has developed a structured training and examination syllabus which is open to medical and non-medical practitioners.

1 Greaves I and KM Porter (eds) (1999). *Pre-Hospital Medicine: The Principles and Practice of Immediate Care*. Arnold, London.

Membership of the Faculty is open to nurses, ambulance service staff, and voluntary aid society members as well as medical practitioners, reflecting the Faculty's commitment to improving pre-hospital care across the whole spectrum of practice and encouraging a multidisciplinary app-roach. The authors are prominent members of the Faculty and serve on its Board of Management. This comprehensive book deals with all aspects of pre-hospital care in a pragmatic down to earth style, which encompasses best practice and is also underpinned by the currently available research evidence. The discerning reader will find numerous pearls which will be relevant to them as doctors, nurses, paramedics, and voluntary aid society members alike.

Rudy Crawford
MBE BSc (Hons) MB ChB FRCS (Glasg) FCEM
Consultant in Accident and
Emergency Medicine and Surgery
Glasgow Royal Infirmary and Chairman
St Andrew's Ambulance Association
September 2006

Foreword

By Fionna Moore

The publication of an Oxford Handbook has to be a defining moment in the recognition of the specialty of Pre-hospital Care, which has existed, often unsung and practiced by a relatively small number of enthusiasts, for many years. This handbook joins a comprehensive list of publications covering almost forty very diverse specialities. It is perhaps unique in that it covers an area which is increasingly recognized as a vital part in the continuum of patient care, even by doctors who still treat patients as if they had collapsed or received injuries just outside the doors of the Emergency Department. It is an area of care often practiced in difficult circumstances when compared to hospital medicine, with a sometimes inadequate history, poor lighting, inclement weather, hostile conditions, and limited assistance, both in terms of personnel and equipment.

Pre-hospital care is an environment well known to ambulance services, historically regarded as the health arm of the emergency services but increasingly regarded as the emergency arm of the health service. With increasing integration between primary and secondary care ambulance staff and other pre-hospital care practitioners have opportunities to assume even greater responsibility for delivering care outside hospital, as highlighted within the recent Ambulance Service Review *Taking Health-care to the Patient.*[1]

The emphasis of the specialty has changed from having a purely trauma focus to include all the conditions which might present to the pre-hospital practitioner. The concept of such a practitioner is an inclusive one covering individuals from a medical, nursing or paramedic background, whether working for an Immediate Care scheme, for the Armed Services or an ambulance service, whether from the statutory, private, or voluntary sector. The settings include primary care emergencies, sporting and mass gathering events but also cover the less common but very challenging areas of CBRN and major incident management The conditions covered include not only those commonly dealt with in the emergency hospital setting, such as acute medical, surgical, and trauma emergencies, paediatrics, obstetrics, and gynaecology but also the less common and unique pre-hospital areas of mass gatherings and sporting events.

Given the variety of clinical settings that may arise, many of the existing sources of written advice are too large and unwieldy to be of much help in the emergency setting. Hospital doctors are very familiar with the assistance afforded by the small, easily referenced and robust handbook which is small enough to fit in the pocket of a white coat, the Emergency Department scrubs, or to keep nearby the phone. This Handbook will fill an important role both as an educational tool well as an aide-memoire when the practitioner might most need it. This is due to the authors

1 Department of Health (2005). *Taking healthcare to the patient: Transforming NHS ambulance services*. DH, London.

being well known within the pre-hospital care community, being at the leading edge of pre-hospital training and education, and having immense credibility through their practical day-to-day involvement in the specialty. With its succinct style, comprehensive contents, and practical advice, this book will find its way into the Hi Viz jacket pockets, Thomas packs, and the vehicles of pre-hospital practitioners. It will be an invaluable quick reference guide both in the emergency setting, for those in training within the specialty and those working towards the Diploma and Fellowship examinations set by the Faulty of Pre-hospital Care.

Fionna Moore
Medical Director
London Ambulance Service
September 2006

Contents

Note: the content of individual chapters is detailed on each chapter's first page

Abbreviations

AAA	abdominal aortic aneurysm
ac	alternating current
ACCOLC	access overload control
ACE	angiotensin converting enzyme
ADI	acute decompression illness
A&E	accident and emergency
AED	automated external defibrillator
AF	atrial fibrillation
AIS	abbreviated injury scale
ALS	advance life support
ALSO	advanced life support obstetrics
AOC	air operations centre
AP	anteroposterior
APLS	advanced paediatric life support
ARDS	acute respiratory distress syndrome
ATLS	advance trauma life support
AV	atrioventricular
AVLS	automatic vehicle location system
AVNRT	AV nodal re-entrant tachycardia
BA	biological agent
BASICS	British Association for Immediate Care
BLS	basic life support
BP	blood pressure
BTLS	basic trauma life support
CAA	Civil Aviation Authority
CAD	computer aided dispatch
CBRN	chemical, biological, radiological, and nuclear
CCS	casualty clearing station
cm	centimetre
COPD	chronic obstructive pulmonary disease
CPP	cerebral perfusion pressure
CPR	cardiopulmonary resuscitation
CSF	cerebrospinal fluid
CVA	cerebrovascular accident
DAI	diffuse axonal injury

dc	direct current
DipIMC	Diploma in Immediate Medical Care
DKA	diabetic ketoacidosis
DNR	do not resuscitate
DVT	deep vein thrombosis
ECG	electrocardiogram
EMD	electromechanical association
EMJ	*Emergency Medicine Journal*
EPO	emergency planning officer
ERL	emergency reference level
ET	endotracheal
FIMC	Fellowship in Immediate Medical Care
FPOS	first person on scene
GCS	Glasgow Coma Scale
GTN	Glycerol trinitrate
HAZCHEM	hazardous chemical
HAZMAT	hazardous material
HEMS	helicopter emergency medical service
hr	hour
ICP	intercranial pressure
IHCD	Institute for Health Care Development
IHD	ischaemic heart disease
ILMA	intubating laryngeal mask airway
im	intramuscular
iv	intravenous
JRCALC	Joint Royal Colleges Ambulance Liaison Committee
JVP	jugular venous pressure
kg	kilogram
l	litre
LMA	laryngeal mask airway
LSD	lysergic acid diethylamide
m	metre
MAC	military aid to the civil powers
MAOI	monoamine oxidase inhibitor
MAP	mean arterial pressure
MCA	Maritime and Coastguard Agency
mcg	microgram
MDI	metered dose inhaler
mg	milligram
MI	myocardial infarction
MICP	mean intracranial pressure

MIMMS	major incident medical management and support
min	minutes
ml	millilitres
mm	millimetres
MRCC	Maritime Rescue Co-ordination Centres
MRSC	Maritime Rescue Sub-centres
NAIR	National Arrangements for Incidents involving Radioactivity
NPIS	National Poisons Information Service
NRPB	National Radiological Protection Board
NSAID	non-steroidal anti-inflammatory drug
ORCON	operational research consultantancy
PASG	pneumatic antishock garment
PCI	percutaneous coronary intervention
PE	pulmonary embolism
PEA	pulseless electrical activity
PEFR	peak expiratory flow rate
PEPP	paediatrics for pre-hospital professionals
PHEC	pre-hospital emergency care
PHPLS	pre-hospital paediatric life support
PHTC	pre-hospital trauma course
PHTLS	pre-hospital trauma life support
PPE	personal protective equipment
PR	per rectum
PTS	paediatric trauma score
RCSEd	Royal College of Surgeons of Edinburgh
RED	Russell extrication device
RICE	rest, ice, compression, and elevation
RNLI	Royal National Lifeboat Institution
RSI	rapid sequence induction
RTC	road traffic collision
RTS	revised trauma score
RVP	rendezvous point
SAH	subarachnoid haemorrhage
sc	subcutaneous
sec/s	second/s
SIDS	sudden infant death syndrome
SSRI	selective serotonin reuptake inhibitors
stat	immediately
SVT	supra ventricular tachycardia
TCA	tricyclic antidepressant
tds	three times daily

TED	Telford extrication device
TIA	transient ischaemic attack
TREM	transport emergency
TRISS	trauma score – injury severity score
v	volts
VF	ventricular fibrillation
VT	ventricular tachycardia
WRVS	Women's Royal Voluntary Service

Chapter 1

An approach to pre-hospital care

Why bother?

There are very few prospective randomized clinical studies proving the value of immediate medical care and its impact on morbidity and mortality. Whilst there are reported series on the value of pre-hospital basic life support and defibrillation, there are very few reports relating to trauma. Yet many people continue to sacrifice their free time to provide medical care everywhere from racecourses to oil rigs, from country cottages to tower blocks. Every active immediate care doctor can recount an incident where a life was saved or a tragic future avoided by early acute medical intervention at scene. Whether the life-saving intervention is the establishment of a patent airway, the splintage of a shattered pelvis, the rapid extrication of an entrapped patient, or defibrillation of a VF arrest, we can all recollect an incident where being there *did* make a difference. In addition, although in many cases intervention alters neither long-term morbidity nor mortality, there can be no doubt that it greatly improves the patient's comfort and confidence, thereby making a potentially dreadful experience slightly less so.

For all these reasons, pre-hospital care is supremely worth doing. It is also a hugely challenging (and sometimes frustrating) speciality which demands a great deal of its practitioners. Despite the difficult situations in which it is practiced, there can be no excuse for anything but the highest professionalism. '*Better than nothing*' is no justification for getting involved: the keys to effective pre-hospital care are education, practice, experience, and revalidation—and enthusiasm. These are the keys to one of the most challenging branches of modern medicine.

IG
KP
North Yorkshire, 2006

Getting started

Like any other subject, the secret of success in pre-hospital care is preparation. This chapter will help anyone beginning to work in the pre-hospital care environment. Having acquired the interest and enthusiasm, attention must be given to the following:

- Training
- Reading
- Equipment
  - Personal
  - Medical
- Transport
- Insurance
- Joining a scheme
- Validation (and revalidation).

Each of these subjects is discussed in this chapter.

Training and education

As in any other branch of medicine, appropriate training is essential. Experience is important, but knowing how to 'do it right' is crucial. The Faculty of Pre-hospital Care of the Royal College of Surgeons of Edinburgh, BASICS (the British Association for Immediate Care), and BASICS Scotland organize or accredit a range of courses (for contact details see p.66). These courses are designed to be relevant to a wide range of different professional backgrounds and skill levels.

Pre-hospital Emergency Care (PHEC)

The three-day *Pre-hospital Emergency Care* course and certificate is organized jointly by BASICS, BASICS Scotland, and the Faculty of Pre-hospital Care of the Royal College of Surgeons of Edinburgh. Advice regarding the content of the course is also taken from ambulance service representatives and representatives of the Royal College of Nursing.

This course is open to anyone who may be called upon to deal with emergency situations including general practitioners, practice nurses, emergency services personnel, paramedics, voluntary aid society members, and those involved in sports medicine. Successful completion of the course and end-of-course assessment leads to the awarding of the PHEC certificate.

The course covers all aspects of emergency care in a pre-hospital setting in relation to adults concentrating on medical and trauma emergencies with an introduction to paediatric emergencies and trauma and major incident management. Course details can be obtained from BASICS Education or BASICS Scotland (see p.66).

First Person on Scene (FPOS)

The *First Person on Scene* awards have been developed by the Institute for Health Care Development (IHCD) and the Faculty of Pre-hospital Care. Two awards are currently available:

- First Person on Scene (Basic)—10 hours' training (including assessments).
- First Person on Scene (Intermediate)—30 hours' training (including assessments).

The content of the two levels is designed to reflect how long responders are likely to have to deal with a patient before the arrival of an ambulance. For the Basic Award this is up to 20 minutes; for the Intermediate Award, up to 40 minutes. Additional skills can be added to both levels of award to accommodate specific responder requirements.

To achieve the FPOS award (at either level) both knowledge and practical assessments have to be successfully completed. Questions are selected from central question banks and training can only be delivered at IHCD accredited centres. Clinical endorsement of the FPOS awards, assessment, and training support materials are the responsibility of the Faculty of Pre-hospital Care. Further information is available from Edexcel or the Faculty of Pre-hospital Care (see p.66).

Pre-hospital Trauma Course (PHTC)

This is a two-day course with 19 hours of highly practical educational activity. Topics include scene safety, triage, clinical assessment, and treatment. There is an emphasis on entrapment and extrication. Candidates are individually assessed on the practical aspects of pre-hospital trauma care. Further information is available from the Faculty of Pre-hospital Care (see p.66) or from *www.basics.org.uk*

Basic Trauma Life Support (BTLS)

Basic Trauma Life Support courses were developed in the USA. BTLS aims to provide pre-hospital responders with a structured approach to the rapid assessment, appropriate treatment, and evacuation of injured patients. The 'advanced' version of the course is aimed at paramedics and other advanced-level providers (such as trauma nurses) permitted to provide invasive treatment. There is also a 'basic' course, aimed at providers of pre-hospital care such as ambulance technicians and fire-fighters, which is limited to non-invasive skills. Both versions of the course are 16 hours in duration and are endorsed by the American College of Emergency Physicians and the (USA) National Association of Emergency Medical Services Physicians. Contact details of BTLS chapters that run courses worldwide (including the UK) can be found at *www.btls.org/organ/chapters.htm*

Pre-hospital Trauma Life Support (PHTLS)

Pre-hospital Trauma Life Support training was also developed in the USA and, like BTLS, offers basic and advanced courses, each of two days' duration and aimed at similar audiences. The USA National Association of Emergency Medical Technicians oversees PHTLS in conjunction with the Committee on Trauma of the American College of Surgeons. The courses have similar aims to BTLS, providing a structured approach for the rapid identification, treatment, and extrication of time-critical trauma patients. The strategies taught are designed to integrate with the Advanced Trauma Life Support (ATLS) approach to trauma management, facilitating seamless care between the pre-hospital and emergency department settings. In the UK, PHTLS courses are accredited by the Royal College of Surgeons of England. Details of courses run in the UK can be obtained from *www.rcseng.ac.uk*

Pre-hospital Paediatric Life Support (PHPLS)

Pre-hospital Paediatric Life Support aims to provide paramedics, nurses, and doctors with the skills to identify and manage seriously ill and injured children in the pre-hospital setting. Although its content is strongly allied to the Advanced Paediatric Life Support (APLS) course, it differs in addressing the practical restrictions on treatment in the out-of-hospital setting and stresses the importance of identifying patients requiring early and rapid transport to hospital. The course is accredited by the UK Advanced Life Support Group and details can be obtained from *www.alsg.org/main_paed_resus.htm*

Paediatrics for Pre-hospital Professionals (PEPP)

Paediatrics for Pre-hospital Professionals was developed in the USA by the American Academy of Pediatrics and is offered in two-day 'advanced' and one-day 'basic' versions, the former being aimed at paramedics, doctors, and nurses. Training may also be delivered on a modular basis. The aims of PEPP are similar to those of PHPLS, although at the time of writing PEPP is yet to be Anglicized and is not directly accredited by a UK professional body. Courses are currently run by BASICS (see p.66). Details of the PEPP programme can be found at *www.peppsite.com*

Advanced Life Support (ALS)

Advanced Life Support is a UK-developed Europe-wide course which teaches the management of cardiac arrest and peri-arrest arrhythmias, including the skills of manual defibrillation, drug administration, and endotracheal intubation. It is aimed at doctors, nurses, and paramedics and, whilst it emphasizes in-hospital care, the principles taught may be easily adapted to an out-of-hospital setting. Details of courses can be obtained from *www.resus.org.uk/pages/alsinfo.htm*

Advanced Life Support Obstetrics (ALSO)

Advanced Life Support Obstetrics aims to teach advanced providers who may be involved in emergency obstetric care. Although based on in-hospital scenarios, the principles taught may be adapted for use in an out-of-hospital setting. Details of courses can be found at *www.also.org.uk/providercourses.asp*

Madingley Immediate Care Course

Run by BASICS Education, this five-day course is primarily for those with experience in immediate care and has the aim of developing and enhancing their skills in dealing with medical and other emergencies encountered in all fields of pre-hospital medicine. The course is an effective preparation for the Diploma in Immediate Care Examination. Contact: BASICS Education (see p.66).

Major Incident Medical Management and Support (MIMMS)

Developed by the Advanced Life Support Group, the MIMMS course is now internationally accepted as the standard training programme for all those likely to be involved in the medical management of a major incident. The three-day course consists of two days of lectures, tabletop exercises, and practical skill stations such as radio voice procedure and triage. This is followed by a written and practical assessment. The final day consists of two major incident exercises, each based at a location near the course venue which might be considered at risk of a real major incident. These venues have included football grounds, industrial plants, and transport facilities. A one-day 'introductory' MIMMS course and a specialist chemical incident course are also now available. Contact: Advanced Life Support Group (see p.66).

Diploma in Immediate Care Preparation Course

This intensive five-day course for the Diploma in Immediate Care is run by the Department of Academic Emergency Medicine of the University of Teesside at the James Cook University Hospital Middlesbrough. It is designed to prepare candidates for the diploma examination. Contact *www.teessideEM.org.uk* for details or see p.67.

A similar course is offered by the West Midlands CARE Team based in Birmingham (details from *www.wmcareteam.org.uk* or from the Faculty of Pre-hospital Care).

Qualifications in pre-hospital care

Diploma in Immediate Medical Care (DipIMC.RCSEd)

In addition to the courses listed above, those who intend a serious and long-term commitment to pre-hospital care should consider taking the *Diploma in Immediate Medical Care* run by the Royal College of Surgeons of Edinburgh. Indeed, in certain areas of professional pre-hospital practice, such as medical support at league football matches, possession of the diploma is mandatory. The diploma is open to doctors, nurses, and registered paramedics (including those holding the highest level of military paramedic qualification).

Entry requirements

Paramedics

Any paramedic wishing to take the Diploma in Immediate Medical Care must show evidence of state registration as a paramedic in the UK (or non-NHS equivalent). Alternatives, such as armed services training, may be recognized by the Royal College. Candidates must show documented evidence of clinical experience in the area of pre-hospital care for a period of 18 months post registration.

Nurses

Nurses must hold registration with the Nursing and Midwifery Council (or its equivalent) and must have been engaged in the practice of their profession for not less than two years thereafter. They must also show documented evidence of clinical experience in pre-hospital emergency care for a period of at least one year and of completion of training of not less than three months in hospital posts approved by the College, including emergency medicine.

Doctors

Doctors must have been engaged in the practice of their profession for not less than two years after registration. Candidates must show documented evidence of clinical experience in the field of pre-hospital emergency care for a period of one year. They must also show evidence of completion of training of not less than three months full time or equivalent part time in hospital posts approved by the College in the management of the seriously ill or injured patient. This may include participation in a vocational training scheme.

Candidates who do not fulfil the normal requirements may apply for special consideration. Such candidates should submit details of their experience and a CV and will be considered by the Education Committee of the Faculty of Pre-hospital Care.

Examination format

The examination consists of:

- A theoretical paper with the following sections:
  - A projected material paper (30 minutes)
  - Multiple-choice question paper (20 questions, 20 minutes)
  - Short answer question paper (6 questions, 30 minutes)
  - Written incident scenario exercise (15 minutes).

- A practical examination consisting of:
  - Core skills assessment (30 minutes)
  - Clinical incident scenario and viva examination (30 minutes).

Candidates who fail the core skills assessment cannot pass the examination.

Further details about the Diploma are available from the Examinations Department of the Royal College of Surgeons of Edinburgh (see p.67).

Fellowship in Immediate Medical Care (FIMC.RCSEd)

The FIMC is open to medical practitioners who have successfully obtained the Diploma in Immediate Medical Care, have at least 4 years' pre-hospital experience, and have completed a training programme in pre-hospital care which has been approved by the Faculty of Pre-hospital Care.

It is first necessary to register an application in order to gain acceptance onto the training programme and to allow the development of a structured programme supervised by a mentor appointed by the Faculty. In the UK, the mentor may, for example, be the medical director of the local ambulance service NHS trust.

During the training programme, each candidate is required to show involvement in the following areas of pre-hospital care:

- Operational experience
- Analysis and audit
- Research activity
- Clinical governance issues
- Major incident management
- Mass-gathering medicine
- Teaching.

These areas, along with three case studies, will form a portfolio of experience and training which must be kept up to date and will be inspected during the FIMC examination.

Examination format

The examination consists of the following components:

- Written examination:
  - Projected material
  - Multiple-choice questions
  - Short answer questions
  - Incident scenario.
- Clinical examination:
  - Core skills
  - Medical skills
  - Trauma skills
  - Major incident scenario.

In addition, there is a viva based on the candidate's personal portfolio of experience case reports and special interests.

It is recognized that non-UK trainees may not follow a conventional UK career progression. This will be taken into consideration in respect of both the training period and the examination.

Further details regarding the FIMC examination may be obtained from the Examinations Department of the Royal College of Surgeons of Edinburgh (see p.67).

Accreditation and re-accreditation

For doctors practising in the UK, the basic accreditation standard is possession of the Pre-hospital Emergency Care (PHEC) Diploma and verification undertaken *by* BASICS. The PHEC certificate is valid for three years and an update one-day course secures re-accreditation.

Medical equipment

The medical equipment carried by an immediate care practitioner is a matter of personal choice and will depend on the skill level of the practitioner, the situations that are likely to be encountered, and the equipment which is likely to be readily available from other sources. There are, however, a number of key principles which must always be followed:

- Only use equipment with which you are thoroughly familiar.
- Only use equipment which is compatible with the emergency services equipment.
- Make sure you are familiar with specialist equipment carried by the emergency services.
- Ensure that equipment is regularly maintained and out-of-date disposables are replaced.
- Ensure that equipment is securely stored.
- Ensure that the packaging is robust and appropriate.

Choice of equipment

A suggested list of basic and advanced equipment is given in Table 1.1 Individual items are discussed using the ABC sequence. The notes that follow do not refer to every individual piece of equipment but are designed to highlight particular points with regard to pre-hospital practice.

Table 1.1 Suggested pre-hospital care equipment

Airway
Hand-operated suction unit
Yankauer suction catheters
Oropharyngeal airways 00–4
Nasopharyngeal airways sizes 6, 7, 8 (with safety pins)
Laryngeal mask airways (single use) 3, 4, 5
Laryngoscope handle, size 3 Mackintosh blade
Spare batteries and bulb for laryngoscope
Magill's forceps
Gum elastic bougie
Lubricating jelly
50ml syringe for cuff inflation
Set of cuffed (uncut) endotracheal tubes with connectors
Tape and ties for securing tubes
Pulse oximeter
End-tidal CO_2 monitor
Cervical spine control
Set of semi-rigid collars*
Breathing
Oxygen cylinder and reservoir/flow control
Oxygen tubing
Oxygen mask with reservoir (trauma/Hudson mask)
Controlled flow oxygen masks
Oxygen-powered nebulizer
Pocket resuscitation mask with one-way valve and oxygen port
Bag valve mask with oxygen reservoir
Flexible catheter mount connector
Wide-bore IV cannula (for needle thoracocentesis)
Asherman® chest seal
Circulation
Wound packs
Pressure dressings
Cling film
IV blood-giving sets
IV fluids
IV cannulae (range of sizes)
Tourniquet (arterial)
Tourniquet (vascular access)
IV dressings and tape
IV arm immobilizing splint
Specimen and X-match tubes and labels
Intraosseous needles
Three-way tap and extension tube
Syringes and needles
Alcohol swabs

Table 1.1 (*Contd.*)

Diagnostic pouch
Stethoscope
Pen torch
Sphygmomanometer
Blood glucose analyser
Peak flow meter
Reference charts
Drug pouch
See pp.307–58.
Paediatric equipment
Paediatric equipment is best packed separately but in the same sequence as adult equipment
Child sizes of ABC kit
Paediatric sizing and dosage guides
Miscellaneous
Plastic gloves
Tough cut scissors
Sharps bin
Triage cards and triage count check sheet
Ancillary equipment
Defibrillator/monitor with manual override and ECG data recorder
Defibrillation pads, electrodes, razor
12-lead ECG machine
Portable ventilator
Additional oxygen cylinders
Entonox apparatus
Fluid warmer/IV insulation jacket
Pressure infuser
Immobilization equipment
Rescue board (as appropriate)
Straps
Extrication device (as appropriate)
Limb splintage
Traction splintage
Maternity/delivery pack (as appropriate)
Plastic ground sheet
Blankets
Plastic waste bags

* Adjustable collars may be used, but provision must be made for all sizes from paediatric to adult.

Large items (e.g. trolley cots, vacuum mattresses) will be carried by the ambulance service.

Airway

Endotracheal (ET) tubes

ET tubes should not be pre-cut to length in case nasal intubation is required.

Laryngeal mask airway (LMA)

The LMA does not offer the same degree of airway protection as a cuffed ET tube, but is easier to insert and skill retention appears to be longer for the occasional user. The LMA should not be used in the obtunded but not unconscious patient. There is increasing evidence to support its use pre-hospital, and a fully equipped medical bag should probably contain a set.

Cricothyrotomy kit

A number of surgical airway kits are available containing all the necessary equipment for insertion. Whichever is chosen, it should have a minimum lumen of 6mm.

The necessary equipment for needle cricothyrotomy should be pre-prepared and carried. A number of options are illustrated in Fig. 1.1.

Breathing

Face masks

Both adult and paediatric face masks should be carried for use with a bag valve ventilator. Such devices MUST have an oxygen reservoir.

Ventilators

A number of portable oxygen-driven ventilators are available. The majority of practitioners are likely to prefer to continue manual ventilation but automatic ventilators offer an alternative during long transfers or if there is more than one patient.

Oxygen

A conventional D-sized cylinder will provide 15L of oxygen per minute for no more than 20 minutes. A spare should always be carried. Refills can usually be arranged through the local ambulance service. Oxygen should always be administered via a Hudson re-breathing mask with reservoir bag. Modern lightweight cylinders are also available. Ambulance services now regularly use CD cylinders with a capacity of 460L.

Chest drain kits

A number of complete intercostal drain kits are available which contain everything needed for drain insertion but NOT skin prep, needles, syringes, and local anaesthetic.

Circulation

Intravenous cannulae

A wide range of sizes of cannula should be carried in adequate numbers. Fluids are best given via a blood administration set. Appropriate means of securing the line after insertion should be co-located with the cannulae, and should include a two-inch crepe bandage.

Fluids

At least 4L of crystalloid should be available.

Intraosseous needles

Screw-in needles are preferable and should be stored with a three-way tap and 50ml syringe for fluid administration. Adult intraosseous needles are now available, although their use is not fully established. A number of automatic intraosseous devices are now available, of which the most commonly used are the FAST® (sternal) and the EZ-10®.

Check the use-by date of disposables on a regular basis.

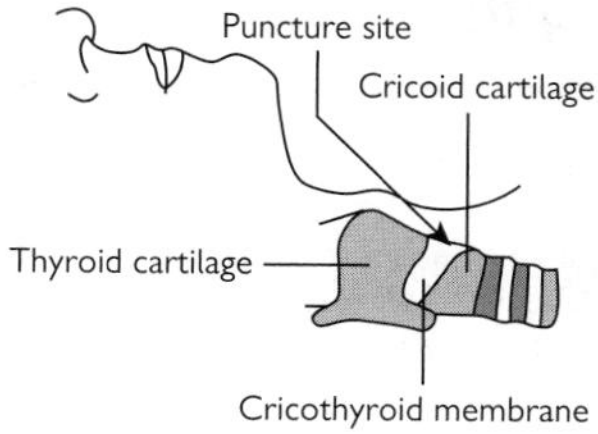

Fig. 1.1 Possible arrangements for needle cricothyrotomy.
Reprinted with permission from Greaves I, Porter K, Hodgetts T, *et al.*, (2006). *Emergency care—a textbook for paramedics*, 2nd edn W.B. Saunders Ltd.

Personal protective equipment

Appropriate personal protective equipment is absolutely vital for the safe practice of pre-hospital care. Essential items are shown in Table 1.2.

Helmets

Industrial 'bump hats' are not acceptable. An appropriate helmet will meet British Standard BS prEN 443. The shell should be made from a strengthened material such as Kevlar and a visor should be fitted. A mounting for a head torch and clear labelling with 'doctor' or 'paramedic' are essential.

Eye protection

Conventional glasses do not provide adequate eye protection in high-risk situations. Appropriate eye protection which will accommodate spectacles (if worn) is recommended. This should meet BS EN 166.

High-visibility jackets and waistcoats

Medical personnel should wear a yellow jacket with green shoulder yolks. There should be two reflective strips around the chest, two round the arms, one around the bottom of the jacket, and a strip on each shoulder. Jackets should be appropriately labelled with the status of the wearer and should conform to BS EN 471 class 2 or preferably class 3. Many modern jackets have a detachable quilted 'inner' which can be removed in warm weather. High-visibility waistcoats are not a substitute for an appropriate jacket and should only be used in hot weather and limited situations, since they offer little if any protection. They should comply with BS EN 471 class 1 standards.

Overalls

Many immediate care schemes have their own 'uniform' overalls. They should include padded elbows and knees and have labels indicating the professional group of the wearer. Overalls should be flameproof or flame-retardant and have two reflective strips on each limb.

Waterproofs

High-visibility waterproof trousers should be carried.

Gloves

Leather debris gloves are essential. Good quality gardener's gloves are a suitable alternative. Non-sterile latex gloves and sterile surgeon's gloves should also be carried.

Boots

Robust footwear with a rubber sole which offers a good grip should be worn. Metal reinforced toecaps are useful. 'Wellington boots' offer very little protection and are not usually appropriate.

Identity cards

All pre-hospital care practitioners *must* be able to produce proof of identity. BASICS produces a membership card for all its accredited practitioners, as do some of the larger schemes. An identity badge with a photograph from an NHS trust is a less satisfactory alternative.

Table 1.2 Essential items of personal protective equipment

- Fluorescent Saturn yellow waterproof, wind-resistant jacket with reflective flashes and identification panel
- Overtrousers (as appropriate)
- Protective (Kevlar) helmet with polycarbonate visor
- Splash protection goggles
- Gloves
  - Waterproof, thermal
  - Debris
  - Neoprene chemical-resistant (as appropriate)
  - Disposable procedure
- Boots with non-slip, spark-free soles
- ID badge with photograph
- Whistle
- One-piece disposable CBRN protection suit (as appropriate)

Packaging

A wide range of types of packaging is available. The two main types are rigid boxes and soft-skinned grip bags. The authors' preference is for the latter.

A pre-hospital formulary

The choice of drugs is a personal one and only familiar drugs should be carried. A suggested drug list for a pre-hospital care doctor is given in Table 1.3. Anaesthetic drugs should neither be used nor carried by those who are not competent and trained in their use. The legal aspects of pre-hospital care drugs are considered on p.26.

Because of the limited amount of available space in bags designed to be carried by one person, each class of drugs should ideally only be represented by one carefully chosen example. Multiple drugs whose effects are equivalent or nearly equivalent should not be carried.

Individual drugs are discussed in detail in Chapters 4 and 5.

Table 1.3 Suggested drugs for pre-hospital care

Cardiac arrest drugs
Adrenaline 1 in 10,000 100mcg/ml 10ml pre-filled syringe
Adrenaline 1 in 1000 1mg/ml 1ml pre-filled syringe
Amiodarone 300mg in 10ml pre-filled syringe
Atropine 3mg in 10ml pre-filled syringe
Cardiac drugs
Buccal nitrate 2mg tabs
Frusemide 10mg/ml 5ml ampoule
Glyceryl trinitrate spray 400mcg/metered dose
Lignocaine 20mg/ml 5ml pre-filled syringe
Aspirin soluble 300mg tabs
Thrombolytic (depending on local protocol) drugs
Tenecteplase
Respiratory drugs
Salbutamol nebulizer solution 1mg/ml 2.5ml ampoule*
Hydrocortisone 100mg vial with 2mg water
Other drugs
Chlorpheniramine 10mg ampoule
Dextrose 50% 50ml pre-filled disposable syringe
Dextrose 10% 500ml bag**
Diazemuls 5mg/ml 2ml ampoule
Diazepam (rectal) 2mg/ml 5mg tube
Glucagon 1ml vial with water
Hypostop
Analgesics
Diamorphine 10mg ampoule
Ketamine 10mg/ml 20ml vial
Morphine 10mg/ml 1 or 2ml ampoules
Antiemetics
Cyclizine 50mg/ml 1ml ampoule
Metoclopramide 5mg/ml 2ml ampoule
Antidotes
Flumazenil 100mcg/ml 5ml ampoule
Naloxone 400mcg/ml 1ml ampoule
Gases
Nitrous oxide/oxygen 50:50 (Entonox)
Oxygen
Obstetric drugs
Syntocinon 10 units/ml 1ml ampoule
Anaesthetic drugs
Ketamine (see above)
Midazolam 2mg/ml 5ml ampoule
Fluids
Normal saline 4x1L bag
Water for injections 5ml ampoules

* If a nebulizer is not carried, salbutamol may be given by metered dose inhaler via a spacer device.

** For paediatric use.

Drug security

Prescription-only drugs must be kept in a locked container in a locked compartment of the vehicle in which they are carried.

Things to take to a call or keep in your vehicle

Inevitably, the departure for an incident tends to be somewhat rushed. It is helpful, therefore, to have a checklist of items which may be helpful or necessary at an incident scene. The following lists may be useful.

Items to be prepared in advance

- Maps—ideally, a customized 'map book' should be prepared using a book of see-through polythene pockets into which appropriate sections of Ordnance Survey and local street maps have been inserted. Use of an A3 folder (opening to A2) allows extensive areas to be covered and avoids difficulties with large map sheets in the car. Satellite navigation is increasingly utilized.
- Satellite navigational equipment (GPS) if available.
- Foul weather clothing—robust waterproofs and boots. Wellington boots can also be carried but may be punctured and should only be used when conditions are appropriate.
- Warm clothing/change of clothing.
- Helmet, gloves, and goggles.
- Warm fluids in electric warmer in boot.
- Medical equipment (see pp.15–21).
- Drugs—in a separate locked container in the boot.
- Extrication equipment (if carried)—this will depend on the nature of likely calls, the operating environment, and the availability of equipment from the ambulance service.
- Blankets.
- Spade—only necessary when snow is lying or expected.
- De-icer (cold conditions only).
- Note pad and paper.
- Torch and batteries.
- Adequate fuel supplies—in icy weather, it is essential to begin defrosting the windscreen and rear window as soon as a call is received. It may be necessary to wait until it is safe to drive. It is never permissible to drive looking through a letter-box-size clear patch in the ice on the windscreen.
- This book!

Items to be prepared before departure

- Overalls/jacket and trousers—where possible, put them on in a warm, light environment.
- Identity card—provided by BASICS or the local ambulance service.
- Mobile phone.
- Spare car keys.

- Cash—small amount for snacks or unforeseen events such as return fares after helicopter evacuations.
- Credit cards.
- Snacks—chocolate bars, Kendal Mint Cake, boiled sweets (take a bag—handing them round is always a popular move!) or other items of choice will always be welcome.
- Flask of tea/coffee—if there is time and the call is expected to be prolonged.

Transport

The majority of pre-hospital care providers will respond in their own vehicles; a few may use vehicles provided by the ambulance service (or other agencies). In any event, the driver is responsible for the maintenance and safety of the vehicle. The following checks *must* therefore be carried out at regular intervals:

- Tyres (pressure and treads).
- Oil.
- Windscreen washers and wipers (blades and washer fluid—do not forget regular antifreeze in cold weather).
- Road tax.

The law offers no exemption or leniency to emergency vehicles regarding legal safety requirements.

Lights and sirens

The law allows medical practitioners responding to emergencies to carry green lights. These may be either bar-mounted or magnetic. The Road Vehicle Licensing Regulations 1984 state:

- Any vehicle being used by a registered medical practitioner for the purposes of an emergency may display one or more green lights. The doctor must be fully registered.
- Each green light or warning beacon must be capable of emitting a flashing or rotating beam throughout 360° in the horizontal plain.
- Only those entitled to use a green beacon may have one fitted to their vehicle.
- Each beacon must be visible a reasonable distance from the vehicle, must be mounted not less than 1200mm from the ground, and flash at a rate between 60 and 240 times per minute. Bulbs must not exceed 55watts.

In some circumstances, following successful completion of appropriate driving courses, responders have been granted permission by the police to use blue lights and sirens. This is subject to local agreement. The practitioner must drive within the confines of the relevant road traffic legislation.

The use of high-visibility reflective markings on any vehicle which will be regularly used for pre-hospital care is strongly recommended. The Road Traffic Act 1984 allows the use of red reflective markings on the rear of a vehicle and markings of any other colour on the sides.

Driving law

Drivers of emergency vehicles are not exempt from any of the normal rules of the road, although they are given more discretion than other road users under certain circumstances. These include permission to:

- Exceed the statutory speed limit by 20mph.
- Treat red traffic lights as a 'give way'.
- Pass on the offside of a keep left sign.
- Turn right where this is not normally permitted.

- Use a bus lane.
- Stop and park on clear ways.
- Stop and park on a pedestrian crossing or its controlled area.
- Park on double yellow lines.

Drivers of emergency vehicles are specifically *not* allowed to:

- Park dangerously.
- Drive without reasonable consideration for other road users.
- Ignore one way signs.
- Ignore stop signs.
- Drive against the flow of traffic at a roundabout (i.e. go the wrong way round).
- Cross double white lines.
- Fail to stop after being involved in an accident.
- Fail to provide information after being involved in an accident.
- Ignore police directions.

The law and pre-hospital care

Consent

Informed consent should always be sought from a patient before any procedure is undertaken. However, in pre-hospital practice where consent can be obtained, it is likely that this consent will be verbal. If possible, witnesses should be sought from amongst other professionals on scene. The patient's decision should be respected and recorded. Refusal of consent must be respected unless the patient is not competent to refuse. In this situation, it is essential that written refusal is obtained, signed by the patient and witnesses.

Treatment without consent

There are circumstances in which treatment without consent may be considered:

- Unconscious patients
- Critically injured patients
- Children (with no legal guardian present)
- 'Incompetent' adults.

The unconscious patient may be treated without their consent if the treatment is necessary to preserve their health or save their life. Similar decisions may have to be taken in cases of critical injury or illness where any delay might adversely effect the patient's outcome. As long as sensible decisions are taken bearing in mind current best practice, it is extremely unlikely that a court would be critical. Nevertheless, it should be borne in mind that, in such circumstances, treatment must be restricted to that needed to save life or prevent serious deterioration. Treatment of physical disorders is not permitted under the Mental Health Act.

'*Gillick competence*' is defined as the possession of sufficient understanding and intelligence to understand fully any suggested treatment. Under 'Gillick rules' children who are considered to be competent may consent *to* treatment without the presence of a guardian; they cannot *refuse* treatment on their own behalf. Such a refusal may be overridden by those with parental responsibility. In an emergency, health care professionals may override the refusal of a Gillick-competent child if no more appropriate person is available. Parents or others with parental responsibility cannot refuse consent to treatment if a competent child has consented. Consent by one person with parental responsibility can not be overruled by refusal by another.

Some adults may be unable to give informed consent, for example due to a mental health condition. Such adults should be treated without consent in their own best interests.

In all situations, appropriate explanation, both to the patient and their relatives, can only have the effect of decreasing distress and increasing co-operation.

Parental responsibility

Parental responsibility is given to the following (Children's Act 1989):

- Both parents, if married at any time since the child's conception.
- The mother alone, if the child is illegitimate, unless the father has obtained agreement from the mother or a court order.
- The local authority, if the child is in care or under a care order.
- An appointed guardian.
- Those with a residence order.
- Adoptive parents.
- Those with an emergency protection order (usually a local authority).

Confidentiality

It is all too easy to break confidentiality in the pre-hospital setting. There is often little, if any, privacy, and a curious crowd all to frequently gathers. In addition, radio and other communications are often overheard and information is passed to other members of the emergency services when this is not appropriate. It is important, therefore, that all responders attempt to maintain confidentiality at all times.

Dealing with the police

Clinicians commit an offence by obstructing a police officer if they dispose of evidence, warn a suspect, or assist a suspect to escape. Good relations should be maintained with the police at all times, bearing in mind the restrictions the law places on doctors and other medical professions.

Negligence

Claims of medical negligence (valid or otherwise) are all too common today. In order to prove negligence, however, it is necessary to establish the following four components of a claim:

- A duty to act.
- A breach of that duty.
- The presence of harm.
- That the harm arose from the breach of duty.

Duty to act means that a professional has a responsibility to act (and act competently) in a clinical situation. Those who put themselves forward to attend emergency situations in a medical capacity accept a *duty to act*. *Breach of duty to act* occurs when a professional fails to perform to an appropriate standard. Breaches of duty may be acts of omission or commission. In order to establish a claim for negligence, it is essential not only to establish that a breach of duty occurred, but also to establish that harm to the patient resulted from that breach. If a mistake was made, but no harm accrued, a claim of negligence will not succeed. Finally, it must be established that the *harm* sustained *resulted from* the *breach of care*.

Living wills

Whilst it is clear that a patient should never be treated against their clearly stated will, the situation is often far from clear in pre-hospital care. If the patient refuses treatment, the situation is clear. However, statements from a relative or friend to the effect that a patient does not wish to receive a certain treatment or to be resuscitated have no legal validity. Similar caution should be applied to documents presented at such times. If there is doubt that a document is genuine, treatment should continue as if it did not exist.

Withholding or terminating resuscitation

Resuscitation may be withheld or terminated if the patient is known to be irreversibly close to death in the short term, if continuing resuscitation would confer no benefit, or if the risks of subsequent brain damage or death at a later stage are unacceptably high. *Advance directives* made by patients should be respected. *Do not resuscitate* orders should not influence any other aspect of treatment.

Pronouncing and certifying death

Following a sudden death due to unnatural circumstances, the attending doctor will not be able to issue a death certificate. *Certification* of death will be delayed until the completion of an autopsy and coroner's inquiry. In such circumstances, the doctor must *pronounce* the patient dead and record this in the medical records. If the patient is known to their general practitioner and has been treated recently by them, and there is no suspicion of unnatural causes, subsequent certification may be carried out.

If the patient has died prior to the arrival of the doctor, it is the doctor's responsibility to pronounce death. In extreme circumstances, it can be very difficult to determine beyond reasonable doubt that death has actually occurred (for example, very cold conditions) or clinical priorities with regard to the living may prevent an adequate assessment. In such circumstances, pronouncement may have to wait until after arrival in hospital.

UK ambulance services now recognize circumstances in which attending paramedics may pronounce death. These are given in Table 1.4. This avoids unnecessary call out of doctors but does not, in any way, replace subsequent certification by an appropriate person.

Table 1.4 Situations in which a paramedic may pronounce death

Finding	Caution
Decomposition	
Rigor mortis	Muscle rigidity as a result of parkinsonism or hypothermia
Dependent lividity (post-mortem staining)	
Expected death from a terminal disease	Presence of a written 'do not resuscitate' order preferred
Decapitation	
Total incineration	Temporary survival may occur in devastating burn injury
Complete separation of the entire heart, lungs, or brain from the body	
Submersion confirmed as being greater than 24 hours	
The duration of the absence of both carotid pulses is confirmed as being greater than 30 minutes, in the absence of any CPR	

Restraint

Health care personnel have no right, beyond those of an ordinary citizen to restrain an aggressive or violent individual, even if the patient is subject to the Mental Health Act. Any attempt to do so constitutes assault, unless a citizen's arrest is being made, in which case it must be clear beyond doubt that an illegal act has been committed. If restraint is necessary, therefore, the assistance of the police should be sought. If violence seems likely, police assistance should ideally be sought before patient contact occurs. Police officers have the right to remove people to a place of safety on their own authority. Personnel who are assaulted are, however, entitled to use 'reasonable force' to defend themselves.

Breaking and entering

Although doctors and paramedics do not have a legal right to force entry into a private address, even if a patient's life appears to be at stake, it is highly unlikely that legal action would ensue in such circumstances.

Insurance

All pre-hospital care practitioners *must* have adequate insurance protection for themselves and their equipment. BASICS and BASICS Scotland have negotiated reasonable insurance rates for members. Providers of motor insurance should be informed that a vehicle is being used for emergency response purposes otherwise a claim resulting from such use may not be honoured. Doctors and nurses should inform their professional indemnity body that they undertake pre-hospital care, although no additional fee is usually raised.

Getting there: safe driving to the scene

Rights and responsibilities

Emergency vehicles have no special rights under the highway code. There is a tendency to get over-excited when driving to the scene of an incident. Unfortunately, this significantly increases the risk of causing an accident. The priority must therefore be SAFETY NOT SPEED. In order to lessen the driving time, whilst minimizing the risk to oneself and other road users, the technique of *defensive driving* is used. This is described in detail in *Roadcraft: the police driver's handbook* (see suggested reading). It should always be remembered that vehicles are not legally obliged to move out of the way of a responding emergency vehicle. It is a matter of courtesy that they do so. It is important to maintain a two-second gap behind the vehicle in front whenever possible, in case it suddenly breaks (sometimes as a response to suddenly seeing lights and sirens in the rear view mirror.) On country roads, appropriate use of the carriageway should be made to maximize visibility at all times (Fig. 1.2).

Other road users may react to emergency vehicles in a number of ways. Hopefully, they will simply move out of the way in a safe manner. Sudden braking, rapid changes of lane, and refusal to give way are also possible. When other motorists do co-operate, this should be acknowledged. Escorted convoys pose particular hazards. Other vehicles may give way to one vehicle before pulling out into the path of those following, confusion may occur when side roads are not blocked as expected, and the situation may degenerate into a race.

Parking at scene

The first vehicle on scene should park in the fend off position (Fig. 1.3). If other vehicles are already present, the new arrival should use the system in Fig. 1.4, or follow the instructions of the police. If the police are in charge of the incident, a (spare) set of keys should be left in the ignition. Otherwise, the vehicle should be locked.

Accidents en route

Green lights do not confer any privileges under the Highway Code. It is essential, therefore, that due care is paid to avoiding accidents. When an accident involving a responding car does occur, the driver is obliged to stop and exchange details as in a 'conventional' collision.

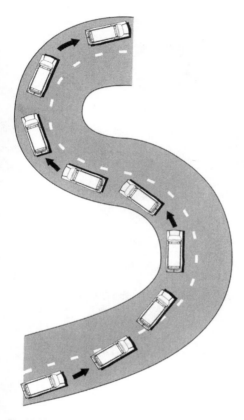

Fig. 1.2 Using road position to maximize visibility on a rural road. Reprinted with permission from Greaves I *et al.* (2006). *Emergency care—a textbook for paramedics*, 2nd edn. W.B. Saunders.

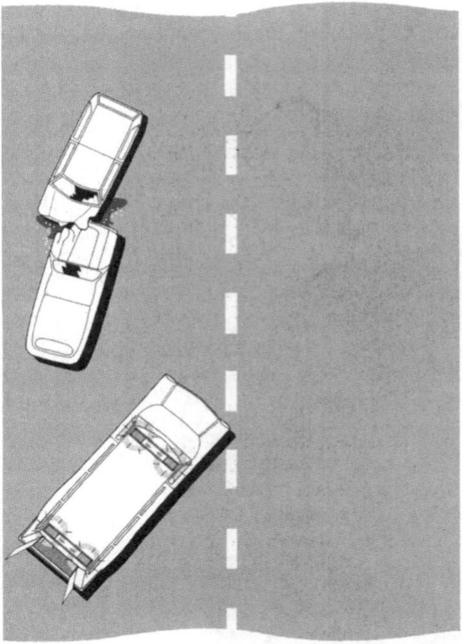

Fig. 1.3 The 'fend off' position. Reprinted with permission from Greaves I *et al.* (2006). *Emergency care—a textbook for paramedics*, 2nd edn. W.B. Saunders.

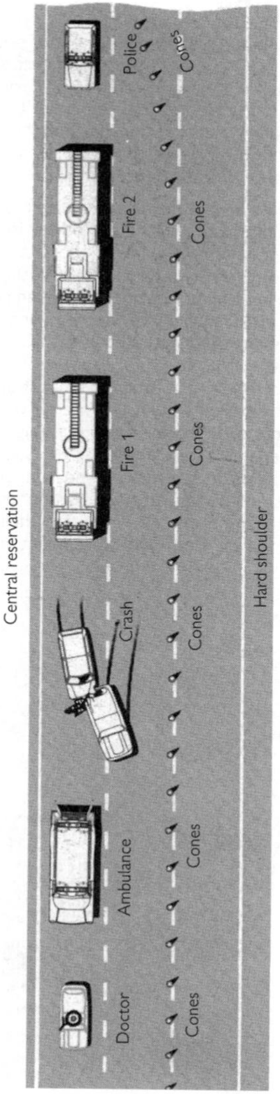

Fig. 1.4 Multi-service parking at scene. Reprinted with permission from Greaves I et *al.* (2006). *Emergency care—a textbook for paramedics*, 2nd edn. W.B. Saunders.

Record keeping

Good record keeping is an essential component of pre-hospital care. However, the lone practitioner cannot be expected to complete records at the same time as assessing and managing a critically ill or injured patient. It is inevitable, therefore, that in some cases notes will be compiled retrospectively, usually after patient handover either to ambulance personnel or in hospital. This is no reason for inadequate or incomplete records. Missing clinical data should not be guessed or estimated!

Good records should be kept for the following reasons:

- They may contain information which will otherwise be unavailable once pre-hospital personnel have left the hospital.
- They will prevent drug errors such as repeat dosing or overdosing (this is particularly important if opiates have been given pre-hospital).
- They will facilitate audit, service development, and research.
- They may offer some protection in the event of a subsequent complaint or inquiry.
- They are legal records in the event of an inquest or criminal case.

All the necessary information should be entered on a pre-printed sheet. Unless there is absolutely no alternative, scribbled notes on scraps of paper are inadequate, amateurish, and bring the speciality into disrepute. Equally, there is little point in every pre-hospital practitioner inventing their own record chart. We suggest that practitioners either use the one provided by the local ambulance service (with their permission) or the *BASICS report form*, available from BASICS (contact details on p.66).

The emergency services: the police

Roles

Duties of the police include:
- Keeping the peace.
- Prevention and investigation of crime.
- Protection of property.
- Law enforcement (including road traffic).
- Major incident management.
- Investigation of sudden death, as agents of the coroner.

Organization

Each police force is under the operational command of a chief constable (commissioner in London). However, police services are required to consult the public they serve and, as a result, are heavily involved in community liaison. A number of authorities and bodies have responsibility for the strategy and efficiency of each individual force. The *Home Office* is responsible for promoting the general efficiency of the police and has ultimate responsibility for levels of funding. In addition, it is responsible for the setting of national performance targets and approves the appointment of chief and assistant chief constables.

The local *police authority* consists of local councillors, magistrates, and independent members. It is responsible for the provision of an efficient police service in its area and has ultimate responsibility for expenditure which is delegated to a greater or lesser extent to the chief constable. The police authority sets local policing objectives and targets and, in consultation with the chief constable, is responsible for the preparation and submission to the Home Office of a local policing plan. Civilian staff are employed by the police authority but, in general, are placed under the operational control of the chief constable.

The *chief constable* directs and controls the police force. S/he is responsible for the financial management of the force under the control of the police authority and directs police officers and civilian staff other than those managed directly by the police authority. The chief constable is responsible for drawing up the draft policing plan for approval or amendment by the police authority. The chief constable is responsible for the operational deployment of his resources.

Rank structure

The rank structure of provincial police forces is shown in Fig. 1.5, and of the Metropolitan Police, in Fig. 1.6. The City of London police force uses the same rank structure as the Metropolitan Police.

Other police forces

The *Royal Parks Police* has responsibility for the London Royal Parks, the *British Transport Police* for railway tracks and train stations, and the *Ministry of Defence Police* for areas of Defence estates. The *Special Constabulary* is a part-time volunteer police force which assists the regular constabulary.

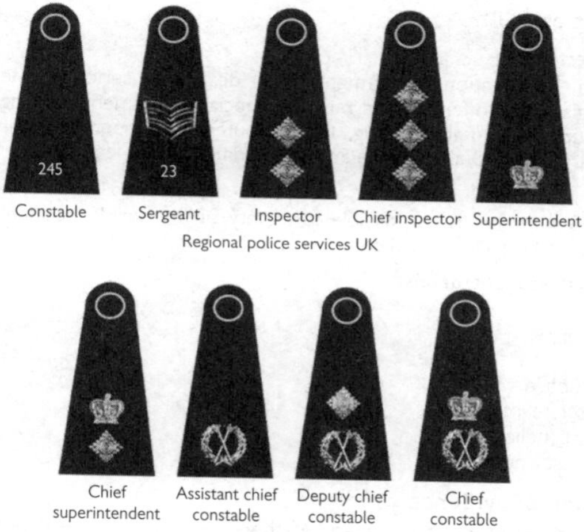

Fig. 1.5 Police service ranks and rank markings—provincial (outside London). Reprinted with permission from Greaves I *et al.* (2006). *Emergency care—a handbook for paramedics*, 2nd edn. W.B. Saunders Ltd.

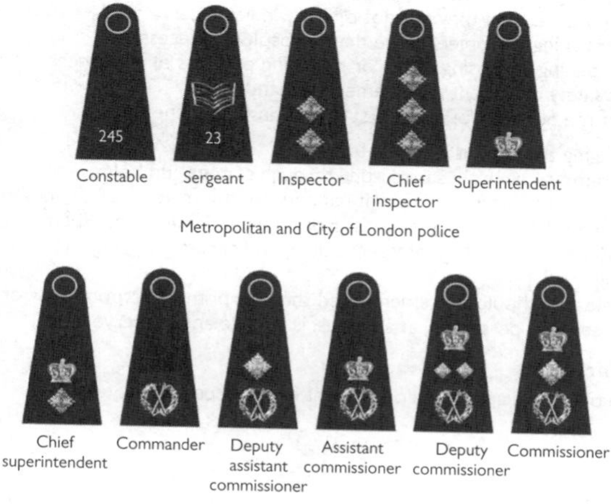

Fig. 1.6 Metropolitan (and City of London) police ranks and rank markings. Reprinted with permission from Greaves I *et al.* (2006). *Emergency care—a handbook for paramedics*, 2nd edn. W.B. Saunders Ltd.

Special duties

Criminal investigation

The Criminal Investigation Department (CID) deals with serious crime such as burglary, sex offences, and murder. Special departments dealing with areas such as child abuse, drug, and computer crime operate under the umbrella of the CID as does the *Scenes of Crime Department*.

Traffic

The *Traffic Department* is responsible for safety on the roads, accident investigation, and vehicle related crime.

Operations (special operations)

These include:

- Firearms teams
- Dog teams
- Mounted police
- Underwater search
- Air support (helicopters)
- Anti-terrorist operations.

Preservation of evidence

Pre-hospital clinicians must be aware of the importance of preserving evidence. Blundering into a crime scene may alter or destroy evidence and render a subsequent successful prosecution impossible. If it is possible that a crime has taken place, great care should be taken to ensure that evidence is not lost. It is important, therefore, to:

- Wear gloves, even if they are not *clinically* indicated.
- Avoid touching any object more than is absolutely necessary.
- Avoid opening or closing doors or switching off lights or appliances (unless safety or patient management demands it).
- Restrict the numbers of medical staff entering the scene.

In managing the patient it is vital to:

- Avoid removal of clothes by cutting through stab or gun holes.
- Ensure that articles from different patients are not mixed.
- Remove articles (including clothes) from the patient and hand them to an identified person (preferably a police officer) for bagging and labelling.

Nevertheless, it should be remembered that the primary responsibility of all health services personnel, at all times, is to save and preserve life.

Major incidents

The role of the police at a major incident is discussed in Chapter 10.

The emergency services: the fire service

Roles

- To save life (including accident rescue and extrication).
- To protect property (fire or flooding).
- To provide humanitarian support.
- To protect the environment (including hazardous material management).

Organization

Fire Services operate under local authority control via *fire authorities*. In England and Wales, ultimate responsibility for all fire services lies with the Home Secretary who exercises this responsibility through the inspectors of the *Fire Department*. Fire authorities have absolute discretion in the day-to-day management of their services. In Scotland, final responsibility lies with the Secretary of State for Scotland.

Each service is headed by a *Chief Fire Officer* (*Firemaster* in Scotland) from a headquarters housing senior officers and support staff. Regionally, most services are divided into divisions each under the control of a *divisional officer*. Every division contains a number of stations each under the control of a *station officer*. Each station is staffed by four watches containing *firefighters* and under the command of a *sub-officer* assisted by a *leading firefighter*. Fire service rank markings are shown in Fig. 1.7.

Officers above the rank of sub-officer have white helmets; below sub-officer have yellow. The greater the width of black banding, the more senior the officer.

Retained firefighters work part-time in the fire service, providing support to full-time colleagues in urban areas or a primary response service where the call level is insufficient to justify full-time manning.

Road traffic accident management

The fire service recognize six phases in the management of a road traffic collision entrapment. These are:

- Scene assessment and safety.
- Stabilization and initial access.
- Glass management.
- Space creation.
- Full access and immobilization.
- Extrication.

Scene assessment and safety

An overview of the incident scene with an assessment of any hazards present and a determination of immediate priorities.

Stabilization and initial access

Stabilization of vehicles and initial approach to trapped casualties. In certain circumstances, hazards may determine the necessity for an immediate snatch rescue of casualties.

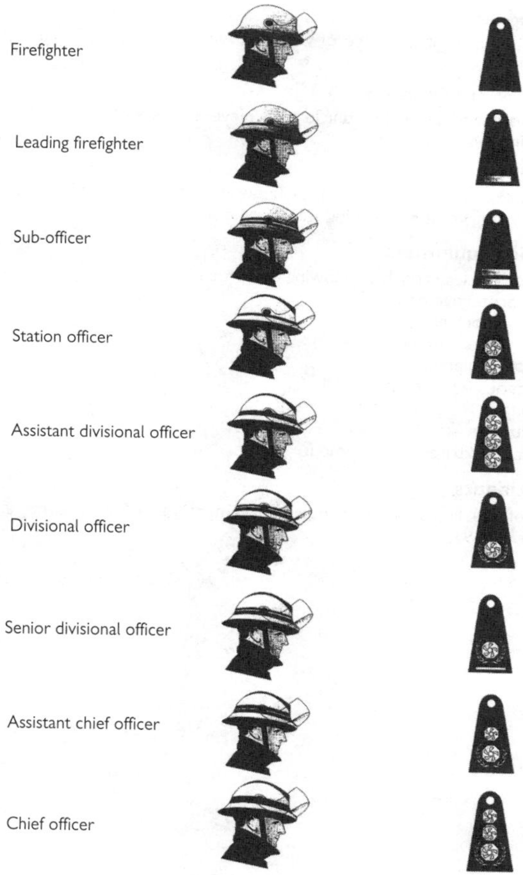

Fig. 1.7 Fire service ranks and rank markings.

Glass management
Controlled removal or breakage of windows with protection of trapped casualties.

Space creation and full access
Systematic dismantling of the vehicle to achieve access to the casualties for treatment and extrication.

Extrication
Controlled extrication of the casualty under the supervision of a paramedic or doctor whilst maintaining spinal immobilization.

Fire service equipment

Fire brigade vehicles carry the following equipment:

- Personal protective equipment
- Communications equipment
- Basic medical equipment
- Extrication equipment
- Miscellaneous equipment
  - Lighting
  - Stabilization
  - Specialist extrication equipment.

Major incidents

The role of the fire services in the management of major incidents is described on p.592.

The emergency services: the ambulance service

Roles

- Emergency patient transfer.
- Routine patient movements.
- Provision of medical support at the scene of major incidents.

Organization

Ambulance services are NHS trusts under the direction of a *chief executive*. Each trust has a *trust board*, the chairman of which is appointed by the Secretary of State. The board contains executive and non-executive directors. The service headquarters provides financial and human resources management. Each ambulance service has a medical director or advisor. In some services, a full time medical director has been appointed.

The operations component of each ambulance service includes:

- Accident and emergency vehicles ('front-line' ambulances)
- Patient transport services
- Support and technical components

Accident and emergency vehicles also undertake specialist transfers of critically ill patients as well as retrieval missions for special categories of patient such as neonatal intensive care. Emergency ambulance response times are governed by ORCON (*Operational Research Consultantcy)* standards. These require an ambulance to reach the patient in 50% of cases within 8 minutes, and in 95% of cases, in 14 minutes in urban areas and 19 minutes in rural areas. There is no clinical rationale for these figures and they are likely to change. In addition to emergency vehicles, the ambulance service also provides the routine transport for outpatient visits, hospital admissions, and discharges and for a variety of other social services agencies. They are also charged with providing a structured response to major incidents (see pp.592–3).

As well as front-line ambulances and patient transport vehicles, ambulance service trusts also provide paramedic response vehicles (cars, four-wheel drive vehicles, motorbikes and cycles), support vehicles (including major incident control vehicles), and helicopters (although air ambulances may also be charitably funded).

Ambulance dispatch

Modern ambulance dispatch is highly technical. Details from 999 calls enter a *computer aided dispatch* (CAD) system which is able to locate the most appropriate vehicle using an *automatic vehicle location system* (AVLS). In order to reduce response times, vehicles are dispatched as soon as the approximate location of the call is known. Protocol-based dispatch systems allow prioritization of calls and data can be passed directly to ambulance crew en route to the incident via a pager or vehicle-based data terminal. These dispatch systems also provide first aid instruction for the caller before the ambulance arrives.

The emergency services: other agencies

Her Majesty's Coastguard

Her Majesty's Coastguard is part of the Maritime and Coastguard Agency (MCA). It is responsible for co-ordinating search and rescue around Britain's coast through six Maritime Rescue Co-ordination Centres (MRCC), twelve Maritime Rescue Sub-centres (MRSC), and sector bases.

The Royal National Lifeboat institution (RNLI)

The RNLI is a charity which provides 24-hour rescue services around the coast of Great Britain and the Republic of Ireland. It operates both in-shore and seagoing rescue services.

The armed forces

Pre-hospital clinicians are unlikely to encounter members of Her Majesty's Forces unless there has been a major incident, when their assistance under the *Military Aid to the Civil Powers* (MAC) scheme may be requested (see p.593).

The voluntary services

St John's Ambulance

St John's Ambulance was founded in 1877. It provides first aid cover at a wide range of public events and sporting fixtures. Although the majority of volunteers are first-aid trained, St John's can also provide doctors and registered nurses. Locally, St John's is divided into divisions, then districts, areas, and counties. Uniform is worn, with a structured rank system. A considerable range of often sophisticated equipment and vehicles is available. St John's Ambulance is a major first aid trainer.

British Red Cross

The British Red Cross is an arm of the international Red Cross Movement founded by Henri Dunant. It aims to provide care to people in their own communities and after major or traumatic incidents but also provides volunteers for service overseas in both peace and war. Each local branch of the Red Cross is run by trustees who are responsible to the National Council.

St Andrew's Ambulance Service

St Andrew's Ambulance Service in Scotland provides first aid provision at sporting fixtures and public events.

Women's Royal Voluntary Service (WRVS)

Founded just before the Second World War, the WRVS plays a wide range of roles in community life from old people's luncheon clubs to hospital tea bars and meals on wheels. Although the emergency services provided by the WRVS have declined in importance since the war, teams are available and can be provided for a wide range of emergency situations from house fires to major incidents. Each area of the UK has a WRVS co-ordinator for these services. Emergency services provided by the WRVS include refreshments, warm bedding, rest centre provision, and support and comfort, not only to victims but also to members of the emergency services.

The Faculty of Pre-hospital Care

The Faculty of Pre-hospital Care of the Royal College of Surgeons of Edinburgh organizes the Diploma in Immediate Medical Care of the Royal College of Surgeons of Edinburgh (DipIMC.RCSEd) and the Fellowship in Immediate Medical Care of the Royal College of Surgeons of Edinburgh (FIMC.RCSEd.) Details of both these examinations can be obtained from the Examinations Office at the College (see useful addresses, p.66).

The Faculty also accredits a wide range of short modular courses such as the *First Person on Scene* (FPOS) *Course* and (jointly with BASICS and BASICS Scotland) *Pre-hospital Emergency Care* (PHEC), and is actively involved in a wide range of joint educational initiatives with other medical bodies.

The provision of expert advice regarding pre-hospital care matters is an important part of the Faculty's role and it works with a wide variety of agencies from airlines to oil-rigs. The Faculty has an active *Pre-hospital Care Research Centre* based at the James Cook University Hospital on Teesside.

Membership of the Faculty is open to paramedics, doctors, and nurses, as well as other emergency personel (for contact details, see p.66). Members receive the *Emergency Medicine Journal* as part of their subscription.

BASICS and BASICS Scotland

The *British Association for Immediate Care* (BASICS) and BASICS Scotland are national charities which represent a wide range of individual pre-hospital providers and schemes. Both organizations are very heavily involved in educational initiatives and, like the Faculty (see p.60), offer advice regarding the provision of pre-hospital care through a wide range of bodies and standing committees. Contact details for BASICS, BASICS Education, and BASICS Scotland are given on p.66. BASICS members receive the *Emergency Medicine Journal* as part of their subscription.

Suggested reading

General texts

Practical pre-hospital care
Ian Greaves, Keith Porter, and Jason Smith (eds) (2009). Elsevier.

Pre-hospital care: a textbook for paramedics, (2nd edn).
Ian Greaves, Keith Porter, and Tim Hodgetts (eds) (2007). Elsevier.

Pre-hospital emergency care secrets.
Peter T Pons and Vincent J Markovchick (eds) (1998). Hanley and Belfus.

More specialised texts

Safety at scene
Vic Calland (2000). Mosby.

Handbook of patient transportation
Terry Martin (2001). Greenwich Medical Media.

Roadcraft: the police driver's handbook
The Stationery Office (1999).

Pre-hospital paediatric life support
Advanced Life Support Group (2000). BMJ Books.

Major incident medical management and support (2nd edn)
Advanced Life Support Group (2002). BMJ Books.

Major incident management system
Timothy J Hodgetts and Crispin Porter (2002). BMJ Books.

Journals

Emergency Medicine Journal (BMJ Publications)
The EMJ is the 'house journal' of BASICS, BASICS Scotland, and the Faculty of Pre-Hospital Care. Mainly concerned with emergency medicine, (A&E) it also includes a significant component of pre-hospital care and publishes most of the important pre-hospital research and practice development.

Useful addresses

Advanced Life Support Group
29–31 Ellesmere Street,
Swinton,
Manchester M27 OLA
www.alsg.org
0161 794 1999

British Association for Immediate Care (BASICS)
Turret House,
Turret Lane,
Ipswich,
Suffolk IP4 1DL
www.basics.org.uk
0870 165 4999

BASICS Education
Turret House,
Turret Lane,
Ipswich,
Suffolk IP4 1DL
www.basics.org.uk
0870 165 4999

BASICS Scotland
Sandpiper House,
Aberuthven Enterprise Park,
Aberuthven PH3 1EL
www.basics-scotland.org
01764 663671

Department of Academic Emergency Medicine, University of Teesside
Academic Centre,
The James Cook University Hospital,
Marton Road, Middlesbrough,
Cleveland TS4 3BW
www.teessideem.org.uk
01642 282898

EdExcel
IHCD Stewart House,
32 Russell Square,
London WC1B 5DN
www.edexcel.org.uk
0870 240 9800

Examinations Office, Royal College of Surgeons of Edinburgh
Examinations Office,
Royal College of Surgeons of Edinburgh,
The Adamson Centre, 3 Hill Place,
Edinburgh EH8 9DS
www.rcsed.ac.uk
0131 527 1600

Faculty of Pre-hospital Care of the Royal College of Surgeons of Edinburgh
Faculty of Pre-hospital Care,
Royal College of Surgeons of Edinburgh,
Nicolson Street,
Edinburgh EH8 9DW
www.rcsed.ac.uk
0131 527 1732

Faculty of Pre-hospital Care Research Unit
Academic Centre,
The James Cook University Hospital,
Marton Road,
Middlesbrough,
Cleveland TS4 3BW
www.teessideem.org.uk
01642 282898

Chapter 2

Acute medical and surgical problems

Approach to the acute medical patient

The initial clinical priority in the management of medical problems in the pre-hospital environment is to ensure that the patient does not suffer a catastrophic deterioration before they reach definitive care. For this reason, the familiar ABC approach is as relevant in medical cases as it is in trauma:

A Airway

Consider C spine immobilization if the patient may have suffered an injury during a collapse.

B Breathing

Patients whose respiratory effort (rate and volume) is inadequate will require ventilatory support. All patients should receive high-flow oxygen unless it is apparent that they are suffering solely from an exacerbation of established chronic obstructive pulmonary disease.

C Circulation

An assessment of the pulse and blood pressure (by palpation of pulses if necessary) provides evidence of inadequate circulation as a result either of dysrhythmia or cardiac failure.

D Disability

AVPU and pupillary assessment may suggest the presence of an intra-cerebral catastrophe or a reduced level of consciousness due to a metabolic problem or poisoning.

E Exposure

Limited exposure may reveal signs of complicating injury, a MEDIC ALERT® bracelet, needle marks, or cutaneous signs of disease.

Many patients who present with pre-hospital medical problems will be suffering from an exacerbation of an existing problem. Similarly, a knowledge of the previous medical history may suggest the current diagnosis. If the diagnosis is not clear, a symptomatic approach must be used.

DON'T FORGET A BM STIX®

A symptom-based approach

Chest pain

Ischaemic chest pain

Angina (see p.114)

Clinical features:

- Typically crushing 'like a weight' 'like a band round my chest'
- Induced by exercise
- Improved by rest
- Often a previous history
- Responds to GTN spray
- More common in smokers.

Myocardial infarction (see p.116)

Clinical features:

- Similar character to angina
- More severe and/or prolonged than 'usual' angina pain
- Onset at rest
- Not relieved by rest/GTN.

Associated symptoms:

- Shortness of breath
- Pallor
- Cold clammy skin.

Chest wall pain

Clinical features:

- Usually 'sharp'
- Worse with coughing, deep respiration (pleuritic)
- Associated with well localized chest tenderness
- May follow minor trauma (may be spontaneous)
- NOT normally associated with shortness of breath
- Respiratory examination normal.

Pulmonary pain

Pneumothorax (see pp.134–6)

- Usually 'sharp'
- Sudden onset
- Pleuritic in nature
- Not usually associated with chest wall tenderness (unless traumatic)
- Associated with shortness of breath
- May be previous history of pneumothorax
- More common in asthmatics and tall young men
- Reduced breath sounds and hyper-resonant percussion note on examination.

Causes of chest pain (see text)

- Ischaemic heart disease
  - Angina
  - Myocardial infarction
- Chest wall pain
  - Minor trauma
  - Costochondreitis
- Pulmonary
  - Pneumothorax
  - Pneumonia
  - Pulmonary embolism
- Gastrointestinal
  - Oesophageal reflux/oesophagitis
  - Peptic ulceration
- Aortic dissection
- Rarer causes
  - Herpes zoster (shingles)
  - Cholecystitis
  - Pancreatitis
  - Pericarditis

CONSIDER PNEUMOTHORAX IN THE DETERIORATING ASTHMATIC

Pneumonia
- Onset usually gradual
- Pleuritic
- Associated with shortness of breath
- Green/brown sputum (worse early morning)
- Patient generally unwell
  - Pyrexial
  - Sweaty
  - Rigors (in systemic infection)
- Haemoptysis may be present
- Commonly complicates COPD.

Pulmonary embolism (see p.132)
- Sudden onset
- Pleuritic
- Associated with shortness of breath
- Haemoptysis (sometimes)
- Dizzness, syncope, collapse (rare)
- Associated with DVT (check the calves!)
- Increased risk with:
  - Oral contraceptive pill
  - Immobility—long journeys, illness
  - Pregnancy and childbirth
  - Previous thromboembolic disease
  - Morbid obesity
  - Recent surgery
- May be a family history of DVT or PE.

Gastrointestinal causes of chest pain

Oesophageal reflux/oesophagitis
- Usually retrosternal
- Burning
- Worse after food
- Associated with particular food types
- May be worse in certain positions
- Associated with trapped wind
- May be a long history
- May respond to antacids.

Peptic ulcer pain
- Usually epigastric
- May be history of aspirin/non-steroidal ingestion
- May radiate to the back (beware aortic aneurysm—see p.154).

Aortic dissection
- Sudden onset central and interscapular/back pain
- Pain may be 'tearing'
- Patient may be hypo- or hypertensive
- Physical examination may reveal absent pulses, new murmurs, neurological signs, or BP differences between the arms.

Herpes zoster—shingles (see p.124)
Shingles may present with pain in the clear distribution of one of the thoracic nerve roots. When the typical vesicular rash is present, the diagnosis is obvious, However, the pain may precede the rash.

Cholecystitis (see p.158).

Pancreatitis (see p.159).

Pericarditis (see pp.122–3).

Shortness of breath

Asthma (see p.128–9)

- Tachypnoea
- Reduced peak flow
- Signs of underlying infection or pneumothorax
- Declining respiratory effort and exhaustion (more severe and late cases)
- Cyanosis
- Hypoxia
- Hypotension (late and severe cases)
- Ventilatory failure /confusion or coma (suggestive of rising $PaCO_2$).

Pulmonary oedema (see p.126)

- Breathlessness (acute or acute on chronic)
- Cough
- Frothy sputum (may be lightly blood stained)
- Collapse
- Shock, sweating, pallor, peripheral coldness.

Other symptoms reflect the underlying cause:

- Chest pain
- Palpitation.

COPD (p.130)

- Wheeze unresponsive to inhaler therapy
- Production of purulent sputum/increased sputum production
- Increasingly severe breathlessness
- Respiratory failure
- Increased respiratory rate (>25/min suggests a significant exacerbation)
- Cyanosis
- Use of accessory muscles
- CO_2 retention flap, confusion (indicative of hypercapnoea)
- Bilateral widespread wheezes (beware the silent chest)
- Peripheral oedema.

Causes of shortness of breath

- Asthma
- Pulmonary oedema
- COPD
- Pneumonia
- Pneumothorax
- Pulmonary embolism
- Hyperventilation syndrome
- Respiratory compensation for a metabolic acidosis

Pneumonia
- Cough
- Tachypnoea
- Purulent sputum
- Pyrexia/rigors
- Pleuritic chest pain
- May be underlying lung disease.

Pneumothorax (pp.134–6)
- Shortness of breath (usually sudden onset)
- Chest pain (non-specific, often pleuritic)
- Acute severe exacerbation of asthma or COPD
- May be previous history
- More common in asthmatics and tall young men
- Increasing difficulty in manually ventilating a patient or deteriorating hypoxia despite effective ventilation.

Pulmonary embolism (see p.132)
- Sudden onset
- Pleuritic
- Associated with shortness of breath
- Haemoptysis (sometimes)
- Dizziness, syncope, collapse (rare)
- Associated with DVT (check the calves!)
- Increased risk with:
  - Oral contraceptive pill
  - Immobility—long journeys, illness
  - Pregnancy and childbirth
  - Previous thromboembolic disease
  - Morbid obesity
  - Recent surgery

May be a family history of DVT or PE.

Hyperventilation syndrome (see p.138)
- Anxiety/panic
- Hyperventilation
- Per-oral tingling
- Carpopedal spasm
- Tinnitus
- Chest tightness.

Respiratory compensation for a metabolic acidosis
- Difficult to diagnose definitively pre-hospital
- May be secondary to:
  - Diabetic ketoacidosis
  - Tricyclic antidepressant poisoning.

Pre-hospital investigations and monitoring

Pre-hospital investigations are only of value if the results will alter patient management. Most investigations can be undertaken more effectively, more comfortably, and more quickly after arrival in hospital. Under no circumstances should the transfer of a critically ill or injured patient be delayed.

All patients with significant injuries or medical problems should have the following monitoring:

- ECG
- Pulse oximetry
- Non-invasive BP (during transfer)

ALL patients whose level of conscious is reduced should have a BM stix® (blood sugar measurement).

Pulse oximetry

The pulse oximeter probe contains two light-emitting diodes (producing red and infrared light) and a light detector which measures the intensity of the light after it has passed through the tissues. Oxygenated and reduced haemoglobins show different light-absorbing properties which affect the relative amounts of light measured by the sensor. Pulse oximetry measures pulse and oxygen saturation; it does not measure PaO_2.

Applications

- Measurement of oxygenation during transport.
- Assessment of limb viability following injury.
- Assessment of pulse and saturation in ill patients.

Limitations

- Does not measure CO_2, therefore may provide false reassurance in respiratory failure or inadequacy with rising CO_2 levels.
- May be ineffective in poor tissue perfusion (including due to cold).
- Effected by bright ambient light.
- Ineffective through *metallic* nail varnish.
- Does not distinguish met- or carboxyhaemoglobins and may, therefore, give a falsely high O_2 reading in carbon monoxide poisoning.

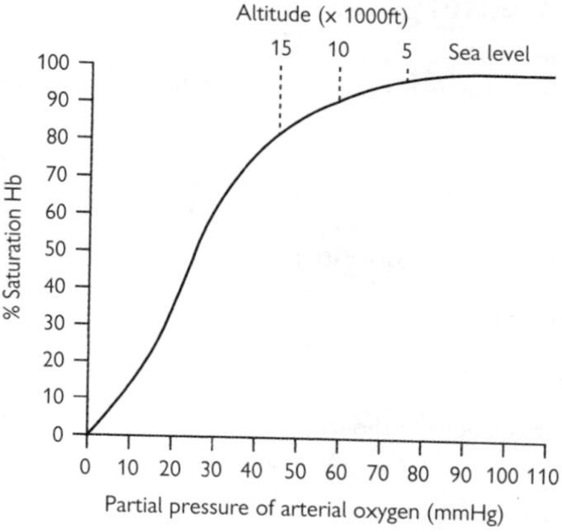

Fig. 2.1 Haemoglobin-oxygen dissociation curve.

Cardiological emergencies

Patient assessment

The assessment of the patient with a known or suspected cardiac problem is as follows:

- Observe
  - Responsiveness
  - Pallor
  - Sweating
  - Dyspnoea **(count the respiratory rate!)**
  - Cyanosis
  - Jugular venous pressure
- Listen
  - Noise of airway obstruction
  - Wheeze
  - Added sounds (crepitations or rhonchi)
  - Heart sounds
- Feel
  - Pulse (volume, rate, and character)
  - Distal pulses where appropriate
  - Chest expansion.

Cardiac arrest

The *most common* arrhythmias associated with cardiac arrest are ventricular fibrillation (VF) and pulseless ventricular tachycardia (pulseless VT). Providing good-quality advanced life support is available, there is little if any justification for transporting patients with one of these rhythms to hospital until cardiac output has been restored. Cardiac arrest may also occur with pulseless electrical activity (PEA) and asystole.

Immediate actions in cardiac arrest:

- Assess response
- Shout for help
- Assess airway
- Assess breathing
  - Call 999
- Expose chest
- Commence CPR
  - 30 compressions: 2 breaths.

As soon as a diagnosis of cardiac arrest is established, professional assistance must be sought if a defibrillator is not available, even if this means leaving the patient for a short period.

Safety

Safety is vital at a cardiac arrest. Careful attention should be paid to ensuring that rescuers are not at risk during defibrillation. Defibrillation may take place in the rain (the patient's chest should be wiped dry first) but is dangerous if the patient is lying in a pool of water (for example, at the side of a swimming pool).

(a)

(b)

(c)

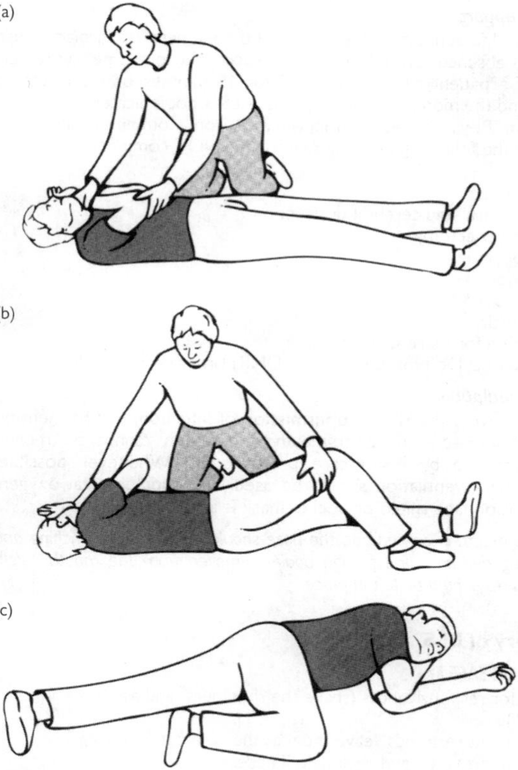

Fig. 2.2 Placing a patient in the recovery position. Reprinted with permission from Greaves I and Porter K (1997). *Pre-hospital medicine—the principles and practice of immediate care*. Edward Arnold (Publishers) Ltd.

Basic life support

Good basic life support is the key to the treatment of cardiac arrest. Prolonged absence of BLS makes a successful outcome extremely unlikely. If a patient has not had BLS for 15 minutes or more after a collapse, and the monitor shows asystole, ALS is not indicated.

The Joint Royal Colleges Ambulance Liaison Committee (JRCALC) recognizes the following as being reasons for NOT commencing resuscitation:

- Decapitation
- Massive cranial and cerebral destruction
- Hemi-corporectomy
- Decomposition
- Incineration
- Hypostasis
- Rigor mortis
- Submersion for more than one hour
- Presence of a 'Do Not Resuscitate' (DNR) order or living will.

Artificial ventilation

In order to avoid the risk of transmission of infection, not to mention for aesthetic reasons, mouth-to-mouth resuscitation cannot be recommended for use by health-care professionals. Whenever possible, mouth-to-mask ventilation should be used with supplemental oxygen. A resuscitation face shield or pocket mask is an alternative.

If mouth-to-mouth is carried out, the nose should be closed by pinching and poorly fitting dentures and foreign bodies removed from the mouth. Well-fitting dentures should be left in place.

Summary of BLS

CHECK FOR SAFETY

- Check for responsiveness (shake the shoulders* and ask 'are you alright?').
- If the patient responds, leave them as they are; attempt to gain further information and seek help if necessary.
- If there is no response, SHOUT FOR HELP.
- Use simple manoeuvres to open the airway.
- If they are breathing normally, put them in the recovery position and obtain help, otherwise:
- Give 30 compressions—DO NOT check the pulse first (for technique, see below).
- Give 2 rescue breaths (for technique, see below).
- Repeat cycle of 30 compressions followed by 2 rescue breaths**.
- Continue until spontaneous breathing recommences or assistance (with a defibrillator) arrives.

NOTES

* Care if there is a possibility of C spine injury.

** Compression only CPR may be used as an alternative in situations where the rescuer is unable or unwilling to provide artificial respiration.

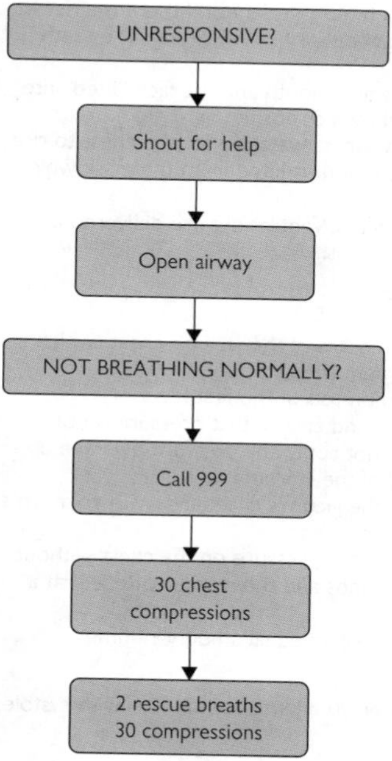

Fig. 2.3 Adult basic life support algorithm. Reprinted wth permission from Resuscitation Council (UK) (2005). *Resuscitation Guidelines*.

Technique of mouth-to-mask ventilation

- The airway is cleared and the chin tilted (ideally not if there is a risk of C spine injury, although it may be necessary). Well-fitting false teeth are left in situ.
- The mask is applied over the nose and mouth and the face 'lifted' into it with the hands in the position shown opposite (Fig. 2.4a)
- Breaths lasting 1 second are given, whilst watching for the chest to rise.
- During the 'expiration' phase, the mouth is lifted from the mask which continues to be held in place
- Irrespective of the number of rescuers, ventilations are delivered at a ratio of 2 breaths to 30 compressions.

Technique of chest compressions (see Fig. 2.4b)

Kneel by the side of the victim

- Place the heel of one hand in the centre of the victim's chest (which is the lower half of the victim's sternum (breastbone))
- Place the heel of your other hand on top of the first hand
- Interlock the fingers of your hands and ensure that pressure is not applied over the victim's ribs. Do not apply any pressure over the upper abdomen or the bottom end of the sternum
- Position yourself vertically above the victim's chest and, with your arms straight, press down on the sternum 5–6cm.
- After each compression, release all the pressure on the chest without losing any contact between your hands and the sternum. Repeat at a rate of 100–120 min^{-1}
- Compression and release should take an equal amount of time

Abandoning resuscitation

Resuscitation may be abandoned after 20 minutes of full ALS with systole, unless:

- The patient is a child.
- The patient is hypothermic.
- The patient is a victim of drowning.
- The patient may have, or is known to have taken an overdose of drugs.
- The situation is in any way 'unusual'.

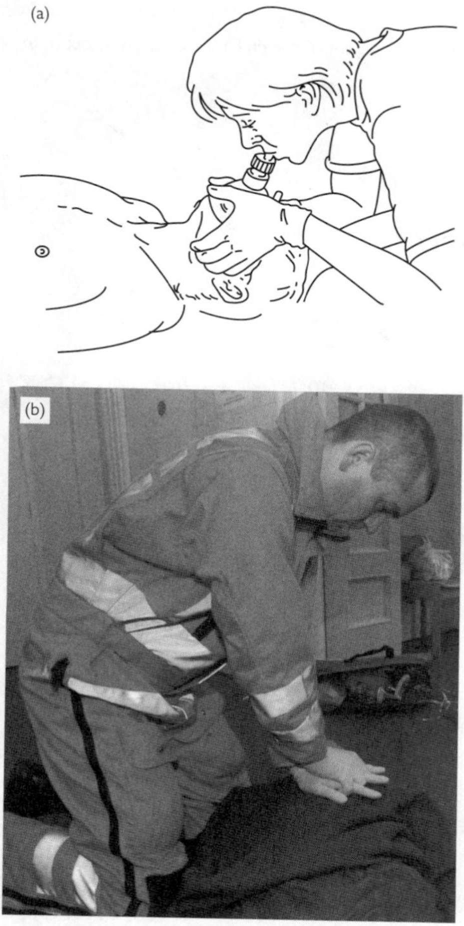

Fig. 2.4 (a) Artificial ventilation and (b) chest compression. Reprinted with permission from Greaves I *et al.* (2005), *Emergency Care—a textbook for paramedics.*

CHOKING IN ADULTS

The algorithm for the management of choking in adults is given opposite in Fig. 2.5.

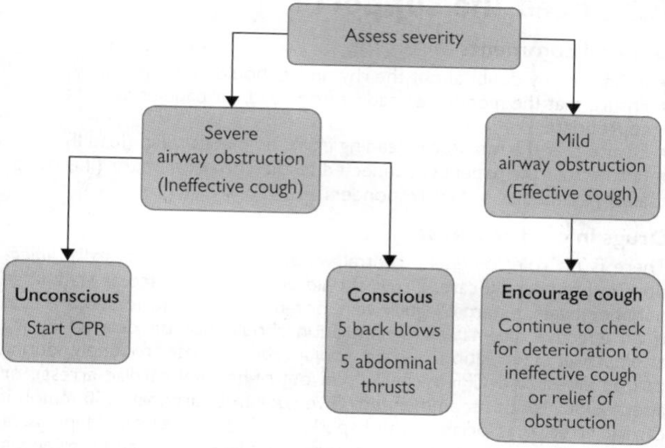

Fig. 2.5 Adult choking algorithm. Reprinted with permission from the Resuscitation Council (UK) (2005), *Resuscitation guidelines*.

Advanced life support

General comments

- If there is any doubt about the rhythm, it should be treated as VF.
- Ensure that the monitor is reading from leads or paddles as appropriate.
- Ensure that the monitor is reading from the correct lead (lead II).
- Ensure that the patient is connected to the correct monitor (if arriving after paramedics or first responders).

Drugs in cardiac arrest

There is no role for either central venous access or intracardiac injections in pre-hospital care. Drugs should be given by IV access via a large peripheral vein, external jugular vein, or femoral vein. Intraosseous access is an effective alternative. Defibrillation should not be delayed during attempts at cannulation. Giving sodium bicarbonate routinely during cardiac arrest and CPR (especially in out-of-hospital cardiac arrest), or after ROSC, is not recommended. Give sodium bicarbonate (50 mmol) if cardiac arrest is associated with hyperkalaemia or tricyclic antidepressant overdose. Although adrenaline, atropine, and lignocaine can be given via the ET tube, this should be considered a last resort.

Patient handover

The following information should be recorded and handed over to medical staff on arrival at the emergency department:

- Presence/absence of bystander CPR and duration.
- Duration of advanced life support.
- Number of defibrillating shocks.
- Duration of cardiac arrest/apnoea.
- Other treatment given.
- Past medical history/drug history.

Following cardiac arrest, no attempt should be made to warm the patient up since moderate hypothermia (32–34°) appears to be beneficial.

Ventricular fibrillation (VF)/pulseless ventricular tachycardia (pulseless VT)

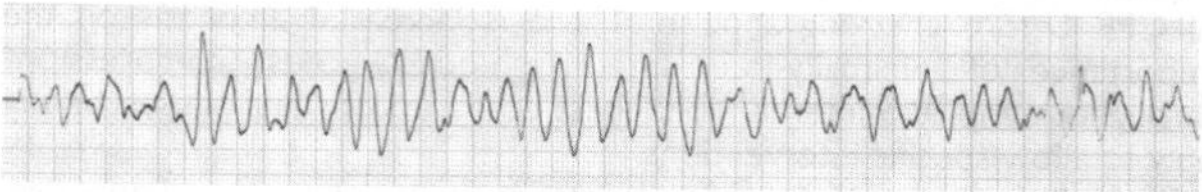

Fig. 2.6 Ventricular fibrillation. Reprinted with permission from Myerson SG *et al.* (2005) *Emergencies in Cardiology*. Oxford University Press, Oxford.

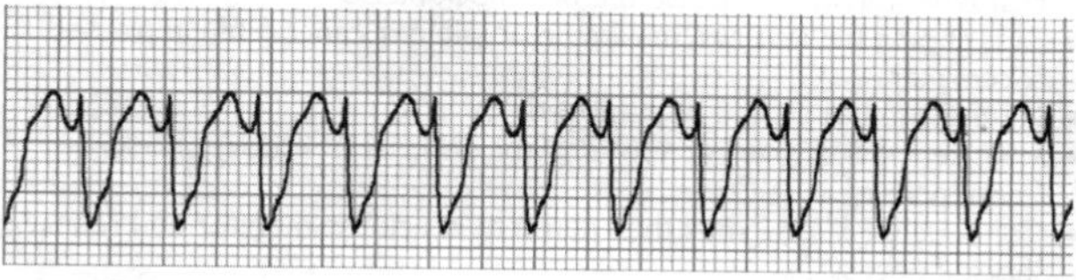

Fig. 2.7 Ventricular tachycardia.

Defibrillation

Rapid defibrillation is the key to optimal resuscitation and offers the best chance of success. Therefore, there is no need to carry out pulse checks between shocks and even if there is a rhythm change complete that cycle of CPR before checking a pulse. There is increased emphasis on the importance of minimally-interrupted high-quality chest compressions throughout any ALS intervention: chest compressions are paused briefly only to allow specific interventions.

- Perform uninterrupted chest compressions while applying self-adhesive defibrillation/monitoring pads
- One below the right clavicle
- The second in the V6 position (cardiac apex) in the midaxillary line
- Chest compressions are now continued while a defibrillator is charged—this will minimise the pre-shock pause
- Pads should be kept at a maximum possible distance from implanted pacemakers
- Nitrate patches should be removed
- A single shock is given at 150–200J (biphasic defibrillator) or 360J (monophasic)
- Continue CPR for 2 min; then pause to check the monitor and repeat shock if necessary
- If an organised rhythm is seen during a 2-minute period of CPR, do not interrupt chest compressions to palpate a pulse unless the patient shows signs of life suggesting ROSC. If there is any doubt about the existence of a pulse in the presence of an organised rhythm, resume CPR
- All subsequent shocks are 150-200J (biphasic) and 360J (monophasic)

If there is doubt about whether the rhythm is fine VF or asystole, DO NOT defibrillate but continue compressions and ventilations.

In out-of-hospital cardiac arrest attended by but UNWITNESSED by health care professionals, 2 minutes of CPR should be given before defibrillation.

In WITNESSED arrest, the first shock is given IMMEDIATELY.

When defibrillating, check:

- That the monitor is set on leads or paddles, as appropriate
- That the leads are connected to the monitor/defibrillator
- That the monitor trace has not changed before each shock

If VF/pulseless VT fails to respond to repeated defibrillation, consideration should be given to:

- Moving the defibrillator pads
- Changing defibrillator

Using an automated external defibrillator AED

Some first responders will use an AED with the result that this type of defibrillator is available before a manual defibrillator.

Notes

- Following the third shock resume chest compressions immediately and then give adrenaline 1mg IV and amiodarone 300 mg IV while performing a further 2 min CPR.
- A further dose of 150mg amiodarone may be given for recurrent or refractory VF/VT.

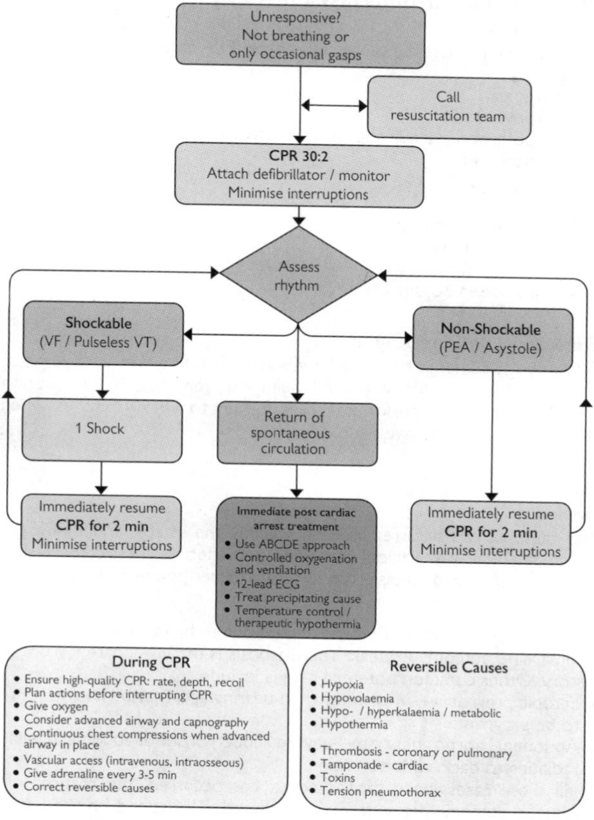

Fig. 2.8 Adult advanced life support algorithm. Reprinted with permission from the Resuscitation Council (UK) (2010), *Resuscitation guidelines.* 1mg adrenaline IV should be given as soon as IV access is obtained and repeated every 3–5 minutes thereafter until return of spontaneous circulation is obtained.

- Give further adrenaline 1mg IV after alternate shocks (i.e. approximately every 3–5 min)
- Do not interrupt CPR to give drugs.
- If the patient has taken an overdose of a tricyclic antidepressant (see p.459), the appropriate treatment of their arrhythmias includes sodium bicarbonate. Unless this is immediately available, rapid evacuation to hospital is essential.

Non-shockable rhythms (asystole/PEA)

4 Hs and 4 Ts

The potentially reversible causes of asystole/PEA arrest are:

'4 H's'

- Hypoxia
- Hypovolaemia
- Hypo/hyperkalaemia and other electrolyte disturbances
- Hypothermia

And:

'4 Ts'

- Tension pneumothorax
- Tamponade (cardiac)
- Toxins (drugs)
- Thromboembolism

Thrombolysis at cardiac arrest

Thrombolysis should be considered when cardiac arrest is thought to be due to proven or suspected pulmonary embolus. Consideration should be given to performing CPR for up to 60–90 minutes when thrombolytic agents have been given.

Notes

Hypoxia

This cause of cardiac arrest is dealt with by the establishment of a protected patent airway, artificial ventilation, and effective chest compressions. Attention can then be transferred to seeking other potential causes.

Hypovolaemia

The most common cause of cardiac arrest due to hypovolaemia is probably trauma. The outcome is bleak. The diagnosis is usually apparent from the history. Other common potential causes include:

- Ectopic pregnancy—women of child-bearing age, may be known to be pregnant
- Abdominal aortic aneurysm—severe sudden onset of abdominal pain radiating to back, with distension

In all these cases, once cardiac arrest has occurred, the chances of a successful outcome are extremely small and will depend on the patient reaching surgery as rapidly as possible. The clinical emphasis must, therefore, be on immediate evacuation to hospital. IV access and fluid resuscitation can be attempted en route.

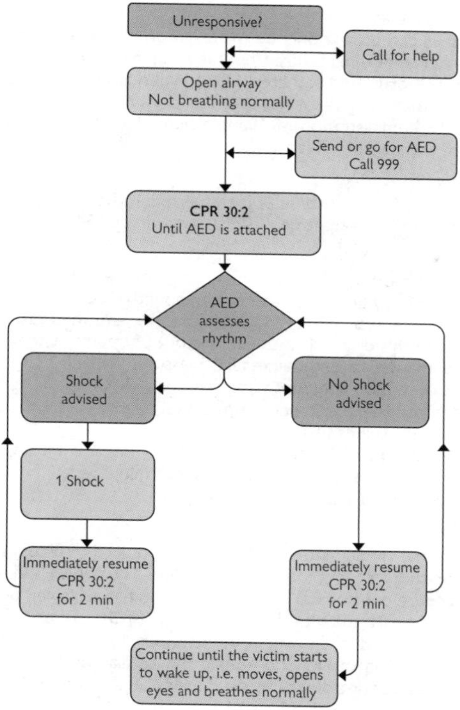

Fig. 2.9 Algorithm for use with an AED. Reprinted with permission from the Resuscitation Council (UK) (2010), *Resuscitation Guidelines*.

Hypo/hyperkalaemia, hypocalcaemia

This diagnosis can usually only be made on presumptive grounds unless there is evidence of renal failure from the examination or history (such as a dialysis shunt or CAPD catheter) when hyperkalaemia can be assumed or it is clear that the patient has taken calcium channel blockers. In any case of EMD, administration of 10ml calcium gluconate or chloride will do no harm and may be effective.

Hypothermia

Hypothermia <35°C. A patient is hypothermic if they feel cold centrally (i.e. on the chest). The treatment is discussed on pp.554–7.

Tension pneumothorax

A tension pneumothorax may be the primary cause of PEA. The diagnosis is made clinically and/or by use of ultrasound. Decompress rapidly by needle thoracocentesis or urgent thoracostomy, and then insert a chest drain. Clues to this diagnosis include a history of trauma, asthma, positive pressure ventilation, or external cardiac massage.

The signs of tension pneumothorax are:

- Hyper-resonant percussion note (ipsilateral)
- Absent breath sounds (ipsilateral)
- Reduced chest movement (ipsilateral)
- Elevated JVP (unless the patient is hypovolaemic)
- Trachea deviation to contralateral side (late)

Cardiac tamponade

In blunt trauma, cardiac tamponade is invariably fatal. Fruitless pericardiocentesis or thoracotomy are NOT indicated. The ONLY indication for either procedure pre-hospital is in a patient who has sustained penetrating trauma to the heart and who loses output *whilst the doctor is present* or who has shown signs of life within the previous 10 minutes. In such rare circumstances, thoracotomy and sealing the cardiac perforation may be lifesaving. Needle pericardiocentesis is valueless in the arrested patient.

Toxins

Unless the toxin is immediately apparent and an antidote is available, there is little that can be done in cardiac arrest due to toxins. Specific antidotes should be used only if the toxic substance is known, although administration of intravenous calcium (10ml gluconate/chloride) is reasonable.

Thromboembolism

The commonest cause of thromboembolic or mechanical circulatory obstruction is massive pulmonary embolus. Thromboembolism large enough to cause cardiac arrest is almost invariably fatal. However, if cardiac arrest is likely to be caused by pulmonary embolism, consider giving a thrombolytic drug immediately. Thrombolysis may be considered in adult cardiac arrest, on a case-by-case basis, following initial failure or standard resuscitation in patients in whom an acute thrombotic aetiology for the arrest is suspected. Ongoing CPR is not a contraindication to thrombolysis. Thrombolytic drugs may take up to 90mins to be effective; only administer a thrombolytic drug if it is appropriate to continue CPR for this duration.

Peri-arrest arrhythmias

Tachycardias

The management of peri-arrest tachycardias depends ultimately on whether the tachycardia is broad complex or narrow complex. The algorithms for broad and narrow complex tachycardias peri-arrest are given on the following pages.

Table 2.1 Potentially reversible causes of asystole/PEA arrest

	Diagnosis	**Management**
Hypoxia	History of inadequate ventilation or perfusion	High-flow oxygen Ventilatory support
Hypovolaemia	History or signs of trauma or other causes of blood loss	Rapid intravenous fluid infusion
Hypo/hyperkalaemia; hypocalcaemia	Medical history of renal failure, presence of a dialysis shunt, clues from medication	Hyperkalaemia—calcium chloride 10ml*
Hypothermia	Feel skin temperature	Patient warming
Tension pneumothorax	Signs of tension pneumothorax (see p.96)	Needle thoracocentesis
Tamponade	Usually penetrating trauma to the pericardium	Urgent transfer
Toxins	Clues from history, scene, or medication	Antidote, if available
Thromboembolism	Clues from past medical history or recent activity	May respond to vigorous cardiac compression. Consider thrombolysis

* or gluconate

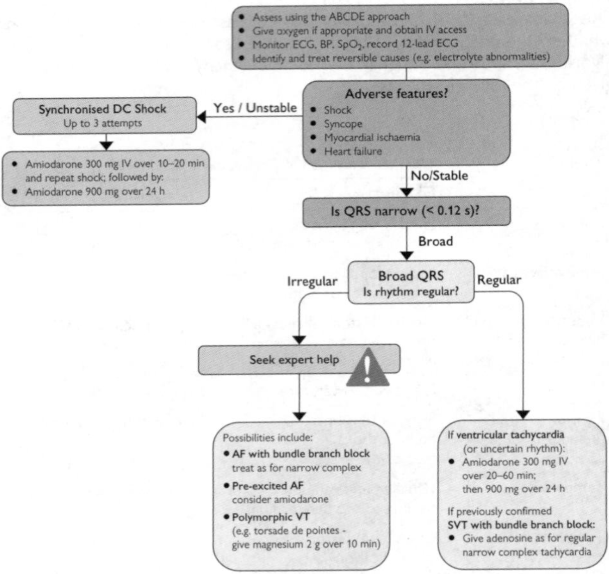

Fig. 2.10 Algorithm for peri-arrest broad complex tachycardia. Adapted with permission from the Resuscitation Council (UK) (2010), *Resuscitation Guidelines*.

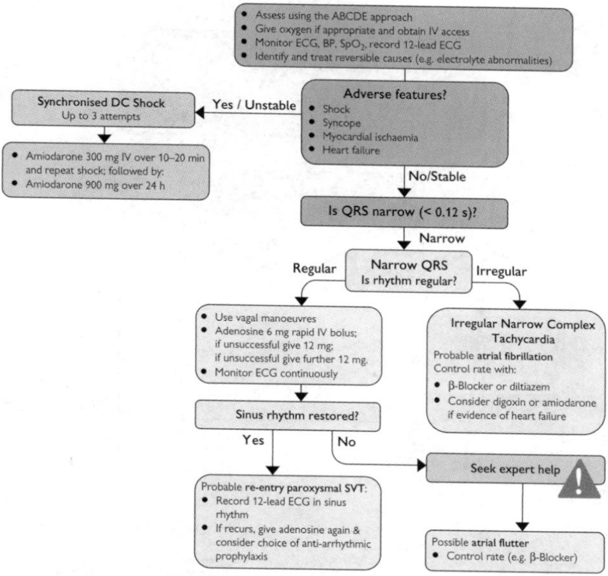

Fig. 2.11 Algorithm for peri-arrest narrow complex tachycardia. Adapted with permission from the Resuscitation Council (UK) (2010). *Resuscitation Guidelines.*

Note: In the majority of cases amiodarone and adenosine use should be restricted to hospital practice. Use may occasionally be justified by medical practitioner of transfer times are prolonged.

Short self-terminating runs of VT do not require any treatment.

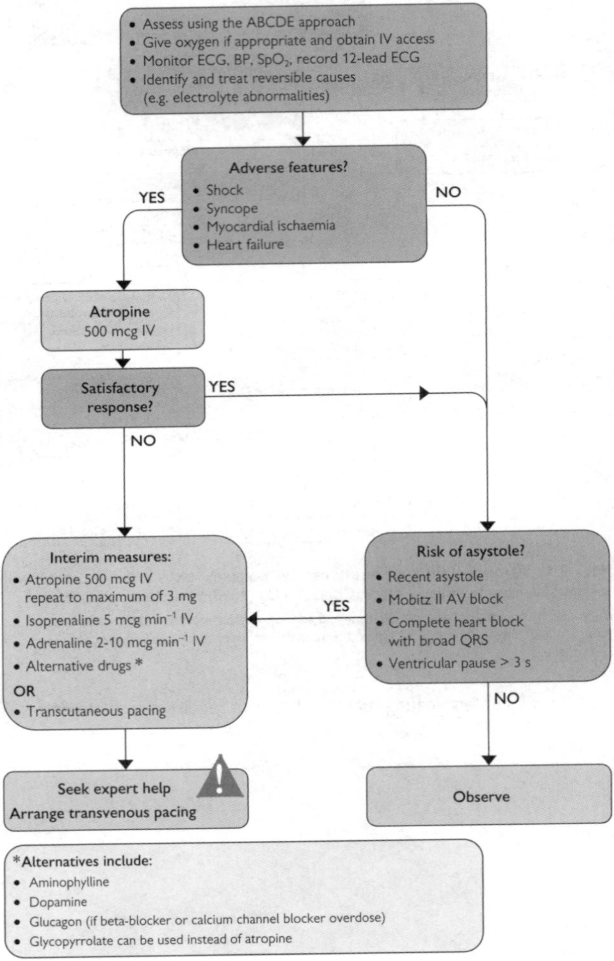

Fig. 2.12 Algorithm for peri-arrest bradycardias. Adapted with permission from the Resuscitation Council (UK) (2010). *Resuscitation Guidelines.*

Bradycardias

Sinus bradycardia

ECG abnormalities

Normal morphology, heart rate <60 bpm.

Clinical features

Patient may be aware of a slow pulse.

Initial management

None required.

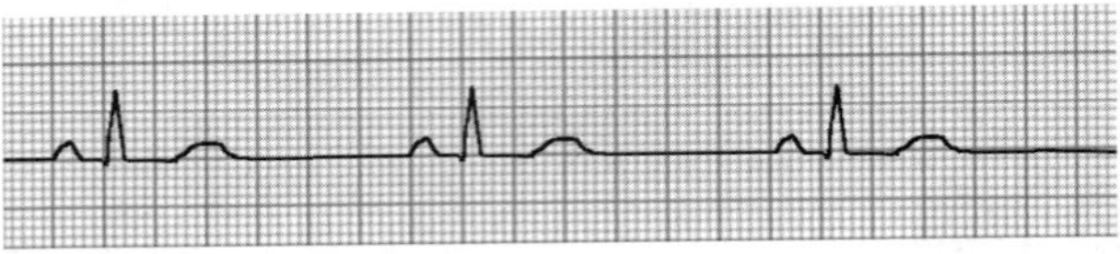

Fig. 2.13 Sinus bradycardia. Reprinted with permission from Myerson SG *et al.* (2005). *Emergencies in Cardiology*. Oxford University Press, Oxford.

1st degree heart block

ECG abnormalities

Prolonged PR interval ≥0.2 sec (5 small squares).

Clinical features

None.

Initial management

None required.

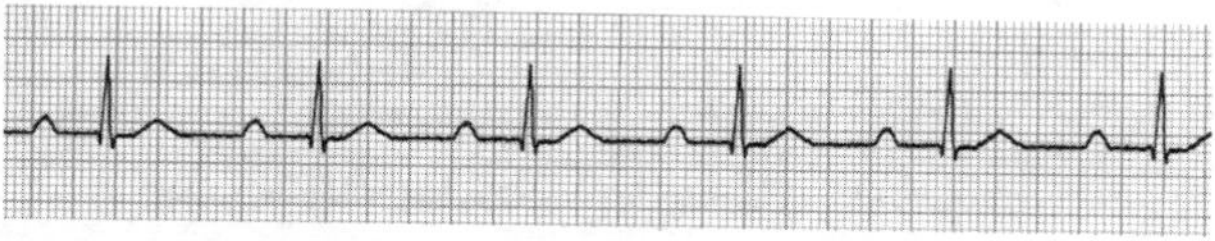

Fig. 2.14 1st degree heart block.

2nd degree heart block:
Möbitz type 1 (Wenckebach)

ECG abnormalities
Progressive lengthening of PR interval with intermittent complete AV block and failure of conduction of P wave.

Clinical features
Usually none.

Initial management
No specific treatment is required pre-hospital.

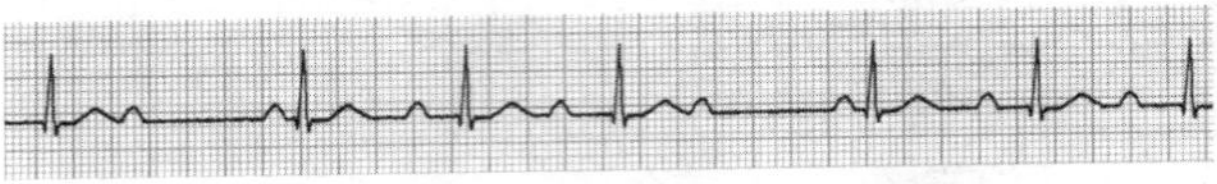

Fig. 2.15 2nd degree heart block: I. Möbitz type 1 (Wenckebach).

2nd degree heart block:

Möbitz type 2 (irregular block)

ECG abnormalities

Normal constant PR interval but intermittent complete heart block (P wave with no corresponding QRS).

Clinical features

Usually none. May develop low output state.

Initial management

- Following myocardial infarction (classically inferior MI), suggests possibility of progression to asystole, therefore administer atropine.
- If haemodynamically stable, no treatment.
- If haemodynamic compromise, atropine 0.5mg repeated if necessary, followed by external pacing if no response.

Transfer to hospital, oxygen, intravenous access, monitor ECG, pulse, BP, and pulse oximetry.

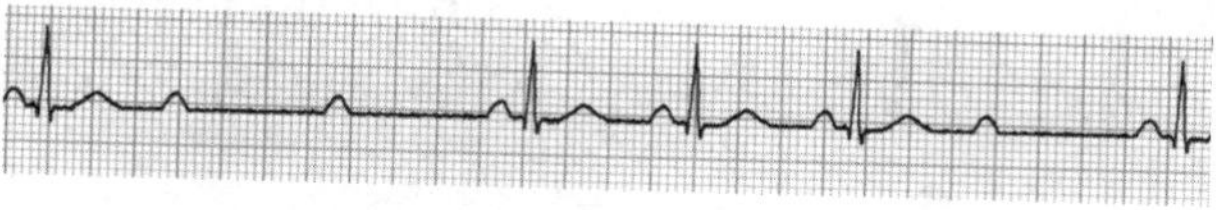

Fig. 2.16 2nd degree heart block: II Möbitz type 2 (irregular block).

2nd degree heart block:

Möbitz type 2 (2:1, 3:1, 4:1 block, etc.)

ECG abnormalities

Constant PR interval but every second, third, fourth (etc.) P wave is not conducted to the ventricles (QRS absent).

Clinical features

Usually none. May suffer palpitation and a low output state.

Immediate management

- If haemodynamically stable, no treatment.
- If haemodynamic compromise, atropine 0.5mg repeated if necessary, followed by external pacing if no response.

Transfer to hospital, oxygen, IV access, monitor ECG, pulse, BP, and pulse oximetry.

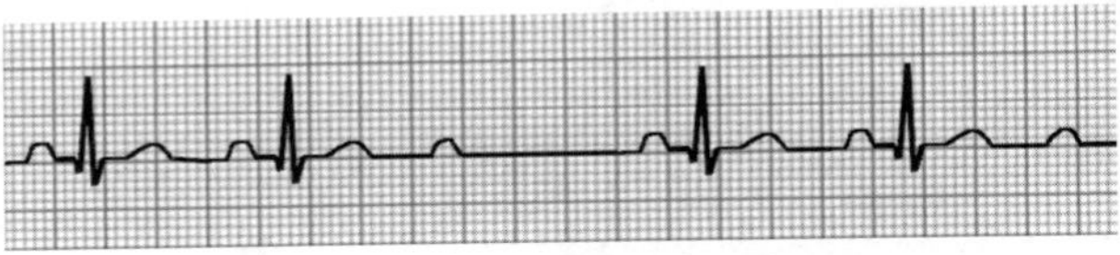

Fig. 2.17 2nd degree heart block, Möbitz type 2: III 2:1, 3:1, 4:1 block, etc. Reprinted with permission from Myerson SG *et al.* (2005). Oxford University Press, Oxford. *Emergencies in Cardiology*.

3rd degree (complete) heart block

ECG abnormalities

Complete failure of conduction from atria to ventricles with independent atrial and ventricular activity.

Presenting features

Will vary with cardiovascular state of patient and the heart rate.

- Palpitation
- Hypotension
- Heart failure.

Immediate management

Rapid transfer to hospital, oxygen, IV access, monitor ECG, pulse, BP, and pulse oximetry.

- If asymptomatic *and* rate >40, no treatment.
- If asymptomatic and rate <40, atropine 0.5mg repeated if necessary.
- If cardiovascular compromise, atropine 0.5mg repeated if necessary.
- If no response to atropine (maximum 3mg), consider external pacing.

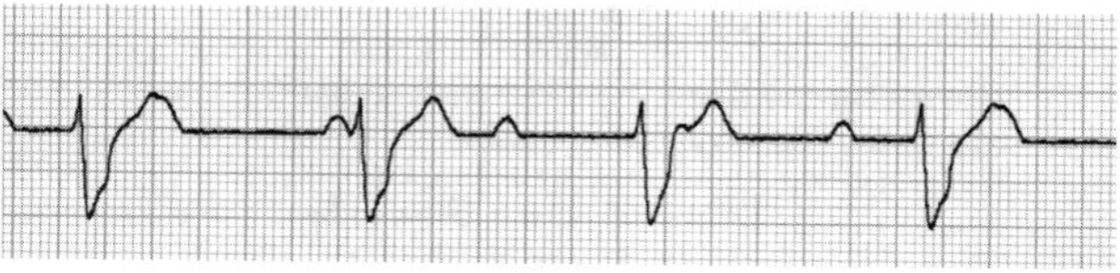

Fig. 2.18 3rd degree (complete) heart block.

Tachycardias

Supraventricular tachycardia: I (AV nodal re-entrant tachycardia—AVNRT)

ECG abnormalities

Regular, rapid, narrow complex tachycardia. P waves not usually visible. Rate 140–200 bpm.

Presenting features

- Palpitation
- Shortness of breath
- Ischaemic chest pain

Note: the symptoms of AVNRT may be remarkably mild in young fit individuals.

Initial management

Vasovagal manoeuvre.
If this fails:

- Urgent transfer to hospital or if transfer likely to be delayed or prolonged and patient is cardiovascularly compromised:
- Adenosine challenge (contraindicated in asthma)
  - Warn patient about chest tightness and a feeling of panic
  - Run a continuous rhythm strip (lead II)
  - Give 6mg adenosine followed by a 10ml flush
  - *If unsuccessful*, give 12mg adenosine followed by a 10ml flush

If this fails:

- Urgent transfer to hospital for further management.
- Oxygen, IV access, monitor ECG, pulse, BP, and pulse oximetry.

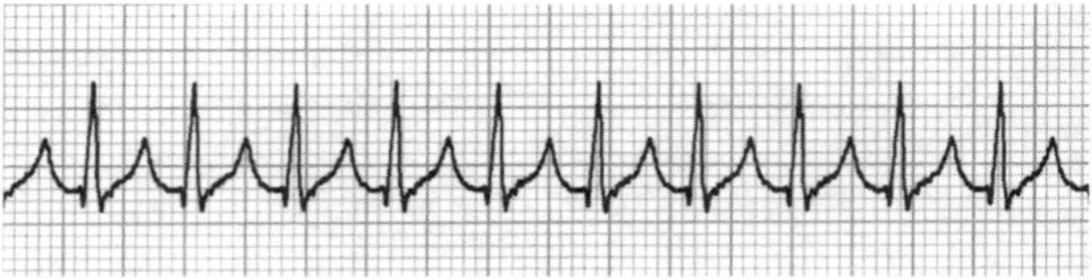

Fig. 2.19 Supraventricular tachycardia: I (AV nodal re-entrant tachycardia—AVNRT).

Atrial fibrillation

ECG abnormalities

Irregular, narrow complex tachycardia. No P waves. Fibrillation waves (not always present). Rate very variable <200 bpm.

Presenting features

May be absent, will depend on cardiovascular status of patient, rate, and time since onset. Chronic AF is less likely to be symptomatic.

- Palpitation
- Shortness of breath
- Heart failure
- Ischaemic chest pain.

Immediate management

- New diagnosis: rapid transfer to hospital, oxygen, intravenous access, monitor ECG, pulse, BP, and pulse oximetry.
- If the patient is cardiovascularly compromised and evacuation is likely to be prolonged or delayed, amiodarone 300mg IV may be given.

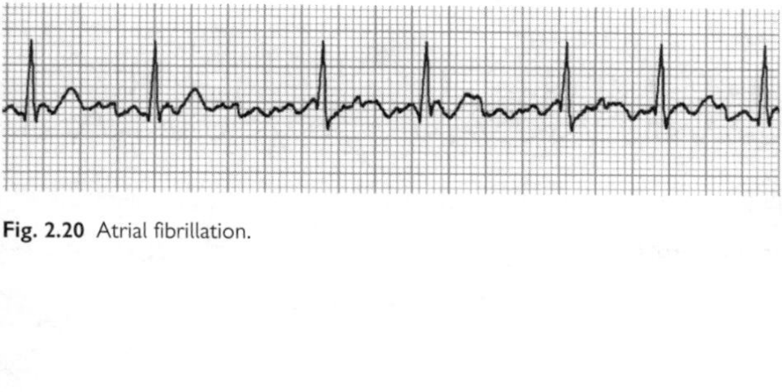

Fig. 2.20 Atrial fibrillation.

Atrial flutter

ECG abnormalities

Saw tooth flutter waves 300 per minute (best seen in II, III aVF, and VI). Rate 75–175 depending on degree of block.

Note: a heart rate of 150 is very strongly suggestive of flutter with 2:1 block.

Presenting features

- Palpitation
- Shortness of breath
- Heart failure
- Ischaemic chest pain.

Immediate management

- Carotid sinus massage may increase the degree of AV block, confirming the diagnosis but is unlikely to terminate the arrhythmia.
- Transfer to hospital, oxygen, IV access, monitor ECG, pulse, BP, and pulse oximetry.

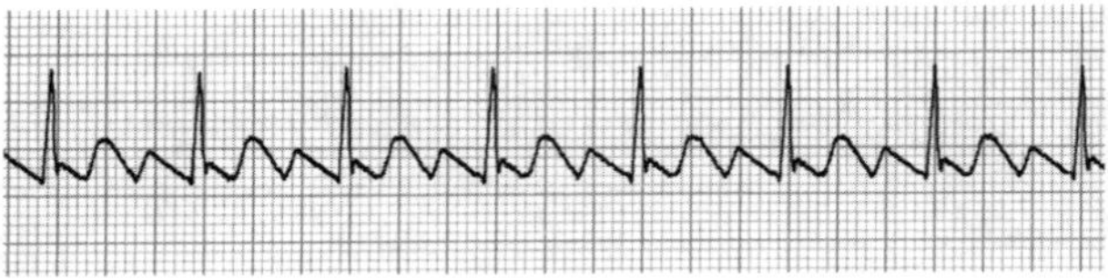

Fig. 2.21 Atrial flutter.

Ventricular tachycardia

ECG abnormalities

Tachycardia with QRS width >120 ms (3 small squares).
Note: without previous ECGs, it is extremely difficult to distinguish SVT with bundle branch block from VT. All broad complex tachycardias with haemodynamic compromise should be treated as VT.

Presenting features

- Palpitation
- Shortness of breath
- Heart failure
- Ischaemic chest pain.

Immediate management

No pulse
Follow cardiac arrest protocol and treat as VF.
Pulse
Short runs (less than 30 sec) should not be treated.
Runs longer than 30 sec:
Amiodarone 300mg over 20–60 min

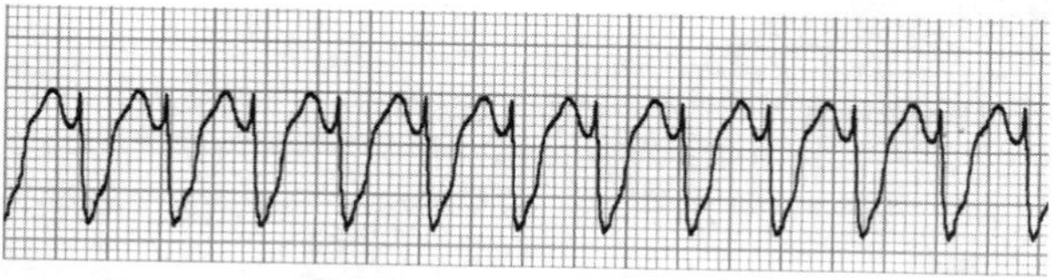

Fig. 2.22 Ventricular tachycardia.

Torsade de pointes

ECG abnormalities

Variation of VT in which appears to twist about the x axis.

Presenting features

- Palpitation
- Shortness of breath
- Heart failure
- Ischaemic chest pain.

Immediate management

Pulseless: manage as VF, otherwise as for VT, consider IV magnesium 8mmol by slow IV injection.

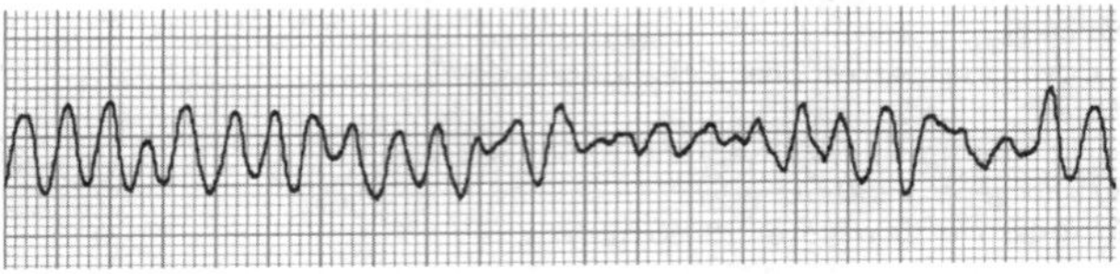

Fig. 2.23 Torsade de pointes.

Myocardial ischaemia

Unstable angina

In the early stages, unstable or crescendo angina is indistinguishable from non-Q wave myocardial infarction.

Crescendo or unstable angina presents with ischaemic pain at rest, sudden onset disabling angina or rapid deterioration in previous long-standing stable angina.

Symptoms

- Crushing/tight central chest pain
- Discomfort/heaviness in the arms (more often the left)
- Discomfort in the neck and jaw
- Nausea and vomiting
- Sweating
- Shortness of breath.

Signs

- Pallor
- Sweating
- Signs associated with complications or precipitants:
  - Palpitation
  - Hypotension
  - Pulmonary oedema.

ECG abnormalities

(See Fig. 2.24)

- T wave flattening or inversion
- ST depression.

Initial management

- Rest
- High-flow O_2
- Monitor pulse oximetry, ECG, pulse respiratory rate, and BP
- Aspirin 300mg (unless recent major GI bleed or aspirin allergic)
- Nitrate (buccal or sublingual—dose varies with formulation)
- Diamorphine up to 5mg with metoclopramide 10mg
- Urgent evacuation to hospital for further management.

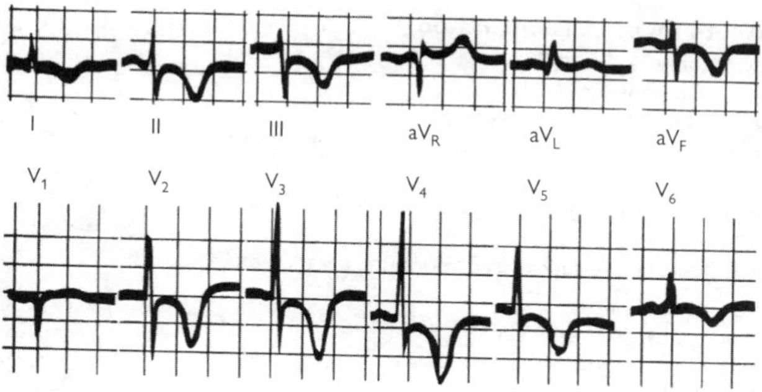

Fig. 2.24 ECG in unstable angina/non-Q wave infarction. Reprinted with permission from Wyatt J *et al.* (2005). *Oxford Handbook of Accident and Emergency Medicine*, 2nd edn. Oxford University Press, Oxford.

Acute myocardial infarction

Symptoms

As for unstable angina, but:

- Pain likely to be more severe
- Sweating, nausea, and vomiting likely to be more marked.

Signs

As for unstable angina, but also:

- Bradycardia/tachycardia
- Cardiac failure/shock (JVP, murmurs, basal crepitations, BP).

ECG abnormalities

May be absent in early stages.

- Peaked T waves and ST elevation.

Followed by

- ST elevation and 'mirror' ST depression.

Followed by

- Development of Q waves.

Followed by

- T wave inversion.

Location of changes:

- *Inferior MI*
  - II, III aVF (may extend laterally or posteriorly).
- *Anterior MI*
  - V_1–V_3 (may extend to V_4, anteroseptal or to V_6, anterolateral).
- *Posterior MI*
  - ST depression and R wave changes in V_1–V_2 (mirror image of anterior changes).

Immediate management

- Rest
- High-flow O_2
- Monitor pulse oximetry, ECG, pulse respiratory rate, and BP
- Aspirin 300mg (unless recent major GI bleed or aspirin allergic)
- Nitrate (buccal or sublingual)
- Diamorphine up to 5mg with metoclopramide 10mg
- CONSIDER thrombolysis (see p.117)
- Urgent evacuation to hospital for further management

Therapy with betablockers or ACE inhibitors should be commenced following arrival in hospital.

Pre-hospital thrombolysis

In the majority of cases, thrombolysis or acute percutaneous coronary intervention (PCI) will be carried out after arrival in hospital and the aim of pre-hospital care must be to expedite arrival at hospital. In some circumstances, geographical location or conditions will mean that pre-hospital thrombolysis is appropriate and thrombolysis is increasingly provided by ambulance service personnel. If this is likely to be the case in a particular area, appropriate protocols should be in place.

Indications

- Ischaemic chest pain (onset within 12 hours)
  AND
- 1mm ST elevation in 2 or more adjacent limb leads
  OR
- 2mm ST elevation in 2 or more adjacent chest leads.

New left bundle branch block is also an indication for thrombolysis in the presence of chest pain, but old notes and ECGs are unlikely to be available in pre-hospital care.

Contraindications

See Table 2.2

Table 2.2 Contraindications to thrombolysis

Absolute	
• Stroke in last six months	• Active peptic ulcer disease
• Trauma with risk of major bleeding	• Recent GI bleeding
• Bleeding diathesis	• Acute pancreatitis
• Severe liver disease	• Oesophageal varices
• Coma	• Known aortic dissection
• Lumbar puncture, visceral biopsy, or dental extraction in last month	• Abdominal, eye, or neuro-surgery in last month
Relative	
• Active menstruation	
• Pregnancy	
• Hypertension (systolic >200mmHg, diastolic >100mmHg)	
• Anticoagulant therapy	
• Abdominal aortic aneurysm	
• Traumatic CPR	

Thrombolytic agents

The thrombolytic agent of choice in pre-hospital care is *tenecteplase* which activates plasminogen to form plasmin which degrades fibrin and breaks up thrombi.

Dose

Weight	Dose	Volume*
< 60kg (< 9st 7lbs)	6,000u	6.0
60–69kg (9st 6lbs–10st 12lbs)	7,000u	7.0
70–79kg (11st–12st 6lbs)	8,000u	8.0
80–89kg (12st 8lbs–14st)	9,000u	9.0
> 90kg (> 14st 2lbs)	10,000u	10.0

*Concentration 1000u/ml

The maximum dose is 10,000u (50mg)

Note: patients receiving thrombolytic therapy will require heparin (up to 4,000u depending on weight).

Side-effects

- Nausea and vomiting
- Bleeding
- Reperfusion arrhythmias
- Hypotension.

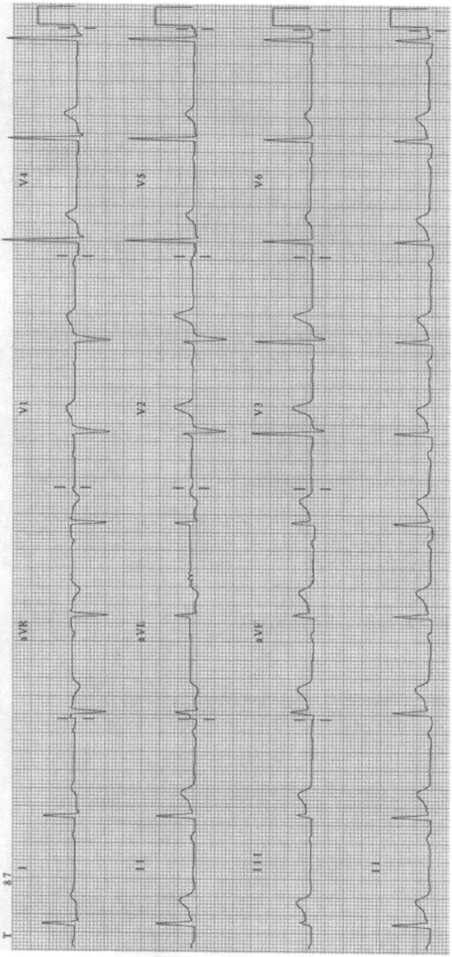

Fig. 2.25 Acute inferior MI. Reprinted with permission from Myerson SG *et al.* (2005). *Emergencies in Cardiology*. Oxford University Press, Oxford.

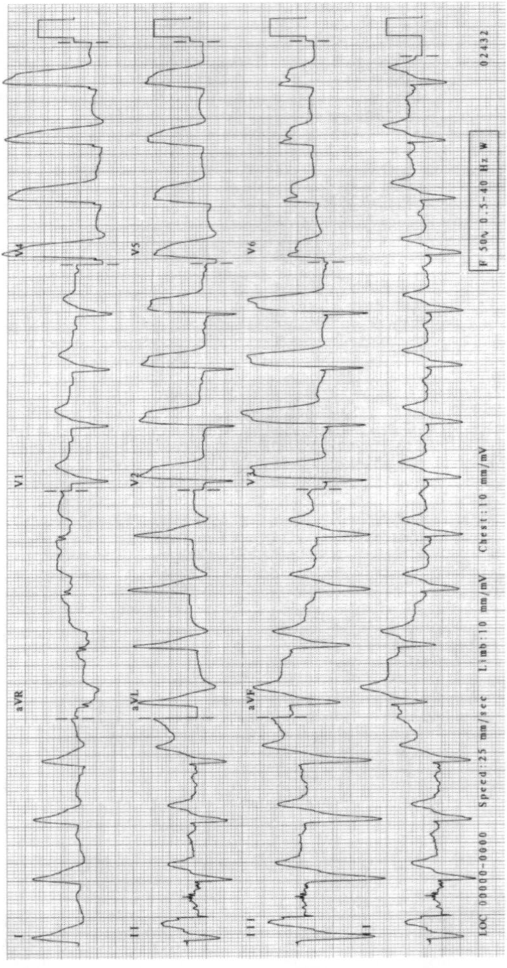

Fig. 2.26 Acute anterior MI. Reprinted with permission from Myerson SG *et al.* (2005). *Emergencies in Cardiology*. Oxford University Press, Oxford.

Pericarditis

Aetiology
Causes include viruses, bacteria including tuberculosis, fungi, malignancy, autoimmune disease, and post myocardial infarction. Many cases are idiopathic. A recent history of a flu-like illness is suggestive of viral pericarditis.

Symptoms
Retrosternal or left-sided chest pain; may be pleuritic. Radiates to neck. Worse with coughing, lying flat, inspiration, or swallowing. May be associated with shortness of breath. Other symptoms may reflect the underlying cause.

Signs
A pericardial rub may be heard in full inspiration or expiration with the patient leaning forward.

ECG abnormalities
Concave upwards ST segment elevation.

Immediate management
Admission to hospital for investigation and management. No other immediate treatment required. In the absence of contraindications, a NSAID can be given for analgesia (ibuprofen 400–600mg tds).

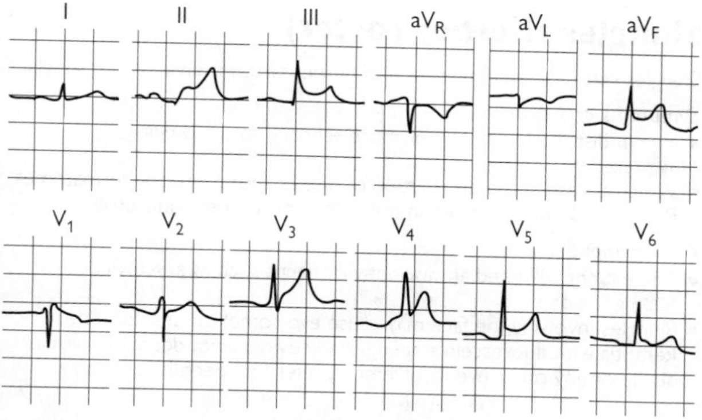

Fig. 2.27 Pericarditis: ECG abnormalities. Reprinted with permission from Myerson SG *et al.* (2005). *Emergencies in Cardiology*. Oxford University Press, Oxford.

Shingles (*Herpes zoster*)

Shingles results from reactivation of herpes virus in sensory root ganglia.

Symptoms and signs

- Pain in distribution of one or more sensory dermatomes

May precede

- Vesicular rash in the distribution of one or more sensory dermatomes. Rash may be disseminated in immunocompromised individuals.

Management

- The patient will need an oral antiviral agent such as acyclovir 800mg 5 x day.
- Shingles involving the face may cause eye complications. Exclude keratitis with fluorescein staining. If any evidence of decreased visual acuity or any other eye involvement, refer for specialist opinion.

Acute pulmonary oedema

Symptoms

- Breathlessness (acute or acute on chronic)
- Cough
- Frothy sputum (may be lightly blood stained)
- Collapse
- Shock, sweating, pallor, peripheral coldness.

Other symptoms reflect the underlying cause:

- Chest pain
- Palpitation.

Signs

- Patient dyspnoeic at rest and sitting upright
- Bilateral basal pulmonary crepitations
- Patient may be cold, clammy, and sweaty in severe cases
- Tachycardia
- Tachypnoea
- Elevated JVP (in congestive failure).

Immediate management

- Rapid evacuation to hospital
- Monitor pulse, respiratory rate, BP, O_2 saturation, ECG
- Give high-flow oxygen (care in COPD)
- Give frusemide 40–120mg IV (40mg boluses)
- Consider morphine 5–10mg IV with an antiemetic
- Consider buccal GTN 2–5mg
- Consider 12-lead ECG to exclude MI.

Signs indicating SEVERE pulmonary oedema

Inability to speak, BP <100mmHg, severe dyspnoea, copious frothy (pink) sputum

Acute exacerbations of asthma

Classification

A classification of asthma (adapted for pre-hospital use) is given in Table 2.3. Transportation to hospital is mandatory if any of the markers of near fatal, life-threatening, or acute severe asthma are present.

Management.

- Sit patient up, administer high-flow oxygen (15L/min)
- Give salbutamol 5mg by nebulizer (on oxygen); repeat if necessary
- Gain IV access and give 200mg hydrocortisone
- Monitor pulse, BP, respiratory rate, and O_2 saturation (maintain above 95%)
- Consider IV magnesium 1.2–2g
- Be prepared to provide ventilatory support if the patient deteriorates
- Evacuate urgently to hospital (warn A&E to call an anaesthetist if required).

Always consider pneumothorax or tension pneumothorax as a cause of deterioration in an asthmatic.

Table 2.3 Classification of asthma for pre-hospital use

Near fatal

- Immediate requirement for ventilation

Life-threatening

- Severe airways obstruction
  - PEF <33% predicted
  - Silent chest
  - Feeble respiratory effort
- Increased work of breathing
  - Exhaustion
  - Systolic BP <100mmHg
  - Bradycardia or arrhythmia
- Ventilation perfusion mismatch
  - Cyanosis
  - Hypoxia (SpO_2 <92%)
- Ventilatory failure
  - Confusion or coma (suggestive of rising $PaCO_2$)

Acute severe asthma

- PEF 33–50% predicted
- Respiratory rate >25/min
- Tachycardia (>110 bpm)
- Inability to complete sentence in one breath

Moderate asthma

- PEF 50–75% predicted
- No features of acute severe asthma
- Increasing symptoms

Chronic obstructive pulmonary disease (COPD)

Presenting features
- Wheeze unresponsive to inhaler therapy
- Production of purulent sputum/increased sputum production
- Increasingly severe breathlessness
- Respiratory failure.

Signs
- Increased respiratory rate (>25/min suggests a significant exacerbation)
- Cyanosis
- Use of accessory muscles
- CO_2 retention flap, confusion (indicative of hypercapnoea)
- Bilateral widespread wheezes (beware the silent chest)
- Peripheral oedema.

Initial management
- Oxygen 24–28% via face mask
- Salbutamol 5mg nebulized
- Consider hydrocortisone 200mg IV
- Consider oral antibiotics if the patient does not require admission
- Be prepared to provide respiratory support in the event of progressive respiratory failure
- In extreme circumstances, institute BVM ventilation with high-flow oxygen.

Pulmonary embolism

Presenting features

- The clinical picture of pulmonary embolism may vary from apparently minor non-specific chest pain to acute cardio-respiratory collapse.
- Sudden onset pleuritic chest pain
- Shortness of breath
- Haemoptysis
- Cardiac arrest, typically with PEA (massive PE).

Signs

- Tachycardia and tachypnoea
- Raised JVP
- Cyanosis
- Pleural rub
- Signs of DVT.

Signs may be of little help in establishing the diagnosis and the history may be of little more than chest pain and mild dyspnoea.

Immediate management

- Have a high index of suspicion; if the diagnosis is a possibility, refer to A&E urgently for further investigation and management
- Give oxygen 15L/min via a non-rebreathing mask
- 12-lead ECG may demonstrate the $S_1T_3Q_3$ pattern but is far more likely to show tachycardia and non-specific ST and T wave changes
- Monitor pulse, BP, respiratory rate, ECG, and pulse oximetry
- Give analgesia (NSAID or *small* dose of opiates).

Cardiac arrest

In the event of cardiac arrest, manage according to appropriate protocol. Vigorous CPR may dislodge embolus and produce effective cardiac output. There is currently no established place for pre-hospital thrombolysis in pulmonary embolism.

Common risk factors for DVT

- Prolonged bed rest
- Prolonged travel
- Recent surgery
- Pregnancy or recent childbirth
- Morbid obesity
- Previous/family history of DVT/PE

Pneumothorax

(See also Chapter 3, Trauma)
Spontaneous primary pneumothorax is rare, with a male to female ratio of 4:1. It occurs in previously normal lungs and is characteristically a disease of young men. Pneumothorax may also occur secondary to pre-existing lung diseases, most commonly asthma and COPD.

Presenting features
- Shortness of breath (usually sudden onset)
- Chest pain (non-specific, often pleuritic)
- Acute severe exacerbation of asthma or COPD
- Increasing difficulty in manually ventilating a patient or deteriorating hypoxia despite effective ventilation.

Types of pneumothorax

Simple
Simple pneumothorax occurs when there is a leakage of air into the pleural space through a hole in the visceral pleura. No valve is formed and the pressure within the pleural space remains atmospheric. Symptoms and signs may be absent or subtle but will be related to the degree of pneumothorax.

Tension
Tension pneumothorax (which is rare in non-traumatic conditions) is a life-threatening emergency and a cause of cardiac arrest. Air enters the pleural space either through a hole in the chest wall or, more commonly, through a hole in the visceral pleura. A flap valve effect develops and air which enters the pleural space is unable to leave during expiration. As a result, an increasingly positive pressure builds up in the pleural space, compressing the great vessels and the heart, shifting the mediastinum, and compressing first the ipsilateral and then the contralateral lung.

Although initially subtle, untreated, the patient will rapidly progress to severe respiratory distress, then cardiorespiratory arrest and death.

Signs
Other signs of tension pneumothorax include a weak thready pulse, elevated JVP, and cyanosis (very late). Tracheal deviation is a late sign.

Table 2.4 Signs of pneumothorax

	Ipsilateral percussion note	*Ipsilateral breath sounds*	*Chest expansion*	*Trachea*
Simple	Hyper-resonant	Reduced	May be reduced	Central
Tension	Hyper-resonant	Reduced or absent	Reduced, then over expanded	Central, then deviated to opposite side

Immediate management

Simple pneumothorax

No pre-hospital treatment is required. Monitor respiratory rate and O_2 saturation and transport to hospital for investigation and management.

Tension pneumothorax

Decompress urgently by inserting a large-bore IV cannula into the second intercostal space, midclavicular line. Once the cannula has been inserted, the needle is removed and the cannula secured in place. Presence of a tension pneumothorax is confirmed by the escape of air under pressure. Even if there is no evidence of a tension pneumothorax, the cannula *must* be left in place until the patient arrives in hospital.

Formal chest drainage (tube thoracostomy)

Insertion of a formal chest drain is very rarely indicated in pre-hospital care. It is a complex, painful procedure with serious complications and, whenever possible, should be carried out after arrival in hospital. Situations when insertion of a chest drain should be considered include:

- Predicted prolonged entrapment
- Very prolonged or delayed evacuation
- Before transfer by air
- In the artificially ventilated patient with a known pneumothorax.

The technique is described on the following page.

Increasing difficulty in manually ventilating a patient or deteriorating hypoxia despite effective ventilation is STRONGLY SUGGESTIVE of the possibility of pneumothorax.

Insertion of a chest drain

1. Prepare the drainage system (a bag/valve system is most appropriate).
2. If possible, position the patient with their arm (on the side of the pneumothorax) abducted with the forearm behind their head.
3. Identify and mark the 5th intercostal space midaxillary line.
4. Clean and prepare the area with antiseptic solution.
5. If the patient is conscious, inject 1% or 2% lignocaine down to the pleura. The needle should be inserted just above the lower rib in order to miss the neurovascular bundle which lies under the lower border of each rib.
6. Fixing the skin firmly between thumb and forefinger, make a 3cm incision along the line of the intercostal space with a scalpel
7. Using the scalpel (carefully!) and then a forceps, create a track down to and through the pleura.
8. Insert a finger (usually the little finger) through into the pleural. space and sweep round the hole to ensure that there is no lung stuck to the inside of the chest wall (care in trauma—there may be sharp ends of fractured ribs).
9. Grip the proximal end of the chest drain (through one of the side drainage holes) with forceps and clamp the distal end of the tube.
10. Using the forceps, insert the drain, directing the tip towards the lung apex.
11. Connect the drain to the drainage bag; check for bubbling.
12. Close the incision with mattress sutures and stitch the drain in place with a 'garter' stitch or equivalent.
13. Dress the wound using 10 cm × 10 cm swabs with a cut in one side to accommodate the drain (making sure it is not kinked) and cover the drain/tube junction with tape.
14. Ensure that the lung is ventilating.

Hyperventilation syndrome

Presenting features

- Anxiety/panic
- Hyperventilation
- Per-oral tingling
- Carpo-pedal spasm
- Tinnitus
- Chest tightness.

Management

Either

Get the patient to breathe slowly and shallowly into a paper (not plastic!) bag

Or

Instruct the patient to take slower and slower breaths

Whilst quietly reassuring them and gradually calming them down. It is often necessary to be firm and insistent on gradual slowing of the breathing whilst ensuring that the breaths become shallower and not deeper.

Once the symptoms have resolved, it may be worth getting the patient to reproduce them by artificially hyperventilating. This confirms the diagnosis and demonstrates to the patient that they have control over their own symptoms.

The unconscious patient

Differential diagnosis

Common causes of loss of consciousness include:

- Hypoglycaemia
- Drug/alcohol intoxication
- Head injury
- Intracerebral catastrophe (subarachnoid haemorrhage, stroke, etc)
- Epilepsy

Approach to the unconscious patient

Responsiveness

The first priority must be to ensure that the patient is unconscious! A gentle shake of the shoulder accompanied by 'Are you alright?' is appropriate.

Airway and breathing

Open the airway, remove any obvious foreign material, consider inserting an airway, and check for breathing. If respiration is absent or inadequate, ventilatory support with high-flow oxygen will be required.

Circulation

Assess the circulation using the pulses; if there is no pulse, commence CPR. Gain intravenous access. Monitor pulse, BP, ECG, and pulse oximetry. **Check the blood glucose.**

Disability

Perform a simple assessment of the conscious level using the AVPU system and assessment of papillary responses. A Glasgow Coma Scale Score can be performed during transfer to hospital, if there is time.

> NEVER forget the blood glucose in an unconscious patient

Table 2.5 Assessment of pupils

	Equal	Unequal
Large		
• Reactive	• Tricyclics • Sympathomimetics • Hypothermia	• Holmes–Adie
• Unreactive		• Tentorial herniation • Mydriatics • Local injury
Small		
• Reactive	• Opiates	• Argyll Robertson
• Unreactive	• Pontine haemorrhage	• Miotics • Horner's syndrome

Diagnostic clues in the unconscious patient

Diagnostic clues from simple assessment of the patient are given in Table 2.6.

Table 2.6 Diagnostic clues in the unconscious patient

Breathing			
Tachypnoea	*Cheyne–Stokes*	*Kussmaul*	*Bradypnoea*
Salicylates	CVA	DKA	Opiates
Hypovolaemia			Raised intracranial pressure
Tricyclic antidepressants			
Circulation			
Hypotension	*Hypertension*		
Opiates	Rising intracranial pressure		
Tricyclic antidepressants			
DKA			
Hypovolaemia			
Tachycardia	*Bradycardia*		
DKA	Rising intracranial pressure		
Hypovolaemia	Beta blockers		
Disability			
Large pupils	*Small pupils*	*Unequal*	
Tricyclics	Opiates	Local trauma	
Hypothermia	Pontine haemorrhage	Head injury (very late)	
General appearance—Look out for:			
Injection marks—opiates			
Urinary incontinence—epilepsy			
Signs of assault or serious injury			
Smell of alcohol			
Smell of ketones			
Medic-Alert® bracelet			
Meningitic rash			

Cerebrovascular events

Cerebro vascular accident (CVA)—stroke

Presenting features

Sudden onset of abnormal cerebral function including:

- Unilateral weakness/paraesthesia
- Dysphasia
- Convulsions
- Headache
- Reduced level of consciousness/coma
- Abnormal respiratory pattern
- Abnormal eye movements.

If the neurological symptoms and signs last less than 24 hours, the diagnosis is *transient ischaemic attack* (TIA). This distinction can rarely be made pre-hospital. An alternative diagnosis (space-occupying lesion, demyelination, encephalitis, etc) is more likely in younger patients

Immediate management

- All patients should be transported urgently to hospital for assessment
- Aspiration is a significant risk, therefore establish and maintain an open airway (use the recovery position)
- Give high-flow oxygen
- Check a BM stix®.

Sub-arachnoid haemorrhage (SAH)

Presenting features

- Sudden onset of occipital headache ('like a blow')
- Neck stiffness
- Nausea and vomiting
- Impaired conscious level/coma
- Fits
- Focal neurological signs.

Notes: onset of headache during sexual intercourse is a classical but rare feature of SAH. Many patients will report lesser headaches in the days leading up to their presentation ('herald bleeds').

Immediate management

- Monitor pulse, BP, respiratory rate, pulse oximetry
- If the patient is drowsy /unconscious, establish and maintain a patent airway (use the recovery position)
- Maintain a quiet environment as far as possible
- Give high-flow oxygen
- Treat fits with diazemuls (p.146)
- Evacuate immediately, preferably to a hospital with neurosurgical facilities
- BM stix®

Status epilepticus

Most patients with epilepsy and their families are experienced at dealing with single seizures. They are only likely to call for help when the fitting appears to be lasting longer than normal. Pre-hospital care personnel may also, more rarely, be asked to treat a patient having their first fit.

Definition

Status epilepticus is defined as fitting lasting 30 min or longer, or multiple short seizures with so little time between them that no recovery occurs before the new attack commences.

Immediate management

- Ensure a safe environment.
- Fits lasting 5 min or less require no treatment.
- Give high-flow oxygen if possible.
- Stop fitting with IV diazemuls (see box).
- Establish and maintain a clear airway (an oral or nasal airway and the recovery position is usually adequate); ensure effective suction is available.
- Transfer urgently to hospital.
- If control is not achieved, transport the patient to hospital for further management. DO NOT give dangerous doses of diazemuls.

Doses

Diazepam/Diazemuls

By IV injection

Neonate: 300–400µg/kg

1 month–12 years: 300–400µg/kg

12–18 years: 10–20mg

Doses repeated after 20 minutes if necessary

By rectum (as rectal solution)

Neonate 1.25–2.5mg

1 month–2 years: 5mg

2 years–12 years: 5–10mg

12–18 years: 10mg

Doses repeated after 10 minutes if necessary

Meningococcal meningitis and meningococcal septicaemia

Meningococcal disease may present with a predominantly meningitic or with a septicaemic picture.

Meningitis

Presenting features

- Neck stiffness
- Pyrexia
- Headache
- Photophobia
- Drowsiness
- Non-specific flu-like symptoms.

Meningococcal septicaemia

Any or all of the above plus:

- Petechial rash
- Ecchymotic/purpuric rash (due to enlargement and confluence of petechiae)
- Non-purpuric maculopapular rash
- Shock
- Respiratory distress.

Notes

A suggestive rash, even in the absence of other symptoms, should be treated as meningococcal septicaemia until proven otherwise. The rash may not always be present on presentation.

Meningism may be absent even in the presence of a rash.

Immediate management

- Intravenous access
- Give benzyl penicillin (see box)
- Commence IV fluids
- Establish and maintain a patent airway
- Transfer to hospital **without delay**.

Consider intramuscular antibiotics if IV access is difficult: DO NOT DELAY TRANSFER. Alternative therapy, suitable also for those genuinely allergic to penicillin, is cefotaxime 2g or ceftriaxone 2g (adult doses).

Benzyl penicillin in meningococcal disease

Adult

1.2g (2.4g in established disease) by IV injection (preferred) or intra-muscular injection

Children

- Under 1 year:300mg
- 1–9 years: 600mg
- 10 years and over: adult dose

Contact prophylaxis in meningococcal disease

The following will need antibiotic prophylaxis:

- Household 'kissing contacts'
- Institutional contacts (nursing home residents, etc)
- Clinical personnel—only if involved in close patient contact (e.g. resuscitation) or risk of body fluid (sputum, blood) contamination

Seek advice from local consultant in communicable disease regarding medication.

Poisoning (including drugs and alcohol)

See Chapter 6.

Hypothermia

See pp.554–7.

Diabetic emergencies

Hypoglycaemia

Presenting features

- Tachycardia/palpitation
- Sweating
- Anxiety
- Headache
- Pallor and cold extremities
- Tremor
- Confusion
- Aggression
- Coma.

Immediate management

If the patient is still conscious and aware of likely diagnosis, consider oral treatment such as hot sweet drinks (milk and sugar, sweet tea, etc), Hypostop®, or confectionery.

If patient unconscious, check BM stix® then give 10% dextrose via a large IV cannula.

If IV access is difficult, give glucagon 1mg by intramuscular injection. Glucagon will not work in cachetic patients, those with chronic liver disease, or alcoholics.

Any BM stix® result of 4 or less should be treated.

Ketoacidosis

Diabetic ketoacidosis is much more insidious in onset than hypoglycaemia. It may result from non-compliance with treatment, be precipitated by infection, or be the presentation of previously undiagnosed diabetes.

Presenting features

- Polyuria, polydipsia
- Weight loss
- Weakness
- Shortness of breath
- Abdominal pain
- Vomiting
- Confusion
- Coma
- Signs and symptoms of underlying infection (eg pneumonia, urinary tract infection).

The diagnosis is made by BM stix® which will usually demonstrate an elevated blood glucose.

Immediate management

- The priority is urgent transfer to hospital.
- Establish and maintain a clear airway (vomiting is a significant risk).
- Give oxygen 15L/min.
- If transfer is prolonged or delayed (or during transit) obtain iv access and give normal saline stat(care in patients with cardiac disease); consider administering a short-acting insulin depending on BM result.

The acute abdomen

The pre-hospital practitioner will not always be able to make a precise diagnosis in the case of a patient with an acute abdomen. Sometimes (e.g. food poisoning) the history will give the probable diagnosis; in other cases, the patient may present the classical history and examination findings of, for example, acute appendicitis or cholecystitis. Very often, however, it will be more useful to answer these two questions:

- Is there a possibility (however small) that this patient has a serious condition requiring operative intervention or further investigation?
- Does the patient require care or symptom relief which cannot be provided at home?

If the answer to either of these questions is yes, the patient requires transfer to A&E for further assessment and management.

Differential diagnosis

Nevertheless, it is often possible to reach at least a working diagnosis for the patient with abdominal pain. This depends on the identification of characteristic symptom patterns for each condition. Use of Table 2.7 allows matching of symptoms and possible diagnoses.

It may also be helpful to consider the age of the patient when attempting to reach a diagnosis (see Table 2.8).

Abdominal aortic aneurysm (AAA)

Presenting features

- Sudden onset abdominal or back pain
- Pulsatile mass (may be tender)
- Hypotension (following rupture)
- Syncope (following rupture)

Notes:

- The aneurysm may be difficult to palpate (especially in the obese).
- Ruptured AAA should always be considered as a cause of syncope in the elderly.
- Any patient with a history and findings suggestive of the diagnosis should be referred urgently for assessment.

Immediate management

- Immediate transfer to hospital
- Oxygen 15L/min
- DO NOT waste time attempting IV access—do this en route.
- If fluids are necessary, maintain a BP of approximately 90mmHg. DO NOT attempt to achieve normotension.

Table 2.7 Matching of symptoms and possible diagnoses

Finding	Possible diagnoses	Page
Severe abdominal pain radiating to back	Aortic aneurysm	154
	Acute cholecystitis	158
	Acute pancreatitis	159
	Peptic ulcer disease	160
	Active labour	664
Flank pain radiating to the groin	Renal/ureteric colic	161
	Pyelonephritis	162
	Testicular torsion	
	Aortic aneurysm	154
Collapse or signs of shock	Aortic aneurysm	154
	Ectopic pregnancy	646
	Gastrointestinal bleed	
	Myocardial infarction	116
Distension	Bowel obstruction	164
	Pregnancy	644
	Ascites	
	Mass	
Abdominal bruising	Trauma	218
	Aortic aneurysm	154
	Acute pancreatitis	159
Pain out of proportion to examination findings	Aortic aneurysm	154
	Mesenteric infarction	165
	Renal colic	161
Haematemesis or melaena	Ulcer	160
	Diverticular disease	166
	Angiodysplasia	
	Malignancy	
	Varices	
Constipation	Bowel ischaemia	275
	Bowel obstruction	164
	Diverticular disease	166

Table 2.7 Diagnosis of the acute abdomen by age. Reprinted from Greaves I and Porter K (1999). *Pre-hospital medicine—the principles and practice of immediate care.* Hodder Arnold

Children under 2 years
Non-specific 61%
Appendicitis 32%
Intussusception 1.3%
Adolescents
Acute appendicitis
Ectopic pregnancy
Adults under 50 years
Non-specific 39%
Appendicitis 2%
Cholecystitis 6.3%
Bowel obstruction 2.5%
Pancreatitis 1.6%
Diverticular disease <0.1%
Hernia <0.1%
Cancer <0.1%
Vascular <0.1%
Adults over 50 years
Cholecystitis 21%
Non-specific 15.7%
Appendicitis 15.2%
Bowel obstruction 12.5%
Pancreatitis 7.3%
Diverticular disease
Malignancy 4.1%
Hernia 3.1%
Vascular 2.3%

Acute appendicitis

Presenting features

- Dull peri-umbilical pain which migrates to the right iliac fossa, becoming sharp
- Anorexia
- Nausea and vomiting
- Right iliac fossa tenderness (signs of peritonitis suggest perforation)
- Mild pyrexia
- Coated tongue and hallitosis.

Other symptoms (variable)

- Previous similar attacks
- Urinary frequency and dysuria
- Diarrhoea.

Notes

Older patients and women tend to present with less 'classical' symptoms.

Immediate management

- Transfer to hospital for assessment and surgery
- Give antiemetic if required.

Gallbladder disease

Gallbladder disease is more common amongst patients who are obese, female, and middle aged, although it can occur in either sex and any age group.

Presenting features

- Biliary colic
  - Short episodes of right upper quadrant pain or epigastric pain which may radiate to the back, usually constant in nature (not truly collicky). Usually less than 30 min duration.
  - Nausea and vomiting (mild)
  - Murphy's sign* usually negative, no abdominal tenderness
  - Fever absent
- Acute cholecystitis
  - Nausea and vomiting (more marked)
  - More prolonged than biliary colic
  - Localized right upper quadrant pain radiating to the epigastrium or scapula
  - Low-grade fever
  - Local peritonism
  - Murphy's sign* usually positive
  - Patient looks 'unwell'.
- Gallbladder perforation
  - Usually in the elderly, infirm, or diabetic
  - Jaundice
  - Fever/rigors
  - Right upper quadrant pain.

These symptoms suggest the presence of ascending cholangitis.

Immediate management

- Urgent transfer to hospital
- Give analgesia (NSAID or opiate), preferably IV
- Give oxygen 15L/min
- Monitor pulse, pulse oximetry, BP, and ECG (myocardial ischaemia is a differential of gallbladder disease).

* Place the hand lightly in the right upper quadrant and ask the patient to take a deep breath. If the patient experiences discomfort (when the inflamed gallbladder jars against the examining hand), *Murphy's sign* is positive.

Acute pancreatitis

A careful history is important in the diagnosis of acute pancreatitis in order to identify potential causes. The most common (>80%) are gallstones and alcohol. Other cause include viral infections such as mumps and hepatitis, drugs, and trauma. Acute pancreatitis can also be familial.

Presenting features

- Severe abdominal pain, usually rapid onset
  - Poorly localized in the epigastrium and left upper quadrant
  - Radiating to back
  - Aggravated by lying down, relieved by sitting forwards
- Vomiting (may be severe)
- Patient looks unwell
- Jaundice
- Shock more common in the elderly
- Abdominal tenderness, usually diffuse; guarding and rebound
- *Rarely*, bruising may be noted in the flanks (*Grey–Turner's sign*) or around the umbilicus (*Cullen's sign*).

Immediate management

- Transfer urgently to hospital
- Establish and maintain a clear airway
- Give oxygen 15L/min
- IV access in transit, commence normal saline. If the patient is not shocked, time may be spent in gaining iv access for analgesia.
- Give antiemetic and analgesia (opiate)
- Monitor pulse, BP, respiratory rate, ECG, and pulse oximetry
- Check BM stix®
- Nil by mouth.

Peptic ulcer disease

Presenting features

- Severe epigastric pain; radiation to the back suggests posterior perforation
- Signs of peritonitis are absent unless perforation has occurred
- If perforation has occurred, the patient will try to lie as still as possible
- Haematemesis and melaena
- Shock (from perforation or bleeding).

Immediate management

- Transfer to hospital for investigation and management
- IV access en route
- IV fluids to maintain a radial pulse if the patient is shocked and transfer prolonged
- Monitor pulse, BP, ECG, and pulse oximetry
- Give high-flow oxygen
- Give analgesia (opiate)
- Nil by mouth.

Ureteric colic (renal stones)

Presenting features

- Often very severe loin and flank pain, radiating to groin and genitalia
- Patient may writhe around in an attempt to gain some ease from the pain
- Nausea and vomiting
- Sweating
- *Frank* haematuria is usually absent
- Loin tenderness (guarding may be present).

Immediate management

- Give analgesia (NSAID, opiate)
- Entonox may be useful whilst other analgesia takes effect
- Refer to hospital for pain control, diagnosis, and further management
- Monitor pulse, BP, ECG, and pulse oximetry
- Recurrent attacks: urgent admission may not be required.

Acute pyelonephritis

Presenting features

- High fever
- Sweating
- Vomiting (not always present)
- Loin pain
- Urinary frequency and dysuria
- Haematuria.

Immediate management

- The decision to refer urgently to hospital will depend on the clinical condition of the patient. Urinary tract investigation will be necessary in all new cases.
- Analgesia
- Increased fluid intake (oral or IV—severe cases will require admission)
- Urine for microscopy culture and sensitivity
- Antibiotic therapy (trimethoprim, amoxycillin, or a cephalosporin are usually suitable).

Gynaecological causes of abdominal pain

See Chapter 12.

Bowel obstruction

Presenting features

Most bowel obstructions are secondary to adhesions from previous surgery. Other causes include malignancy, herniae, and diverticular disease. Examination may reveal evidence of such a cause or features of a careful history may suggest the diagnosis. The common presenting features of bowel obstruction are:

- Abdominal pain
- Nausea and vomiting (vomiting may be absent in distal small bowel and large bowel obstruction)
- Abdominal distension
- Abdominal tenderness
- Constipation and inability to pass flatus (variable)
- The hernial orifices must be carefully examined and note taken of scars from previous surgery.

Immediate management

- Urgent transfer to hospital for assessment and further management
- Give oxygen 15L/min
- Nil by mouth
- During transit, gain IV access and start crystalloid
- Give analgesia (opiate)
- Monitor pulse, BP, ECG, and pulse oximetry.

Mesenteric infarction

Mesenteric infarction with bowel ischaemia and necrosis has a high mortality. The patient is often desperately unwell, but by the time the diagnosis is apparent, it is very often too late to intervene.

Presenting features

- Previous history of cardiac disease such as IHD or atrial fibrillation
- Abdominal pain (sudden onset)
- Nausea and vomiting
- Blood in stool or vomit
- Abdominal tenderness
- Patient looks disproportionately ill
- Shock (may be severe).

Management

- High-flow oxygen
- Urgent transfer to hospital
- IV access en route
- Analgesia
- Nil by mouth.

Diverticular disease

Diverticular disease (which is rare under age 35) is usually relatively benign with little more than cramping left iliac fossa pain which is often improved by passing faeces, in an otherwise well patient. Symptoms of acute diverticulitis are usually more florid, with the patient looking obviously unwell.

Presenting features

- Left iliac fossa pain (may be longstanding)
- History of irregular bowel habit
- Localized peritonism
- Nausea and vomiting
- Fever and tachycardia
- Rectal bleeding (can be massive)
- Mass in left iliac fossa (not always present).

Immediate management (severe or previously undiagnosed cases)

- Urgent transfer to hospital for assessment and management
- Give oxygen 15L/min
- Nil by mouth
- During transit, gain IV access
- Give analgesia (opiate)
- Monitor pulse, BP, ECG, and pulse oximetry.

Medical causes of abdominal pain

A number of medical diagnoses may present with abdominal pain, these include:

- Myocardial infarction
- Pneumonia
- Diabetic ketoacidosis
- Poisoning (more commonly in children)
- Patients with abdominal pain from these causes do not have signs of peritonism.

Chapter 3

Trauma

Patient assessment and treatment

The assessment and management of the trauma victim is divided into the following stages:

- Pre-hospital Primary survey
  Resuscitation
- Hospital Secondary survey
  Definitive care

In time, critical trauma pre-hospital care involves undertaking a rapid primary survey and instituting life-saving measures only. A detailed secondary survey and definitive care can be undertaken at an appropriate time in hospital.

Primary survey

[illegible] assessment designed to identify [illegible] life-threatening [illegible] way. For example:

[illegible] airway obstructive [illegible] opened [illegible]

The [illegible] survey and resuscitation are performed [illegible]. The [illegible] survey follows the following ABCDE sequence:

A Airway with cervical spine control
B Breathing with ventilation and oxygen [illegible]
C Circulation and control of external haemorrhage
D Disability
E Exposure and environment

Airway with cervical spine control

[illegible] airway obstruction produces [illegible] brain damage [illegible] can be complete [illegible] patient [illegible] or partial [illegible] breathing [illegible] obstruction can occur anywhere from the [illegible] to the [illegible] and trachea.

External causes of airway obstruction include:

- Tongue
- Foreign bodies
- Vomit
- Dentures
- Facial trauma
- Upper airway haemorrhage
- Airway burn
- Laryngeal trauma

Management summary

The [illegible] inspected for foreign bodies, vomit [illegible] removed [illegible] suction [illegible] must be [illegible] with [illegible] airway [illegible] undertaken with [illegible] manipulation [illegible] cervical spine [illegible].

[illegible] nasopharyngeal airway placement may be necessary [illegible] above measures do not open [illegible] clear airway. [illegible] may be [illegible] followed by [illegible] definitive airway [illegible] of the individual [illegible] skills and competence [illegible] of an [illegible] without [illegible] of an anaesthetist [illegible].

The airway should [illegible] maintained using the simplest [illegible] advanced [illegible] may [illegible] required for [illegible]:

- [illegible]
- [illegible] and [illegible]
- Manual airway opening manoeuvres—chin lift and jaw thrust
- Airway adjuncts—oropharyngeal or nasopharyngeal airways [illegible] patient [illegible]

Primary survey

The ***primary survey*** is a rapid structured assessment designed to identify injuries which are immediately life-threatening. When a problem is identified, it must be rectified straightaway. For example:

Airway obstruction ⇒ Airway manoeuvre ⇒ Airway opened

Therefore, the primary survey and resuscitation are performed simultaneously. The primary survey follows the following ABCDE sequence:

A **A**irway with cervical spine control
B **B**reathing with ventilation and oxygen therapy
C **C**irculation and control of external haemorrhage
D **D**isability
E **E**xposure and **E**nvironment.

Airway with cervical spine control

Complete airway obstruction produces irreversible brain damage in 3 min. Obstruction can be complete (a silent patient who may be conscious or unconscious) or partial (usually noisy breathing in a conscious or unconscious patient). Airway obstruction can occur anywhere from the mouth to the larynx and trachea.

Potential causes of airway obstruction include:

- The tongue
- Foreign bodies
- Vomit
- Dentures
- Facial trauma
- Upper airway haemorrhage
- Airway burns
- Laryngeal trauma.

Management—summary

The airway must be inspected for foreign bodies, vomit, displaced dentures, or debris. Gloved manual removal or aspiration using suction, followed by a jaw thrust manoeuvre, will open most airways. All airway manoeuvres should be undertaken whilst maintaining in-line cervical spine stabilization.

Oropharyngeal or nasopharyngeal airway placement may be needed if the above measures do not open and maintain a clear airway. Continued airway obstruction may be temporarily relieved by needle cricothyroidotomy and jet insufflation or definitively by a surgical airway or rapid sequence induction of anaesthesia to facilitate orotracheal intubation, depending on the individual practitioner's skills and competence. In some cases, the passage of a laryngeal mask airway (LMA) or orotracheal intubation can be achieved in the unconscious patient without the use of anaesthetic drugs.

The airway should be opened initially and maintained using the simplest steps. A more advanced technique may subsequently be required for longer term management. Stepped airway care can be summarized as:

- Airway inspection
- Airway clearance—manual and aspiration
- Manual airway opening measures—chin lift and jaw thrust
- Airway adjuncts—oropharyngeal or nasopharyngeal airways and pocket masks

- Orotracheal intubation or laryngeal mask airway
- Needle cricothyroidotomy and jet insufflation
- Surgical airway.

Basic airway manoeuvres

Airway inspection

The airway must always be inspected prior to a jaw thrust manoeuvre as a foreign body may move more distally into the airway if the patient inspires on airway opening.

Airway clearance—manual and aspiration

Gloves must always be worn as part of individual personal protective equipment. Broken dentures should be removed, but it is easier to maintain an open airway (and to achieve an effective seal with a face mask) by leaving good-fitting dentures in place.

The 'finger sweep' manoeuvre should be specifically avoided in children and care should always be exercised, even in adults, as foreign bodies may be pushed deeper down the airway. Blind 'poking about' in the airway must be avoided.

Postural positioning may be necessary if suction and manual removal of debris are inadequate to maintain an open airway, or it becomes necessary to leave the casualty alone to go to fetch help. Where possible, cervical spine stabilization should be maintained but this may not always be possible for the lone rescuer, where airway opening takes priority over cervical spine control.

Manual airway opening measures

Chin lift and jaw thrust (Fig 3.1)

The chin lift manoeuvre works in combination with head tilt. Because of the potential risk of spinal cord injury, it should not be used in the trauma patient. Jaw thrust is the procedure of choice. In the presence of bilateral mandibular body fractures, a jaw thrust is ineffective. In these cases, the airway may be opened by gripping the point of the chin and the tongue and lifting upwards, or by postural positioning.

Under no circumstances should the fingers be inserted in the mouth during the chin lift manoeuvre. This is asking for them to get bitten.

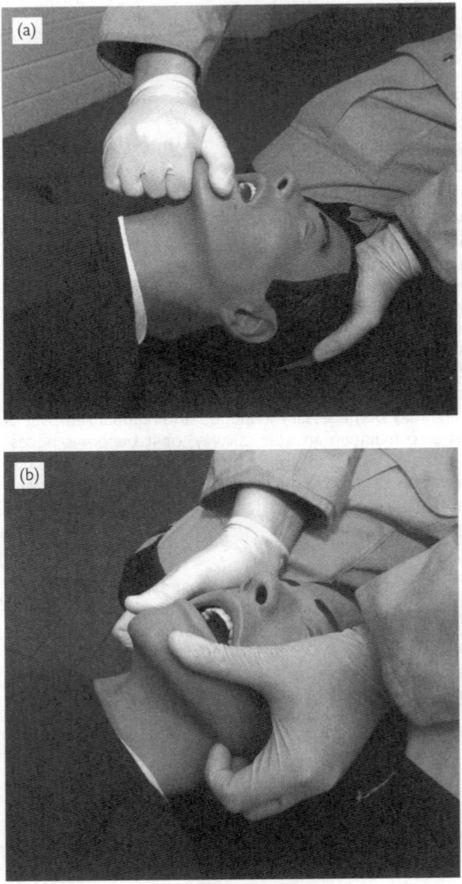

Fig. 3.1 (a) Chin lift and (b) jaw thrust manoeuvres. Reprinted with permission from Greaves I *et al.*, *Emergency care—a text for paramedics*, 2nd edn. W.B. Saunders.

Airway adjuncts—oropharyngeal or nasopharyngeal airway, and pocket masks.

Oropharyngeal airway

Oropharyngeal airways are available in a range of sizes to fit neonates to adults. The appropriate size is determined by measuring the distance from the teeth to the angle of the jaw.

An oral airway will not be tolerated in patients who have a gag reflex in whom it may induce gagging, vomiting, coughing, or laryngeal spasm. In adults, the airway is inserted with the convex side downwards and then rotated through 180 degrees with the flange anterior to the teeth. In children, the airway is inserted under direct vision with the concave side downwards and with the use of a tongue depressor. An oropharyngeal airway is always supported by a manual manoeuvre.

Nasopharyngeal airway

A nasopharyngeal airway can be inserted in the unconscious or semi-conscious patient with a gag reflex. It is of particular value in patients who have sustained head injuries and have clenched teeth. Providing the airway is lubricated and inserted perpendicular to the front of the face, there is no risk of intracranial penetration.

If coughing, laryngospasm, or airway obstruction occurs, the airway should be withdrawn 1–2cm and the patient reassessed. When the airway is in position, a safety pin should be placed through the airway to prevent distal migration. The airway can be placed in either nostril.

The risk of trauma to the nasal mucosa and turbinates is reduced by lubrication, appropriate sizing, and careful insertion which includes gentle rotatory movements backwards (perpendicular to the face) and NOT upwards.

Laerdal pocket mask

The pocket mask facilitates expired air ventilation for the lone rescuer and is easier to use than a bag valve mask. It is best used in combination with an oropharyngeal airway. Oxygen supplementation is achieved through a side port (not on all models).The one-way valve prevents rebreathing and the clear plastic presentation allows earlier detection of vomiting.

Orotracheal intubation

Orotracheal intubation is the gold standard in producing a definitive airway. However, patients rarely die from not being intubated but they do die from misplaced tubes or inappropriately prolonged intubation attempts.

Indications for intubation include actual and potential airway obstruction and patients with a reduced conscious level as a result of a significant head injury. Many of these patients require pharmacological agents to facilitate intubation. Recognition of correct tube placement is mandatory and requires clinical examination, saturation monitoring, and end tidal CO_2 monitoring.

Assessment of tube placement:

- Observation of correct passage
- Chest movement
- Listen in axillae
- Listen over stomach
- End tidal CO_2.

Rapid sequence induction (RSI) should only be attempted by those who are appropriately trained and experienced. Patients who can be intubated without pharmacological agents have an appalling prognosis.

Laryngeal mask airway (LMA)

The LMA is likely to have an increasing role in allowing the non-anaesthetically trained to provide a more definitive airway. A more recent development is the intubating laryngeal mask (ILMA) which allows an endotracheal tube to be passed through an in situ LMA.

The LMA may be used following failure to intubate . There is a recognized risk of aspiration although the risk is small.

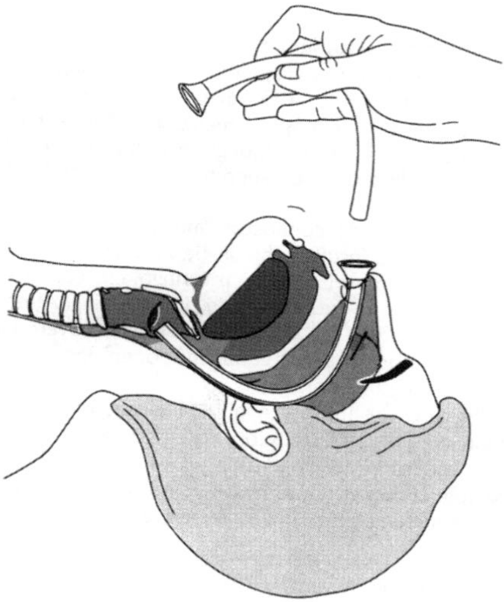

Fig. 3.2 Nasopharyngeal airway size (size 6 is the optimal size for women and size 7 for men). Reprinted with permission from Greaves I *et al.* (2005). *Emergency care—a textbook for paramedics*, 2nd edn. W.B. Saunders.

Technique for orotracheal intubation

1. Check the equipment.
2. Position the patient optimally. Remove the cervical collar and institute manual in-line immobilization.
3. Pre-oxygenate the patient for 30—60 seconds via a face mask
4. Use an assistant (if available) to apply cricoid pressure
5. Insert the laryngoscope (held in the left hand) into the right hand corner of the mouth. Slide the blade backwards and downwards towards the midline, moving the tongue to the left.
6. As the epiglottis comes into sight, lift ALONG THE LINE OF THE LARYNGOSCOPE HANDLE to show the vocal cords.
7. DO NOT LEVER on the teeth.
8. If the cords are visible, insert the tube through them from the right side of the mouth
9. Attach a self-inflating bag and connector to the tube, ventilate, and inflate the cuff until no air leak is heard.
10. Check for position If only one lung inflates, withdraw the tube 1—2cm and reassess.
11. Secure the tube with a tie. Adhesive tape is less effective in the pre-hospital environment.

Surgical airways

Needle cricothyroidotomy and jet insufflation

This is a fallback option when all other means of opening the airway have been unsuccessful. It is a simple technique and involves the placement of a 12–14 gauge cannula through the cricothyroid membrane. The technique can be used in both adults and children, although in children care must be taken as the cricoid ring is the major supporting structure for the paediatric airway.

Jet insufflation requires a specific connector and oxygen supply. A number of systems are available. Insufflation can be achieved by placing bubble oxygen tubing into the barrel of a 2mm syringe and connecting this to the cannula. A hole must be cut in the side of the tubing. Alternatively, a Y connector can be used. In the first case, the hole is covered for one second then open for four; in the second, the 'open' limb of the Y connector is covered for the same period.

Oxygen should be delivered at 15L per minute. There is minimal opportunity for elimination of CO_2 and, therefore, progressive hypercapnia limits the effectiveness and survivability of this procedure to approximately 20 minutes. Needle cricothyroidotomy offers no protection when the airway is being contaminated by bleeding from above.

Surgical airway

The scenario of 'can't intubate, can't ventilate' is fortunately rare. Needle cricothyroidotomy is a temporizing solution, but a definitive airway requires surgical cricothyroidotomy. Very rarely, a surgical airway is the only option when rapid sequence induction would be preferred but is unavailable or not within the skills of the practitioner.

Technique for surgical cricothyroidotomy

- Make a transverse incision in the skin and cricothyroid membrane using a scalpel.
- Use an artery clip to enlarge the hole (the handle of the scalpel can be used but risks injury to the operator and is best avoided).
- Pass a bougie into the trachea.
- Pass a size 6mm cuffed endotracheal tube into the trachea over the bougie.
- If circumstances allow, local anaesthetic may be infiltrated down the front of each sternocleidomastoid muscle.

There are a number of commercially available devices, most of which, however, take longer to insert than the above.

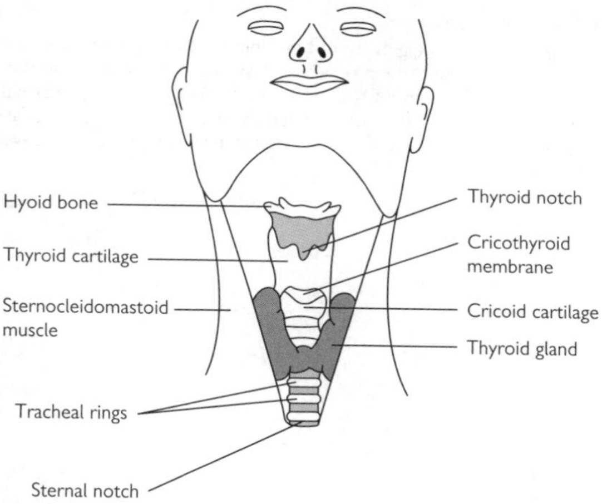

Fig. 3.3 Anatomy of the cricothyroid membrane.

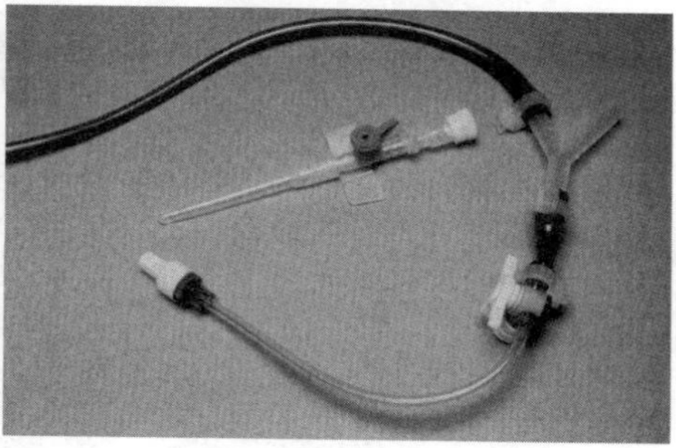

Fig. 3.4 Needle insufflation system. Reprinted with permission from Greaves I and Porter K (1997). *Pre-hospital medicine—the principles and practice of immediate care.* Edward Arnold.

Oxygen therapy

For optimal oxygenation, oxygen should be delivered at a rate of 15L per minute through a non-rebreathing reservoir bag and mask which, with an effective seal, can produce an FiO_2 of 85% (100% oxygen is only possible with a closed system via an ET tube). Oxygen should be administered in all cases of significant trauma even if the patient has chronic obstructive pulmonary disease.

Dilemmas in spinal immobilization

Securing an open airway takes priority over cervical spine immobilization. In unconscious trauma patients, the risk to the cervical spine and spinal cord is approximately 5%. A lone rescuer will be unable to maintain in-line stabilization and complete a primary survey. Simple measures to support the neck should be considered.

Cervical spine immobilization may be impossible in the confused or combative patient when hypoxia, hypovolaemia, and hypoglycaemia should be excluded. Forced application of a cervical collar and securing to a spinal board often worsens the situation. The neck should be supported as well as possible and appropriate documentation of these difficulties made. Some of these patients will tolerate a collar without further immobilization.

Breathing

Following successful opening of the airway spinal stabilization, and oxygen administration, breathing should be assessed as the next component of the primary survey.

Assessment

An open airway does not imply adequate breathing and ventilation. Breathing MUST be assessed by exposing the chest and examination must be systematic in order to identify immediately life-threatening problems. Time saved by not exposing the chest will be regretted later.

Life-threatening breathing problems

The six immediately life-threatening breathing problems are listed below. The mnemonic 'ATOMIC' may be helpful:

- **A**irway onstruction
- **T**ension pneumothorax
- **O**pen chest injury
- **M**assive haemothorax
- Fla**I**l chest
- **C**ardiac tamponade.

Inspection	• Rate of breathing • Distended neck veins • Adequacy/depth of chest movement • Symmetry of chest movement • Flail segments • Bruising or pattern bruising • Chest wounds
Palpation	• Chest wall tenderness—rib fractures • Paradoxical movement—flail chest • Tracheal position • Surgical emphysema • Laryngeal crepitis
Percussion	• To detect hyper-resonance—pneumothorax • To detect (dullness) hypo-resonance—haemothorax
Auscultation	• To determine the presence of breath sounds bilaterally

Management summary

- All patients with significant chest trauma require supplementary oxygen with a non-rebreathing reservoir mask and an oxygen flow rate of 15L per minute.
- Inadequate ventilation (in adults a rate of <10 breaths per minute or > 29 breaths per minute) requires assisted ventilation.
- Supplementary ventilation requires a bag valve mask reservoir device emptied to a maximum of 700–1000ml per breath at a rate of 15 breaths a minute.
- A tension pneumothorax should be decompressed immediately by needle thoracocentesis.
- Open chest wounds should be sealed with an Ashermann® chest seal.
- Major flail segments should be stabilized by direct pressure.
- Patients with a diagnosable haemothorax require judicious fluid replacement but drainage can wait until hospital.
- All patients with life-threatening chest trauma require prompt transfer to hospital.

Circulation

Shock

Shock is defined as *inadequate tissue perfusion which results in hypoxia and ultimately in cell death*. The common causes of shock are:

- Hypovolaemia (blood loss, plasma loss, severe dehydration)
- Cardiogenic (myocardial infarction, myocardial contusion)
- Obstructive (tension pneumothorax, cardiac tamponade)
- Septic (bacterial, viral, or fungal infections)
- Neurogenic (following head or spinal injury)
- Anaphylactic.

In pre-hospital care, the most common type of shock is hypovolaemic due to blood loss. The clinical features of hypovolaemic shock are:

- Tachycardia
- Changes in blood pressure
- Tachypneoa
- Cool, clammy skin
- Altered mental status
- Prolonged capillary refill time

Pathophysiology

The cardiac output is the volume of blood pumped around the body per minute.

Cardiac output = Stroke volume x Heart rate

In response to blood loss, tissue perfusion can only be maintained by increasing the cardiac output. This is achieved by increasing the stroke volume (the amount of blood ejected from the heart each cycle) and, secondly, the heart rate, in response to sympathetic stimulation.

These compensatory measures will begin to fail at a point when the heart muscle is maximally stretched and the heart rate cannot rise further. The effect of a rapid heart rate is an inadequate filling time and a fall in cardiac output.

As a pre-terminal event, if blood loss continues and venous return to the heart decreases, distortion of the heart chambers occurs and activation of cardiac C fibres stops. This produces vagal stimulation and slowing of the heart. Together with vasodilation, this causes a profound drop in blood pressure, progressing to cardiac arrest.

Splanchnic and peripheral vasoconstriction occurs due to sympathetic stimulation. This is designed to redirect flow to vital organs, for example the heart, brain, and kidneys. As a consequence, the patient will look pale. In addition to vasoconstriction, venoconstriction occurs, reducing the amount of pooled blood. The net effect of this action will be an initial increase in the end diastolic pressure. Relative hypoxia as a result of loss of circulating volume will cause an increase in the rate and depth of respiration.

Other physiological compensatory mechanisms include the release of aldosterone from the adrenal gland and antidiuretic hormone from the pituitary gland. Both function by reducing urine output.

Clinical features of hypovolaemia

In a healthy adult, the normal circulatory blood volume is 7% of the lean body mass. For a 70kg man, the total circulating blood volume is

Table 3.1 Grading of shock and its clinical features

Grade	Blood loss	Signs and symptoms
Grade I	Up to 750ml <15%	Minimal Blood pressure unchanged Slight tachycardia may occur
Grade II	750–1500ml 15–30%	Pallor Tachycardia: >100 per min Decreased pulse pressure Anxiety
Grade III	1500–2000ml 30–40% Minimum volume loss that leads to a fall in blood pressure	Pallor Sweating Altered mental state Tachycardia: >120 per min Tachypnoea Hypotension
Grade IV	>2000ml Life-threatening	Pulse weak and thready Tachycardia deteriorating to bradycardia Marked hypotension Drowsiness progressing to unconsciousness

approximately 5000ml. Clinical features of shock depend on the percentage of circulating volume loss. The grading of shock and its clinical features are summarized in Table 3.1.

This classification serves as a clinical guideline in the assessment of shock. Pitfalls in the assessment include:

- Age (the elderly are less able to compensate)
- Fitness
- Medications (for example, betablockers)
- Co-morbidity
- Pregnancy.

Patients at the extremes of age have different abilities to compensate for blood loss. The elderly have less physiological reserve, whereas children will compensate and maintain their blood pressure until the point of a catastrophic deterioration. Fit athletes may have a resting pulse below 50 and may have few physical signs even when significantly hypovolaemic. Cardiovascular medication such as betablockers may modify or restrict the patient's response to trauma. Co-morbidity, in particular heart disease, means that the patient has limited cardiovascular reserve and will cope less well with the effects of trauma. The pregnant woman nearing term has an increased circulatory volume up to 50% of normal and even in severe shock will display minimal signs.

Treatment

Treatment follows the normal ABCDE system (See p.172). External haemorrhage should be controlled, where possible, using direct pressure, elevation, packing, indirect pressure, or tourniquets to arrest haemorrhage. Limbs should be rapidly realigned and immobilized.

The source of blood loss may not be so obvious. The common sites of blood loss are:

- External
- The chest
- The abdomen
- The pelvis and retroperitoneum
- Multiple long bone fractures.

Blood on the floor and four more

The management of blood loss depends on the site of bleeding. For example, compressible, controllable bleeding such as occurs in limb fractures can be managed by splintage and attention to bleeding wounds. Non-controllable, non-compressible blood loss (in the chest, abdomen, retroperitoneum or the pelvis) requires prompt hospital treatment and, in many cases, surgery. In these circumstances, use of a tournequet may be lifesaving. In these patients, IV fluids should be given to restore and maintain a radial pulse only. This equates to a BP of 80–90mmHg and, therefore, essential organ perfusion. There should be no time delay in transfer to a hospital with the necessary assessment and surgical facilities. Additional measures include limb elevation and external pelvic splintage.

Intravenous cannulation

In time-critical trauma, the time spent on scene should be as short as possible. The airway should be opened, breathing and ventilation secured, external haemorrhage controlled, and the patient rapidly transported to hospital. To avoid delay, intravenous cannulation should be undertaken en route to hospital. These patients are often cold and shut down, and obtaining vascular access is difficult. The volume of fluid given pre-hospital is invariably small and only those patients that require restoration of a radial pulse are likely to benefit, providing there is no time delay.

Vascular access is usually via a peripheral vein using the largest cannula that the vein will accommodate. In children under 6 yrs of age, vascular access can be gained using an intraosseous needle. Intraossseoud needles are also available for adult use. The experienced practitioner may be trained in using the Seldinger® technique for femoral vein access, or in extreme cases, a large conventional cannula over needle can be used. Subclavian access carries the risk of pneumothorax, and internal jugular access requires the head to be turned to one side. Both of these techniques should, therefore, be avoided in trauma.

Choice of intravenous fluids

There is a great deal of published data in support of both crystalloid and colloid as resuscitation fluids. The Faculty of Pre-hospital Care has produced a consensus document taking all the available evidence into consideration and has concluded that normal saline in aliquots of 250cc, subject to patient review and the maintenance of a radial pulse, is at the present time the best choice in uncontrolled haemorrhage.

Cardiogenic shock

Cardiogenic shock is failure of the pump mechanism due to compromise of cardiac function. Whilst this may be seen following myocardial infarction, it also occurs following blunt trauma which produces cardiac contusion and as a result of penetrating trauma to the heart.

Obstructive shock

In obstructive shock, cardiac output is compromised by external compressive forces. This occurs in cardiac tamponade and tension pneumothorax. Following a penetrating heart wound, blood may collect within the pericardial space, compressing the heart chambers. Needle pericardiocentesis is not effective and is not recommended in the pre-hospital environment.

In tension pneumothorax, due to the progressive air leak, pressure (tension) in the pleural space increases and the heart is displaced away from the side of the tension pneumothorax, obstructing venous return.

Neurogenic shock

This results from an injury, to the spinal cord and loss of sympathetic tone. Distal to the level of injury, blood vessels dilate and the peripheries are warm. The patient is hypotensive and bradycardic. In major trauma, even in the presence of a spinal injury, shock is more likely to be due to hypovolaemia from associated injuries.

Septic shock

This results from cellular mediators producing vasodilatation and capillary leak. The patient, therefore, often appears warm and vasodilated.

Anaphylactic shock

Anaphylactic shock occurs due to an allergic reaction to a foreign protein such as nuts and is also seen following stings, bites, and drugs. The clinical features are:

- Vasodilation
- Hypotension
- Bronchospasm
- Cutaneous erythema.

Disability

Baseline neurological observations should be undertaken as part of the primary survey, in the form of an assessment of pupillary size and reactivity and an AVPU assessment:

A > Is the patient **A**lert?
V > Is the patient responding to **V**erbal response?
P > Is the patient responding to **P**ainful stimulus?
U > Is the patient **U**nresponsive?

Expose and evaluate

The patient should be appropriately exposed to facilitate a thorough examination. In particular, the neck and chest should be visualized. Once the assessment is complete, the patient should be covered up, especially in cold and damp conditions, to maintain their core temperature.

During this part of the examination, a quick visual inspection is made for other obvious musculoskeletal injuries.

Reassessment

If at anytime during the primary survey a patient deteriorates, it is important to return immediately to the beginning of the primary survey. In non-critical patients, a secondary survey may be appropriate.

IF THE PATIENT DETERIORATES – ALWAYS GO BACK TO AIRWAY

Secondary survey

The secondary survey is a head-to-toe examination undertaken in non-critical patients (for example, patients with minor injuries who may not require transport to hospital) and is usually carried out in the ambulance. A comprehensive secondary survey is undertaken in the A&E department at a later stage.

Assessment of the head

Look for:
- Lacerations
- Bruising
- Blood or CSF from the nose or ears
- Pupil size and reaction
- Battle's sign and racoon eyes
- Pallor
- Cyanosis
- Inspect the mouth for broken teeth, broken dentures, and debris.

Feel for:
- Scalp wounds
- Scalp haematomas
- Depressed skull fractures
- Facial tenderness and fractures.

Listen for:
- Airway noise suggesting obstruction
- Breathing rate and adequacy.

Assessment of the neck

The cervical collar should be removed and in-line manual stabilization maintained during examination of the neck.

Look and feel for:
- Tracheal position
- Elevated jugular venous pressure
- Laryngeal crepitus (rare)
- Surgical emphysema
- Wounds
- Swelling and tenderness
- Midline cervical tenderness.

Assessment of the chest

Look for:
- Wounds or penetrating injury
- Chest wall deformity
- Symmetry of chest movements
- Flail chest
- Respiratory distress and pain with breathing.

Feel for:
- Tenderness
- Instability of a flail chest
- Surgical emphysema
- Percussion note—hyperesonance in pneumothorax or dullness with a haemothorax
- Feel the posterior chest wall for evidence of injury.

Listen for:
- Presence of equal breath sounds
- Unilateral absence or reduction of breath sounds due to a pneumothorax
- Unilateral reduction of breath sounds (usually posterior and basal) due to a haemothorax.

Assessment of the abdomen

Look for:
- Abdominal wall contusion and penetrating wounds
- Seatbelt contusions and clothing imprints
- Abdominal distension.

Feel for:
- Tenderness—either generalized or localized
- Guarding

There is no value in assessing bowel signs in the pre-hospital environment.

Assessment of the pelvis

Look for:
- Perineal wounds, swelling, and bruising
- Blood at the urethral meatus.

Feel for:

Tenderness and instability from lateral and antero-posterior compression. Only do this ONCE.

Assessment of lower and upper extremities

Look for:
- Wounds and contusions
- Deformity and swelling
- Voluntary movements.

Feel for:
- Tenderness
- Distal pulses
- Sensation
- Motor function
- Joint movement.

Injuries identified during the secondary survey may be treated immediately or, in some cases, left until after arrival in hospital.

Head and neck injuries

Mechanism of injury

Blunt trauma is the most common mechanism of injury and follows inter-personal violence, falls, sports injuries, and road traffic collisions where, depending on the energy involved ('energy transfer'), the injuries produced range from simple scalp contusions and lacerations to non-survivable intracranial injuries.

Penetrating injuries include gunshot wounds, stab wounds with a knife or other sharp weapon, and, occasionally, impalement (for example, following falls from a height or industrial accidents).

Pathophysiology of injury

The brain consists of three main anatomical components. These areas and their principle functions are:

- The cerebral hemispheres:
  - Responsible for higher function including, sensory, motor, vision, and hearing.
- The cerebellum:
  - Acts as a control centre for balance and co-ordination.
- The brain stem:
  - Contains vital control centres including the cardiac and respiratory centres.

Following injury, the neurological deficit relates to the anatomical area of brain injury which may be further compromised by secondary complications (see below). Because there is no prospect of recovery of damaged nerve cells in the central nervous system, it is essential to provide optimal pre-hospital care in an attempt to minimize or prevent the subsequent manifestation of secondary injury.

The brain is surrounded by the meninges (dura mater, pia mater, and arachnoid mater) with potential spaces within them for extradural and subdural haematoma formation. The brain is suspended or floats in cerebrospinal fluid (CSF) which is found in the subarachnoid space and functions as a shock absorber.

The skull is a rigid box and, therefore, there is minimal space for brain expansion (for example, due to cerebral oedema or haematoma formation) without producing an increase in intracranial pressure (ICP).

The skull base is tiered which makes the brain particularly vulnerable to twisting or deceleration injuries on the bony ridges. Parts of the skeleton are thinner, notably the cribriform plate and the middle ear, rendering these common sites of compound fractures with blood and CSF loss from the nose and ear respectively.

Direct trauma produces both coup and contra-coup injuries including contusion, lacerations, oedema, and intracranial and intracerebral haematomas. Contra-coup injuries occur when the brain strikes the inside of the skull as a result of an impact elsewhere.

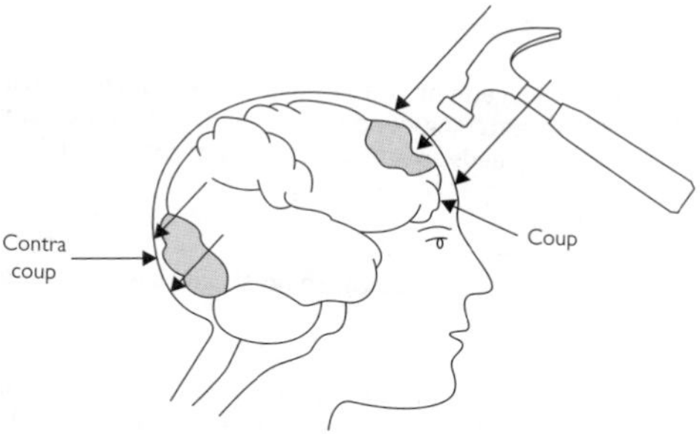

Fig. 3.5 Coup and contra-coup injuries

There are two principle types of brain injury:
- Primary (direct)
- Secondary (indirect).

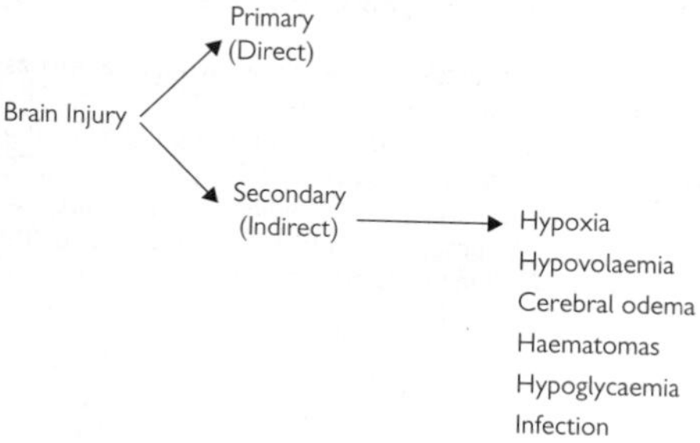

Primary brain injury relates to the mechanical events that occur at the moment of injury and can only be influenced by accident prevention measures. Secondary injury relates to a combination of factors which produce brain swelling.

It is therefore essential that the immediate care practitioner addresses the issues of hypoxia, hypovolaemia, and hypoglycaemia.

Cerebral perfusion must be maintained after a severe head injury where the cerebral perfusion pressure (CPP) is related to the mean arterial pressure (MAP) (normally 80–90mmHg) and the mean intracranial pressure (MICP) (normally 5–10mmHg) by the equation:

$$CPP = MAP - MICP$$

It is desirable to maintain a cerebral perfusion pressure of between 70–80mmHg. Whilst ICP is not measured in the pre-hospital environment, cerebral perfusion pressure can be optimized by the correction of hypoxia and hypovolaemia (good ABC care).

Patient assessment

General assessment

The initial assessment and management of the head-injured patient must begin with a search for life-threatening conditions. Particularly important in head trauma, where the brain needs an adequate supply of oxygen, are:

- A Adequate protected airway
- B Uncompromised breathing
- C Adequate cerebral perfusion.

In patients suffering head trauma, the cervical spine should be protected at all times.

Specific assessment

Neurological assessment during the primary survey follows ABC assessment and is limited to pupillary equality and reaction to light and an AVPU assessment.

- A Alert
- V Response to voice
- P Response to pain
- U Unresponsive.

Patients responding only to pain or who are unresponsive are at risk of airway obstruction and usually have a Glasgow Coma Scale (GCS) of less than 8.

A BM Stix® should always be undertaken to exclude hypoglycaemia as the cause of unconsciousness or as a contributing factor.

A more detailed neurological examination is undertaken during the secondary survey which, in many patients, occurs in hospital. The GCS provides a quantitative score by assessing eye opening, verbal response, and motor response. The painful stimulus should be applied above the neck to ensure that a cervical spine injury is not responsible for a lack of response.

The Glasgow Coma Scale

Eye opening	
Eyes are already open and blinking normally	E = 4
Eyes open in response to speech or specific questions	E = 3
Eyes open in response to pain	E = 2
No response	E = 1
Verbal response	
Fully orientated	V = 5
Confused conversation	V = 4
Inappropriate words	V = 3
Incomprehensible sounds	V = 2
No response to speech	V = 1
Motor response	
Spontaneously moves limbs to command	M = 6
Localizes pain by purpose or motion towards the painful stimuli	M = 5
Withdraws or pulls away from painful stimuli	M = 4
Abnormal flexion, known as decorticate posture	M = 3
Extensor response, known as decerebrate posture	M = 2
No movement	M = 1

Pupillary responses and limb responses to command in the conscious patient or painful stimuli in the unconscious patient are assessed to determine the presence of lateralizing signs or focal neurological deficit. Pressure over the supraorbital nerve is a useful painful stimulus.

During the secondary survey, the scalp is inspected. Simple abrasions and lacerations often need no specific treatment pre-hospital. Large scalp lacerations can bleed profusely and should be controlled by direct pressure. Should this prove ineffective, the edges of the wound can be inverted and direct pressure applied to secure haemostasis, or a number of large sutures can be inserted for temporary haemorrhage control. Hypotension should never be attributed to scalp bleeding in an adult and alternative sites of blood loss should be sought. In children, however, bleeding from large scalp wounds can produce clinical shock.

Assessing the conscious level with the GCS provides a quantitative measurement, which acts as a baseline for further observations. A deteriorating GCS may be the first indication of neurological deterioration. When reporting the GCS, the scores for the individual components should be given.

The history of injury is important and, in the case of unconscious patients, onlookers may have important information regarding the mechanism of injury which should be passed onto the staff of the emergency department.

All patients with a history of unconsciousness should be transported to hospital, although the majority will have a transient loss of consciousness lasting a few seconds only. A measure of the degree of concussion is determined by the retrograde amnesia (last recollection before the accident) and the post traumatic amnesic period (first recollection after the accident).

Helmet removal

If there are a limited number of trained personnel available and the airway is clear, there is no urgency to remove the helmet. The only absolute and immediate indication for helmet removal is an inability to open and maintain a clear airway.

The removal of a motorcycle helmet should be a two-person technique and is undertaken as follows:

- Undo the chin strap.
- The first rescuer supports the neck from the front and progressively moves their hands up the back of the patient's neck during the procedure.
- The second rescuer, at the head of the patient, carefully expands the helmet laterally and tips the helmet forwards in a vertical plane, to clear the occiput, and then backwards, to clear the nose.
- Throughout the procedure, the rescuer controlling the neck ensures that they have firm control of the neck at all times.

In an emergency, a lone rescuer may remove a motorcycle helmet as follows:

- Kneel above the patient's head.
- Undo the chin strap.
- Expand the helmet laterally.
- Tilt the helmet forward until the occiput is clear.
- Tilt the helmet backwards to release the chin from under the chin bar.
- The rescuer maintains in-line immobilization by placing their hands either side of the patient's head and face and uses their forearms to complete removal of the helmet.

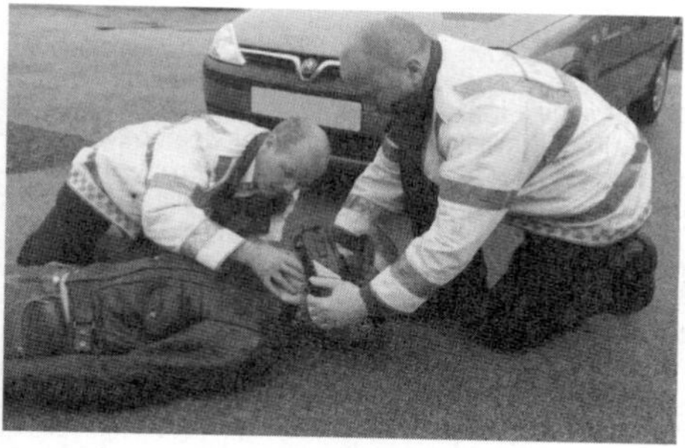

Fig. 3.6 Helmet removal: two-person technique. Reprinted with permission from Greaves I *et al.* (2005). *Emergency care: a textbook for paramedics*, 2nd edn. W.B. Saunders Co. Ltd.

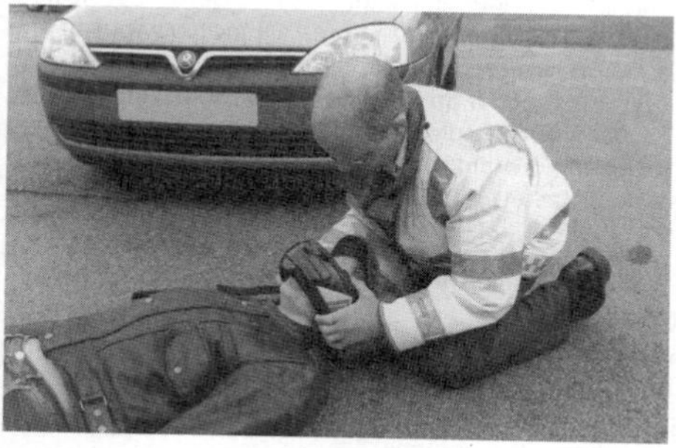

Fig. 3.7 Helmet removal: one-person technique. Reprinted with permission from Greaves I *et al.* (2005). *Emergency care: a textbook for paramedics*, 2nd edn. W.B. Saunders Co. Ltd.

Skull fractures

The presence of a skull fracture is a reflection of the magnitude of force producing the head injury and, therefore, the degree of violence to which the underlying brain has been subjected. This may be seen as an alteration in the level of consciousness. The risk of intracranial bleeding is significantly higher in patients with a skull fracture.

Linear fractures

These are common and are of particular relevance when they cross blood vessels (for example, the middle meningeal artery in the parietal area), when they are often associated with extradural haematoma. The fracture itself requires no specific treatment and is only diagnosed on X-ray in hospital.

Compound fractures

These occur in the cranial vault and are associated with overlying wounds which will require surgical debridement and, in the case of CSF leak, a neurosurgical opinion. Many compound fractures are not obvious at the outset when only a simple laceration may be visible. The diagnosis may be made on X-ray. Where there is an obvious compound skull fracture, consideration should be given to direct transfer to a hospital with a neurosurgical facility, bearing in mind the patient's other injuries.

A number of base skull fractures are also compound, as manifested by blood and CSF leak from the nose or ear. Antibiotics should only be given if there is a significant delay in the transfer to hospital.

Basal skull fractures

Weak points in the skull structure include the cribiform plate and the petrous temporal bone and these are both sites of basal skull fractures, the common features of which are:

- CSF leakage from the nose (rhinorrhoea)
- CSF leakage from the ear (otorrhoea)
- Bleeding from the ears
- Panda (raccoon) eyes (periorbital bruising) in anterior cranial fossa fractures
- Swelling and bruising over the mastoid process (Battle's sign).

Panda eyes and Battle's sign develop over a number of hours and are not usually seen at the outset. No specific treatment is necessary following blood and CSF loss in the pre-hospital environment.

Depressed skull fractures

Blunt weapons or strikes against protruding objects may fracture the skull pushing bone inwards. The dura is often torn and there is an associated underlying brain contusion or laceration. Treatment includes the application of a dressing and, if necessary, surrounding pressure to stop bleeding. In cases where there is a significant delay to hospital, a broad spectrum antibiotic should be given.

Localized brain injury

Localized brain injuries include:
- Bruising or contusion
- Intracranial haemorrhage
- Laceration and penetrating injury.

Contusion

Cerebral contusions result from direct injury and their size will depend on the magnitude of the force involved. Most patients suffer a period of concussion. The diagnosis is made on a CT scan in hospital. Pre-hospital management follows the ABCDE regime.

Intracranial haemorrhage

Intracranial haemorrhage may be:
- Extradural
- Subdural
- Intracerebral
- Subarachnoid.

Extradural haematoma

This is an uncommon and sometimes rapidly fatal condition. Classically, it occurs due to a tear in the middle meningeal artery produced by an overlying parietal skull fracture. The patient recovers from an initial period of unconsciousness (concussion) but following a lucid interval lapses into unconsciousness as the intracranial pressure rises due to the enlarging haematoma in the extradural space. Complete recovery is possible with prompt surgical intervention.

The classical features of raised intracranial pressure are:
- Decreasing level of consciousness
- Increasing blood pressure
- Falling pulse rate
- Falling respiratory rate
- Pupillary dilatation.

Specific additional features may include weakness on the opposite side of the body to the head injury. The pupillary dilatation initially occurs on the same side as the injury but then becomes bilateral. The diagnosis is confirmed by CT scanning.

Subdural haematoma

These are more common than extradural haematomas and result from damage to blood vessels in the subdural space. Because they are due to venous bleeding, the haematoma may collect more slowly. Acute subdural haematoma presents with the same features as extradural haematoma and should be treated by surgical intervention. The diagnosis is made in hospital by CT scan. Chronic subdural haematoma is an occasional cause of progressive confusion in the elderly.

Intracerebral haematoma

Bleeding may occur within the cerebral hemispheres and may present with evidence of raised intracranial pressure. In contrast to extracerebral haematoma surgery is not normally an option.

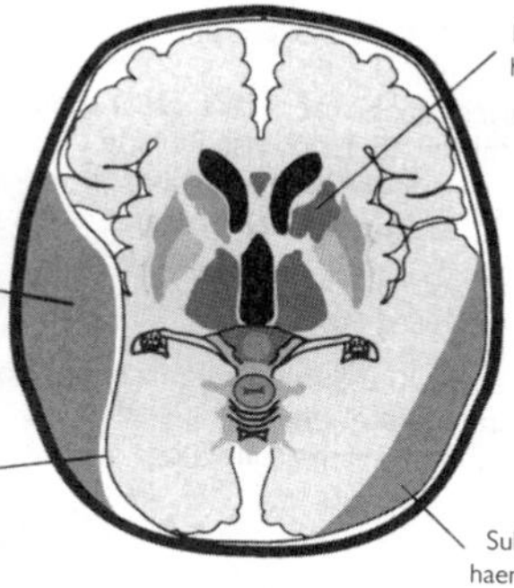

Fig. 3.8 Anatomy of intracranial bleeding. Reprinted with permission from Greaves I *et al.* (2005) *Emergency care: a textbook for paramedics*, 2nd edn. W.B. Saunders Co. Ltd.

Subarachnoid haemorrhage

Subarachnoid haemorrhage is a fairly common feature in severe brain injuries and is associated with a poor prognosis. The diagnosis is made on CT scanning.

Serial neurological observations are essential in order to detect progressive changes in the patient's neurological status, for example early deterioration in the level of consciousness following a lucid interval in a patient with an extradural haematoma. As much clinical history as possible should be given to the receiving staff in the emergency department.

Lacerations and penetrating head injuries

Cerebral lacerations result from tearing of brain tissue due to shearing forces and cause intracranial bleeding. Such injuries are associated with a high mortality rate.

Intracerebral haemorrhage may also be caused by penetrating injuries. Causes include low velocity implements such as knives, industrial impalement, and road traffic accidents. The orbits and temporal regions are common sites of penetration since the bone in these areas is relatively thin.

Gunshot wounds to the head are becoming increasingly common in the UK and follow distinct patterns, depending on the energy transfer. Both high- and low-energy transfer wounds lacerate and crush brain tissue. However, high-energy transfer wounds damage tissue extensively by generating shock waves, temporary cavitation, and sucking contaminated debris into the wound. Such injuries are almost invariably rapidly fatal. Injuries are also produced by bomb and grenade fragments.

Treatment follows the normal ABCDE philosophy. Clean dressings should be applied to the entry and exit wounds.

Generalized brain injury

Diffuse axonal injury (DAI) results from major shearing injuries and commonly results in coma, which may last days, weeks, or be permanent. The diagnosis is made in hospital, based on clinical assessment and CT scanning.

Neck injuries

Blunt or penetrating injuries to the neck are associated with significant morbidity or mortality. Vital structures at risk include the:

- Trachea
- Larynx
- Jugular veins
- Carotid artery
- Oesophagus
- Cervical spine
- Spinal cord and nerve roots
- Thyroid gland
- Thoracic duct.

The priority in management in the pre-hospital scene is to establish and maintain an open airway and control external blood loss.

The neck should be examined for the following:

- Tracheal position
- Neck vein distension
- Laryngeal crepitus
- Surgical emphysema
- Wounds
- Swelling
- Posterior midline bony tenderness.

Immobilization

Any patient who has suffered major trauma or who has evidence of injuries above the clavicle should be considered to be at risk of cervical spine injury and appropriate measures must be taken to prevent any further damage.

The cervical spine can only be cleared if:

- The patient is fully conscious
- There is no history of alcohol or drug abuse
- There are no painful distracting injuries
- There is no past history of significant neck injury
- The patient does not suffer from rheumatoid arthritis or ankylosing spondylitis
- There is no midline posterior bony tenderness
- There is no evidence of motor weakness or sensory deficit.

Patients at risk of cervical spine injury should receive inline manual stabilization followed by the application of an appropriately sized semi-rigid collar. They should be transported to hospital on a spinal board complete with head blocks and straps, unless the journey is likely to be prolonged, in which case transfer to a vacuum mattress is more appropriate.

Penetrating neck injuries

Many structures may be damaged. The priorities are an open airway and arrest of haemorrhage. The wound should be left undisturbed and if necessary direct pressure applied to arrest haemorrhage. Foreign bodies or embedded weapons should be left in situ. Airway compromise due to bleeding may require, depending on clinical competencies, intubation or a surgical airway. Some support to the neck and retention of dressings may be afforded by the application of a cervical collar even in the absence of potential spine injury.

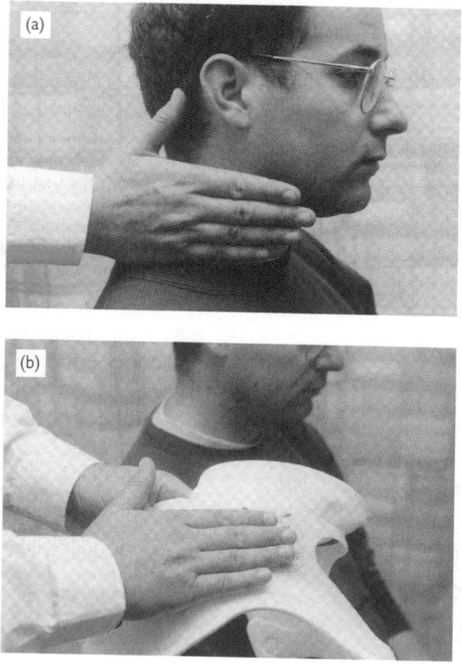

Fig. 3.9 Sizing a cervical collar. Reprinted with permission from Greaves I and Porter K (1997). *Pre-hospital medicine—the principles and practice of immediate care.* Edward Arnold.

Blunt trauma to the upper airway

Injuries to the larynx may present with:

- Hoarseness
- Stridor
- Tachypnoea
- Surgical emphysema
- Laryngeal crepitus.

The patient should be left in the most comfortable position for breathing and oxygen therapy should be administered. In the event of clinical deterioration and airway compromise a surgical airway may be necessary. This may be made simpler by the presence of a hole in the larynx and access to the airway may simply require a skin incision.

Faciomaxillary injuries

Faciomaxillary injuries may occur in isolation or in association with other injuries. They may be immediately life-threatening due to airway obstruction or severe haemorrhage.

Anatomy

The mandible is connected to the base of the skull by the narrow condyles at the temporo-mandibular joint. The condyles are attached to the ramus of the mandible and, in turn, to the body which joins in the midline at the mental symphysis. The teeth are attached to the bone at the dentoalveolar margin. In a similar way, the maxilla supports the upper dentition and constitutes part of the orbital margin and lateral margin of the nose.

The zygoma forms the outer margin of the cheek and orbital margin. The nose consists of a cartilaginous framework and a bony component that articulates with the frontal bone and the maxilla. Deep to the nose are the ethmoid sinuses and beneath the maxilla is the maxillary sinus.

The facial skeleton has a rich blood supply from the facial artery, maxillary, artery, and ethmoidal artery which may account for potentially life-threatening haemorrhage following injury.

Mechanism of injury

Blunt trauma from road traffic accidents, assaults, falls, and sports injuries constitute the most common mechanisms of injury. Drink driving legislation and seat belt laws have reduced the number of facial injuries due to road accidents. However, facial trauma due to interpersonal violence is increasing and is related to unemployment and alcohol consumption. Penetrating trauma and burns are less frequent causes of facial trauma.

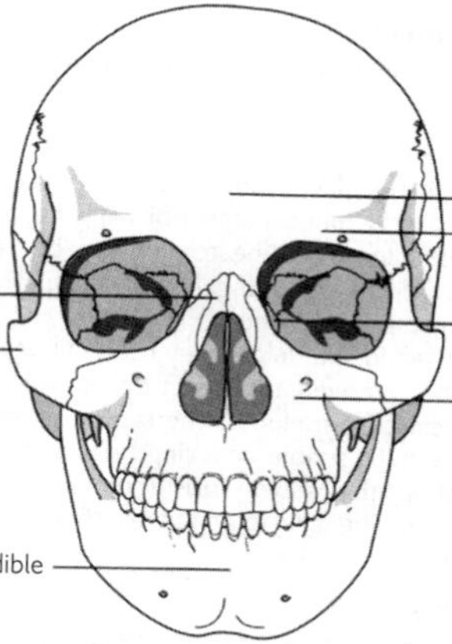

Fig. 3.10 Anatomy of the bony skeleton of the face. Reprinted with permission from Greaves I *et al.* (2005) *Emergency care: a textbook for paramedics*. 2nd edn. W.B. Saunders Co. Ltd.

Immediate management

In facial maxillary trauma, the airway may be compromised by:

- Inhalation of foreign bodies
- Posterior impaction of a fractured maxilla
- Loss of tongue control in a case of fractured mandible
- Haemorrhage
- Intra-oral swelling
- Direct trauma to the larynx.

In addition, haemorrhage can be severe and produce hypovolaemic shock. 2% of patients with facial injuries have cervical spine injury and manual stabilization, followed by a semi-rigid collar, head blocks, and tape should be used, with the patient positioned on a spinal board. However, in the case of significant bleeding the supine position may result in airway obstruction. These patients may require manual spinal protection, whilst in the lateral position, to permit postural drainage of blood. The patient with bilateral mandibular fractures may have no control over their tongue and will sit up and lean forwards to maintain an open airway. Major bleeding may be controlled by the use of nasal Epistats™, Foley catheters, or anterior or posterior nasal packing. In most cases, however, immediate transfer to hospital will be more appropriate.

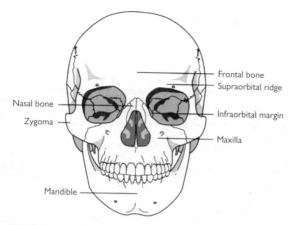

Soft and hard tissue injuries

Facial injuries may be divided into soft tissue injuries, including the eyes, and hard tissue injuries, including the teeth.

Soft tissue injuries

These include cuts and grazes, lacerations, and penetrating wounds. Bleeding from the skin and oral mucosa can normally be controlled by direct pressure; profuse bleeding from the tongue can be controlled by pulling the tongue forward using a piece of gauze or alternatively by using a large suture and the application of traction.

Foreign bodies should be left in situ unless they cause airway obstruction, in which case they should be removed and direct pressure applied.

Injuries to the eye may result from blunt, penetrating, or chemical injury. Most serious eye injuries require simple covering (without pressure) and transportation to hospital in the supine position. Penetrating foreign bodies should be left in situ. The eye exposed to chemicals should be thoroughly irrigated with water.

Hard tissue injuries, including teeth

The mouth should always be inspected during the primary survey since broken teeth and broken dentures may be inhaled, especially in the unconscious patient. Avulsed teeth in children should be replaced and held until appropriate splintage can be applied in hospital. Should the child have an altered level of consciousness, the tooth should be transported to hospital in a container of milk.

Mandibular fractures occur most commonly following assault. A blow to the right side of the jaw, for example, may produce a fracture of the angle of the jaw on the right side and a condylar neck fracture of the left side. The patient may complain of pain and swelling, difficulty opening their mouth, and malocclusion. In addition, the patient's teeth may be fractured or displaced or missing. Treatment for this type of fracture is usually unnecessary in the pre-hospital situation.

The patient sustaining bilateral fractures of the body of the mandible may be unable to maintain an open airway as the tongue has lost structural support. This patient will not tolerate a supine position. A jaw thrust manoeuvre will not work and, if necessary, the tongue and symphysis should be pulled forwards using a gloved hand. The patient may need positioning in the recovery position to facilitate postural drainage of blood and saliva. The patient is often found sitting forwards to allow natural drainage and should not be forced to lie supine.

Fractures of the maxilla commonly follow blunt trauma and can present as airway obstruction if the maxilla is impacted backwards. This can be relieved by hooking a gloved finger around the soft pallet and pulling forwards.

Fractures of the orbit and zygomatic complex are associated with periorbital bruising and swelling and, if displaced, the patient may complain of diplopia and infra-orbital nerve anaesthesia.

Fractures of the nasal complex present with swelling and epistaxis which will usually respond to direct pressure. Midface fractures may be associated with significant haemorrhage which may require the use of nasal Epistats™.

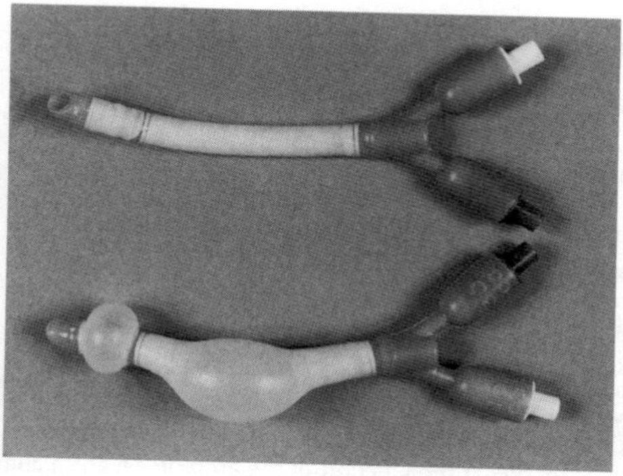

Fig. 3.11 Nasal Epistats®

Chest injuries

Injuries to the chest are responsible for up to a quarter of all trauma deaths usually as a result of acute hypoxia or hypovolaemia.

Mechanism of injury

Blunt injuries

Blunt trauma is the most common mechanism of chest injury, the clinical consequences of which depend upon the amount of energy involved. These injuries commonly follow road traffic collisions, falls, assaults, and sports injuries. The forces involved are shear forces due to a change of speed (deceleration) and compressive forces. In a frontal impact road traffic collision, the driver may sustain a chest injury by direct contact with the steering wheel. At the time of impact, mobile organs continue to move forwards whereas fixed organs remain stationary. An example of this type of injury is tearing at the junction of the arch of the aorta and the descending aorta. Compressive forces produce damage to the underlying structures. For example, a lateral chest compression may produce chest wall contusion, rib fractures, a flail chest, and pulmonary contusion.

Penetrating injuries

The damage produced by a penetrating injury depends on the energy of the weapon, the anatomical site, and the posture of the patient. Any wound between the umbilicus and the male nipple level equivalent may enter both the abdominal cavity and the plural cavity.

Penetrating wounds below the clavicle and above the costal margin, which lie within the mid-clavicular boundary, are likely to inflict critical mediastinal trauma.

Blast injuries

Primary blast injury results in alveolar haemorrhage and consolidation, pneumothorax, haemothorax, and air embolism. Penetrating injuries may also occur due to fragments and displacement of the body.

Anatomy and surface landmarks

The trachea is a 2.5cm diameter tube made up of a number of incomplete fibro-cartilagenous rings, which is lined by a mucous membrane. It begins at the cricoid cartilage and ends at the carina where it bifurcates into the left and right main bronchi. The carina is at the level of the sternal angle (second rib). The trachea is a midline structure, the position of which can be checked in the suprasternal notch. The larynx can be palpated above the trachea.

The right main bronchus is more vertical than the left and, therefore, aspirated foreign bodies are more likely to enter the right side, although this will depend on the position of the patient at the time of the foreign body inhalation.

The bronchial tree branches, becoming progressively smaller towards the periphery where it reaches the terminal bronchioles and alveoli. Gas exchange is by diffusion, facilitated by the close proximity of the alveoli and pulmonary capillaries.

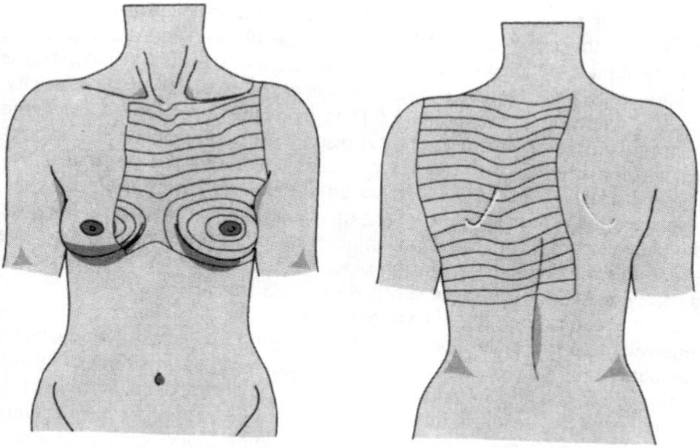

Fig. 3.12 The danger area for thoracic and abdominal stab wounds. Any stab wound within the marked area may penetrate the pericardium. Reprinted with permission from Landon BA *et al.*, (1994). *An Atlas of Trauma Management: The first hour.* Taylor & Francis.

The outer surface of the lung is covered by visceral pleura and the inner surface of the chest is lined by the parietal pleura. These surfaces are closely applied by virtue of a negative pressure in the plural cavity. This is produced as a consequence of the tendency, by virtue of tissue elasticity, for the lung and chest wall to pull in opposite directions. During the inspiratory phase of respiration, the diaphragm descends and the antero-posterior diameter of the chest increases, increasing the negative intra-thoracic pressure. In the presence of an open airway, inspiration occurs.

If there is an opening in the lung or chest wall, air will be sucked into the pleural space, producing a pneumothorax. In the presence of a flap-valve effect, this may become a tension pneumothorax, especially if the patient is receiving positive pressure ventilation or assistance.

During expiration, the diaphragm reaches the fifth intercostal space (equivalent to the male nipple level), although it can reach even higher if the patient is in a crouched position. The heart is positioned slightly to the left of the midline and is covered by the pericardium. Stab wounds to the heart may result in bleeding into the space within the pericardium, producing cardiac tamponade. The heart, major blood vessels, trachea, and oesophagus are positioned in the central part of the chest (mediastinum) and trauma to this region is often life threatening or rapidly fatal.

Pathophysiology

Normally, respiratory physiology relies on a concentration of oxygen flowing into the alveoli (ventilation), where it is separated from blood flowing in the pulmonary capillaries (perfusion) by a thin membrane that facilitates oxygen (O_2) and carbon dioxide (CO_2) transfer (diffusion) between the alveoli and the capillaries. To maintain normality, the balance between ventilation and perfusion is important. Impairment will lead to hypoxia and hypercarbia.

Ventilation

In a normal fit adult, 7–8ml/kg of air (approximately 500ml) is taken into the lungs with each breath. This amounts to approximately 5L per minute for a 70kg patient at rest. Only 70% (350ml) of each tidal volume reaches the terminal bronchioles where gas exchange occurs. The remaining 150ml remains in the upper airway and constitutes the anatomical dead space. In addition, areas of ventilation without perfusion with blood constitute the physiological dead space. In healthy adults, the anatomical and physiological dead space are approximately equal.

Pulmonary perfusion

There is a difference in blood flow between the apex and base of the lung because the pressure in the pulmonary circulation is much lower than the systemic circulation. This results in under-perfusion of apical alveoli and over-perfusion of basal alveoli. At the bases, therefore, there is inadequate elimination of CO_2 and uptake of oxygen. This blood is known as shunted blood. The effects of this are compensated by hypoxic pulmonary vasoconstriction which diverts blood to better ventilated areas.

Diffusion

The close proximity of the alveoli and pulmonary capillaries facilitates gas exchange by passive diffusion due to a pressure gradient across the respiratory membrane.

pO_2 (alveoli) 100mmHg → pO_2 (capillaries) 40mmHg
pCO_2 (pulmonary capillaries) 45mmHg → pCO_2 (alveoli) 40mmHg

The partial pressure is much smaller in relation to carbon dioxide exchange but this is not a problem because carbon dioxide is 20 times more soluble than oxygen. In the healthy adult, exchange of both gases takes place at the same rate. The lung has a pulmonary membrane surface equivalent to half a tennis court, making it ideal for gas exchange. Lung function may be compromised by poor ventilation (smoke inhalation, pain inhibition), reduced diffusion (pneumothorax), or increased thickness of the respiratory membrane (pulmonary oedema).

Patient assessment

There are six immediate life-threatening conditions (ATOMIC) that should be detected in the primary survey. These are:

- **A**irway obstruction
- **T**ension pneumothorax
- **O**pen chest wound
- **M**assive haemothorax
- Fla**I**l chest
- **C**ardiac tamponade.

All patients with chest trauma require high-flow oxygen and this should be administered at 15L per minute after ascertaining that the airway is clear. A mask and non-rebreathable reservoir bag should be used. Examination of the neck may reveal important physical signs suggestive of time-critical injury and must, therefore, take place before a collar is applied. The neck is examined for:

- Tracheal position
- Neck vein distension
- Wounds
- Surgical emphysema
- Laryngeal crepitis
- Spinal tenderness.

Depending on clinical urgency, it may be more appropriate to maintain inline cervical stabilization whilst completing the primary survey and to apply a collar after it has been completed.

Examination of the chest

Where possible, the chest should be exposed, although this may be difficult in entrapments. A systematic examination should follow the sequence:

- Inspection
- Palpation
- Percussion
- Auscultation.

DO NOT FORGET THE BACK

The specific determents of the primary survey are summarized in Table 3.2. The back should always be checked for evidence of injury. In victims of assault, posterior stab wounds are relatively common. If it is impossible or untimely to turn the patient onto their side to inspect their back, the gloved hand of the rescuer should be run down the back of the patient's chest whilst in a supine position and then inspected for blood. Extreme care should be used if there are fragments of broken glass about.

Tension pneumothorax

A tension pneumothorax may arise following blunt or penetrating trauma. Air is sucked into the plural space either through a hole in the chest wall or through a perforation in the visceral pleura, and a pneumothorax is produced. Should a flap be formed, from pleura or other soft tissue, a one-way valve may result. This may allow air to pass into the pleural space during inspiration but prevent it from leaving during expiration. The pneumothorax therefore increases in size, and the pressure inside the thorax rises. This situation is worsened by coughing and positive pressure ventilation. Eventually, the patient becomes shocked because of impeded venous return and diminished cardiac output. The classical features of a tension pneumothorax are:

- Rapid respiratory rate
- Decreased air entry
- Hyper-resonant hemithorax
- Rapid, weak pulse
- Decreasing level of consciousness
- Deviated trachea (late sign)
- Raised jugular venous pulse (if there is no accompanying hypovolaemia)
- Cyanosis (very late).

This condition can be rapidly fatal and the rescuer should have a high index of suspicion for the diagnosis. The treatment is a needle thoracocentesis using a 16 gauge cannula connected to a 10ml syringe. This is inserted into the second intercostal space in the midclavicular line. A rapid release of air confirms the diagnosis. The syringe and needle should be removed and the cannula left in situ and secured in position. This cannula may become blocked or dislodged, particularly during patient transfer. If the patient deteriorates, reassessment using the primary survey is necessary. If it appears that a tension pneumothorax is re-accumulating, a second cannula should be immediately inserted.

Depending on clinical competence, the clinical situation, and the distance to a hospital, it may (rarely) be necessary to consider a formal tube thoracocentesis. Thoracostomy with an Aschermann® chest seal is an alternative. If needle thoracocentesis fails to demonstrate a tension pneumothorax, the needle should still be left in place. If it is likely that the needle may not have reached the pleural cavity and the possibility of tension pneumothorax is high, a second cannula can be inserted behind the pectoralis in the anterior axillary line high in the axilla.

Table 3.2 Primary survey for chest injury

Inspection	Palpation	Percussion	Auscultation
Respiratory Rate	Crepitus or surgical emphysema	Increased resonance (pneumothorax)	*Listen*: axilla—lower half, upper half
Depth of respiration	Rib tenderness	Decreased resonance (haemothorax, lung contusion)	Determine: air entry Symmetry of air entry
Effort of breathing	Rib crepitus		
Symmetry of movement	Flail chest		
Bruising			
Abrasions			
Wounds			

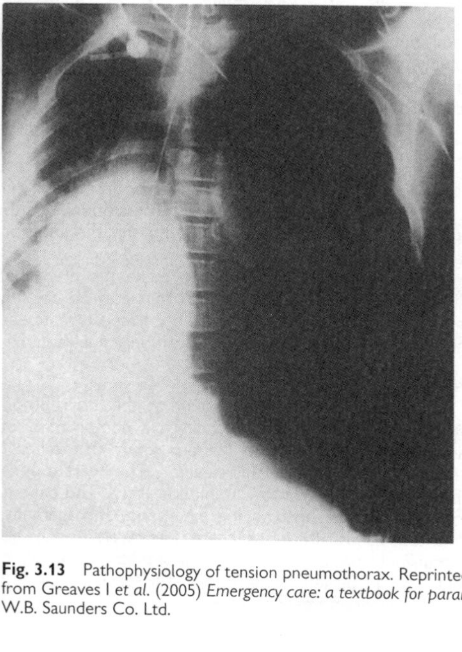

Fig. 3.13 Pathophysiology of tension pneumothorax. Reprinted with permission from Greaves I *et al.* (2005) *Emergency care: a textbook for paramedics*, 2nd edn. W.B. Saunders Co. Ltd.

Open chest wound

Open chest wounds commonly follow stab and gunshot wounds, although they can occur following road traffic and industrial accidents. An open chest wound will produce an open pneumothorax on the side of the injury. If the size of the wound is greater than two thirds the diameter of the patient's own trachea, air will preferentially pass through the hole in the chest wall during inspiration (a 'sucking wound'). The open wound may be preventing the accumulation of a tension pneumothorax and should not, therefore, be sealed. The best treatment is the application of an Aschermann® chest seal, although a dressing, sealed on three sides only, may be used.

Massive haemothorax

A massive haemothorax may complicate both blunt and penetrating trauma. The clinical features are:

- Decreased air entry on the affected side
- Dull percussion note over the affected side
- Clinical features of shock
- Low jugular venous pulse.

The management includes high-flow oxygen and judicious fluid replacement to maintain a palpable radial pulse. If other injuries allow, the patient should be positioned with the injured side uppermost (to optimize gas exchange) and rapidly transferred to hospital. Tube thoracocentesis should not normally be undertaken in the pre-hospital environment as this may result in catastrophic uncontrollable bleeding.

Flail chest

This occurs when two or more adjacent ribs are broken in two places, resulting in a flail segment which moves paradoxically on inspiration (*in* on inspiration, *out* on expiration). It occurs after compression injuries to the chest and, in frontal impacts, may involve the whole of the anterior chest wall. Massive anterior flail segments are often missed and a detailed and specific look at the chest wall is required to make the diagnosis. Looking tangentially at the chest from the patient's feet may be helpful. Lateral flail segments are usually more obvious. The pre-hospital treatment includes oxygen therapy, analgesia, and manual or positional stabilization.

Cardiac tamponade

This occurs most commonly following a stab wound to the heart. Blood collects within the pericardial sac and this leads to a compromise of ventricular filling and a fall in cardiac output. Venous return to the heart is reduced and the jugular venous pressure is elevated. The heart sounds are muffled and an ECG may display a low amplitude trace. The patient requires urgent transportation to hospital for emergency management. Needle pericardiocentesis is usually inneffecitive. However, it may be considered if the transfer time is likely to be prolonged. If blood is aspirated, the cannula should be left in the pericardial space, aspirated periodically, and allowed to drain freely.

Penetrating weapons or foreign bodies still in situ MUST NOT be removed. No attempt should be made to stop a weapon or foreign body which is moving with the heart cycle, as doing so this may worsen cardiac damage.

Table 3.3 Clinical signs in life-threatening chest injuries

	Position of the trachea in relation to the side of injury	Chest wall movement on the side of injury	Percussion note on the side of injury	Breath sounds on the side of injury
Flail chest	Central	Paradoxical movements	Decreased with pain on palpation	Decreased
Massive haemothorax	Central/away	Normal/ decreased	Decreased	Decreased
Open pneumothorax	Central	Decreased	Increased	Decreased
Tension pneumothorax	Away	Decreased	Increased	Decreased

The secondary survey

Re-examination of the chest forms part of the detailed head-to-toe secondary survey. Immediately, life-threatening injuries should have been identified during the primary survey, although their development can be delayed. The secondary survey may pick up potentially life-threatening conditions including:

- Simple or closed pneumothorax
- Pulmonary contusion
- Diaphragmatic rupture
- Fractured ribs
- Fractured sternum
- Surgical emphysema.

Simple or closed pneumothorax

This commonly occurs in blunt trauma and is often associated with damage to the lung from a fractured rib. It is more often than not a diagnosis made on X-ray in hospital as the clinical signs may be difficult to detect. They include:

- Reduced chest movement in the affected side
- Decreased air entry
- Decreased breath sounds
- Hyper-resonance to percussion.

Importantly, the trachea is not deviated and the jugular venous pressure is not elevated. Pre-hospital management includes oxygen therapy, analgesia, appropriate patient positioning, and transfer to hospital.

Pulmonary contusion

Pulmonary contusion is often a diagnosis that is made in hospital and on X-ray. In cases of prolonged entrapment, it is a diagnosis to consider. Alerting features include the mechanism of injury, the presence of chest wall contusion, rib fractures, and flail chest. The patient is often tachycardic and tachypnoeic with decreased air entry but a normal percussion note. There are no features to suggest a pneumothorax or a haemothorax.

Diaphragmatic rupture

Diaphragmatic rupture commonly follows blunt or penetrating trauma; the latter following stab wounds. Blunt trauma to the abdomen may lead to a rupture of the left hemidiaphragm through its central tendon (weakest point). Clinical features include increasing respiratory distress and a decreasing abdominal girth.

Fractured ribs

These commonly occur following blunt trauma, producing localized areas of pain, tenderness, and sometimes crepitus. Pre-hospital treatment includes manual splintage and analgesia. The patient should be observed for the development of intrathoracic complications, in particular pneumothorax.

Fractured sternum

Sternal fractures follow blunt trauma to the front of the chest. The most important clinical feature is pain which is often severe but can be treated by manual support and analgesia. Complications are unusual but can include cardiac dysrhythmias.

Surgical emphysema

Surgical emphysema is indicative of an air leak and may suggest an underlying pneumothorax. No treatment is necessary but the patient should be assessed carefully for an obvious pneumothorax and the risk of developing a tension pneumothorax.

Pain relief

The common feature of all chest injuries is pain. Appropriate analgesia is essential to ensure adequate breathing, which will reduce the risk of subsequent chest infection and facilitate patient handling and packaging for transport to hospital. Entonox® should not be used because of the risk of worsening an occult pneumothorax. The analgesia of choice is an opiate titrated to clinical response.

Abdominal and genitourinary trauma

The abdomen has three main regions:

- The peritoneal cavity
- The retroperitoneum
- The pelvis.

The peritoneal cavity can be divided into intra-thoracic and intra-abdominal components. The intra-thoracic component is the area under the costal margin and lower ribs; its upper thoracic boarder is the mobile diaphragm. The size of the intra-thoracic component, therefore, varies with respiration—increasing in expiration and decreasing during inspiration. It contains the diaphragm, liver, spleen, stomach, and transverse colon.

The relaxed diaphragm may reach the fifth intercostal space during expiration. Therefore any blunt or penetrating injury at or below this region may produce intra-abdominal trauma. Transdiaphragmatic stab wounds from higher in the chest are uncommon. Fractures of the lower ribs may damage the underlying organs, particularly the spleen on the left and the liver on the right side.

The abdominal compartment contains the small and large intestine. These are particularly at risk from shear forces which may tear the bowel or its blood supply. Penetrating injuries may produce multiple gut perforations.

Behind the abdominal compartment is the retroperitoneal space which contains the following structures:

- Ascending and descending colon
- Duodenum
- Pancreas
- The kidney
- Ureters
- Aorta
- Inferior vena cava.

These structures receive some protection from the anterior organs and injuries in this region may, therefore, be occult.

The pelvis contains the bladder, rectum, and iliac blood vessels in addition to the uterus, ovaries, and vagina in the female and the prostate in the male. Whilst the pelvis may offer some protection, the underlying organs are frequently damaged by displaced bony pelvic fragments.

Mechanism of injury

Blunt trauma, particularly from road accidents, significant falls, and industrial trauma are the main causes of abdominal injuries. Penetrating trauma, particularly from stabbing and gunshot, is on the increase in the UK and USA.

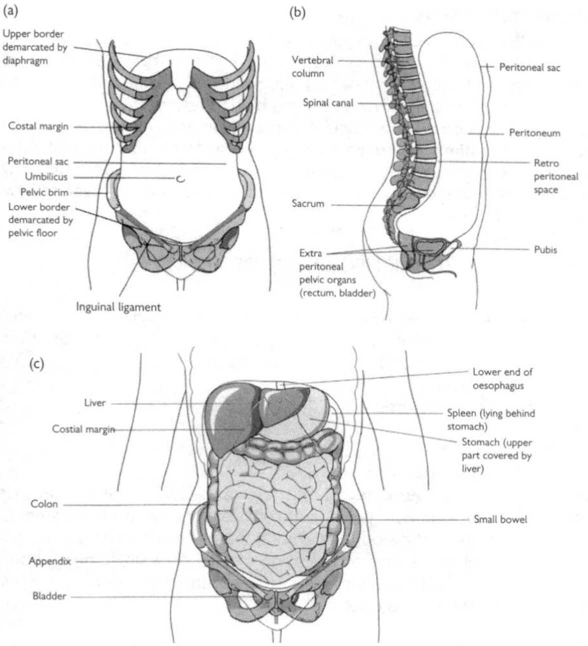

Fig. 3.14 Anatomy of the abdomen: (a) front view; (b) side view; (c) the peritoneal cavity. Reprinted with permission from Greaves I *et al.* (2005) *Emergency care: a textbook for paramedics 2nd edn.* W.B. Saunders Co. Ltd.

Blunt trauma

Blunt trauma may result from compression, crush, and shear forces. Sudden compressive forces may increase intra-abdominal pressure resulting in bowel rupture. This type of injury may follow lap belt injuries. Direct crushing may rupture the underlying organs, for example, the liver, spleen, pancreas, and the fixed retroperitoneal structures. Shear forces, commonly due to sudden deceleration, produce injuries at the interface of fixed and mobile structures including vascular pedicles.

Penetrating injuries

Penetrating injuries may occur through the anterior and posterior abdominal wall, the flanks, buttocks, and perineum and also through the diaphragm from above. Multiple stab wounds are not uncommon. Gunshot wounds are traditionally divided into low-energy and high-energy transfer wounds. The latter are associated with cavitation and contamination with a high incidence of morbidity and mortality. Any penetrating injury which perforates the bowel wall will result in faecal soiling and peritonitis.

Patient assessment

It is vital that the carer remembers that they are not concerned with establishing a specific anatomical diagnosis but that their priority is to decide, based on the mechanism of injury and clinical findings, whether there is a possibility of abdominal trauma being present.

Clinically significant solid organ trauma (liver and spleen) and major blood vessel trauma (aorta and inferior vena cava) may present with severe shock at the outset. Trauma producing hollow viscus injury may lead to an insidious development of peritonitis, sometimes over several hours or days.

THINK MECHANISM OF INJURY

Assessment follows the ABCDE system. The first suspicion of abdominal trauma may occur during the circulatory assessment. Hypotension must be explained. Sources of major blood loss include:

- External haemorrhage
- Major long bone fractures
- The chest
- The abdomen
- The pelvis and retroperitoneum.

In the absence of obvious external bleeding, major long bone fractures or chest injuries, the abdomen, pelvis, and retroperitoneum are implicated as the possible location of blood loss. During the primary survey, the detection of abdominal tenderness to palpation or pain on a single pelvic bony assessment is significant. It must be remembered that abdominal viscus and solid organ trauma may not initially be associated with any abnormal physical signs.

The assessment is made more difficult in the unconscious patient or patient with head trauma, spinal cord injury, major distracting injuries, or who has ingested drugs or alcohol.

Penetrating wounds are an obvious indicator of abdominal injury. In blunt trauma, bruising and contusion to the abdominal wall may be pathomnemonic of internal injury. Blood per urethram confirms renal tract trauma. The classic signs of intra-abdominal trauma include tenderness, guarding, and rigidity. Bowel sounds are frequently absent following trauma, even in the absence of specific intra-abdominal injury.

The clinical examination should include:

- Adequate exposure of the abdomen
- Inspection of the abdomen, lower chest, flanks, pelvis, and perineum
- Inspection and palpation of the posterior abdominal wall
- A single palpation of the pelvis.

Management

Blunt trauma

In the presence of hypotension, fluid replacement should be tailored to maintain or restore the radial pulse (systolic BP 80–90mmHg), ensuring essential organ perfusion.

Excessive fluid resuscitation will lead to accelerated bleeding or rebleeding, dilutional coagulopathy, and hypothermia in patients with non-compressible, non-controllable internal bleeding.

Opiate analgesia titrated to clinical response, preceded by an antiemetic, should be considered. There is NO justification for withholding analgesia pending surgical assessment.

Penetrating trauma

In the case of penetrating trauma, the wound should be covered with a moist sterile pad. This should be large enough to keep extruded bowel (if present) moist. Cling film may help retain dressings by covering the whole abdomen. The hypotensive patient's fluid replacement should follow the controlled hypotension principle.

Impaling injuries

Impaling objects should be left in place as their removal frequently produces major bleeding. External bleeding should be controlled by direct pressure. The object should be supported and prevented from moving during transfer by bulky dressings. Objects which are moving in time with the pulse should not be immobilized.

Evisceration

The passage of part of the intestine or other organ through a wound may occur. The protruding part should be kept moist using sterile pads and saline. No attempt should be made to relocate a protruding organ.

Pelvic fractures

There is a common association between pelvic fractures and abdominal organ trauma. Bleeding from pelvic fractures, particularly open book fractures (diastasis of the symphysis pubis), can be reduced by external splintage. A number of commercially available wrap-around pelvic splints are now available, or an improvised splint can be fashioned from a sheet, FRAC Straps®, or triangular bandages. The pneumatic antishock garment (MAST Suit) has lost popularity as it has been shown to increase morbidity and mortality in patients suffering head and chest trauma and cannot be used in patients with diaphragmatic rupture, those who are pregnant, and those with impalement and evisceration injuries.

Genitourinary trauma

Genitourinary trauma commonly occurs in conjunction with abdominal and pelvic trauma.

Anatomy

The kidneys and ureters lie in the retroperitoneal space gaining some protection from anterior abdominal trauma. The diagnosis of injury is often delayed. Wounds or contusions to the loin or flank area raise the possibility of renal or renal tract trauma.

Injuries to the bladder and urethra are usually more obvious. Bladder trauma is often associated with anterior pelvic fractures. Blood per urethra suggests lower urinary tract trauma. The external genitalia, especially in the male, are at risk from direct injury such as kicks and straddle injuries.

Mechanism of injury

As with abdominal trauma, injuries may be either blunt or penetrating, blunt being the more common. The bladder and urethra are frequently damaged at the time of pelvic fractures when they are exposed to both compression and shear forces.

Urethral injuries

Urethral injuries are commonly associated with direct injuries to the perineum. Injuries to the bulbous urethra are seen in straddle injuries and those to the membranous urethra, in pelvic fractures.

Bladder injuries

Bladder injuries follow both blunt and penetrating trauma. As a result of a compressive force, the intra-vesical pressure is acutely elevated leading to acute bladder rupture which can be intra-abdominal or extra-abdominal.

At the time of displacement of anterior pelvic fragments there may be direct injury to the underlying bladder. This is also seen in abdominal stabbing injuries. An inability to pass urine, lower abdominal tenderness, and blood per urethra are suggestive of significant injury.

Ureteric injuries

Because of its protected position in the retroperitoneal area, a diagnosis of injury to the ureter is normally made following specific investigation in hospital.

Renal injuries

Blunt injuries are most commonly associated with road traffic collisions but are seen in sport (for example, in rugby and football). The patient presents with loin tenderness, and, because of the association with more significant trauma, there may be generalized abdominal tenderness and hypovolaemia. Penetrating injuries are usually associated with stab wounds and gunshot wounds.

Genital injuries

Genital injuries are most commonly due to blunt trauma and the bruised testicle is made more comfortable by an ice pack and good supporting underwear. Severe blunt trauma may rupture the testicle. The pain is severe and the patient requires urgent surgical opinion. Not surprisingly, the patient tends to be extremely anxious.

Skin avulsions to the genitalia and penis require replacement in situ with a supportive dressing and transfer to hospital.

Bone and joint injuries

Limb injuries (including bone and joint trauma) are the most common injuries encountered in pre-hospital care. Although rarely immediately life-threatening, they require careful assessment, appropriate pain relief, realignment, and splintage if necessary, followed by safe extrication and transport.

Mechanism of injury

Fractures occur when the force applied to a bone exceeds its tensile strength. Bone is strongest under loading and weakest if distracted or twisted. The causative force may be direct, as in a kick to the tibia or associated with rotation and twisting as in the majority of ankle fractures. If the force is significant, fractures will occur in normal bones. However, in the elderly, many of whom are osteoporotic. Fractures may occur following relatively minor falls, fracture of the neck of the femur is a classic example.

Fracture classification

Many of the fracture classification systems relate to the X-ray appearances (for example, spiral butterfly oblique). The most important classification in pre-hospital care is:

- Simple (closed)
- Compound (open).

Each limb must be examined for any associated neurovascular deficit. Simple (closed) fractures occur when there is no overlying wound communicating with the fracture. Compound fractures, however, have an overlying or related wound which communicates with the fracture.

Careful patient handling will prevent simple fractures from becoming compound.

Children, by virtue of their immature skeleton and growth potential have different fracture types. These include 'greenstick' fractures and epiphyseal fractures (growth plate injuries). Although biologically and pathologically different, the clinical mode of presentation (pain, tenderness, swelling deformity, and loss of function) are common to both children and adults.

Dislocations

A dislocation is a complete disruption of a joint such that normally congruous joint surfaces are no longer in contact. Incomplete dislocations are known as subluxations. Common examples of dislocations include patella dislocations and dislocations of the shoulder. Fractures may occur in conjunction with dislocations, for example, posterior dislocation of the hip with fracture of the posterior wall of the acetabulum.

Patient assessment

The initial assessment follows the ABCDE system. Fractures can present as immediately life-threatening injuries either directly or indirectly.

Airway compromise
- Skull fractures: the unconscious patient unable to protect their own airway
- Facial fractures, including impacted maxillary fractures and bilateral mandibular fractures
- Laryngeal fracture
- Posterior sternoclavicular dislocation.

Breathing compromise
- Rib fractures and flail chest
- High spinal cord injuries.

Circulatory compromise
- Compound fractures with bleeding
- Multiple long bone fractures
- Pelvic fractures
- Fractures with damage to underlying organs (liver and spleen).

Disability/neurological compromise
- Major skull fractures
- Depressed skull fractures
- Spinal injuries.

Limb-threatening injuries

It may be obvious at the outset that a patient has sustained a catastrophic limb injury with a high risk of subsequent amputation. Examples include extensive soft tissue injuries or soft tissue loss, major compound fractures, or major neurovascular deficit. Optimal pre-hospital care will maximize the chance of limb salvage.

Examination of the musculoskeletal system must be systematic and follow the 'look, feel, and move' system.
- Look—wounds, swelling, deformity.
- Feel—tenderness, swelling, deformity, neurovascular deficit.
- Move—can the patient move the limb (avoid moving limbs that have obvious fractures)?

Limb-threatening complications such as compartment syndrome do not normally occur in the pre-hospital environment unless there is a delay in transfer to hospital.

Principles of management

The principles of management of musculoskeletal injuries are:
- Life-threatening injuries should be identified and treated.
- All patients who have sustained a major long bone fracture require oxygen.
- Unless there are time-critical injuries, all fractures and dislocations should be splinted.
- The joint above and the joint below the injury should be immobilized.
- Appropriate pain relief should be given—Entonox® (care in chest injuries!) or an opiate titrated to clinical response.

Closed fractures

Where possible, significant deformity should be corrected by traction, restoring length, and rotation, followed by limb splintage. Pre-extrication splintage may not be possible other than companion support (broad bandages, FRAC Straps®).

Splintage has a number of important beneficial effects:

- Reduces pain
- Reduces blood loss
- Reduces the risk of neurovascular damage
- Reduces pressure on skin
- Reduces the risk and magnitude of fat embolism
- Facilitates packaging

Compound fractures

Good wound care at the outset will reduce the risk of soft tissue and bony infection. Gross contamination should be removed and the bone ends irrigated with saline and relocated in or as near the normal anatomical position as possible. The wound should be covered with a sterile dressing and splintage applied to the limb. Life-threatening bleeding should be controlled by direct or indirect pressure, wound packing, or a tourniquet.

Dislocations

The treatment of a dislocation is the prompt restoration of joint congruity if the patient's other injuries permit. A good example is fracture dislocation of the ankle where there may be ischaemic skin due to local pressure and major vascular compromise. The timing and place of reduction will depend on the skills of the carer, the availability of drugs, and the transfer time to hospital.

If pre-hospital reduction is impossible or inappropriate, the patient should be given analgesia, the limb splinted as much as possible, and the patient transported to hospital. Reduction under analgesia aims to restore normal anatomical position by reversing the forces which caused the original injury. This may not always be possible, (for example, due to soft tissue interposition) and undue force should not be used. In inexperienced hands, the correct approach is usually to arrange urgent transfer to hospital.

Splintage

The principles of splintage involve

- Padding to protect any vulnerable bony points
- Splintage of the joint above and below the fracture
- Checking the circulation before manipulation and splintage
- Regular reassessment of the neurovascular status.

Methods of splintage include

- Self help, for example, supporting the arm in the presence of a fracture of the clavicle or neck of humerus
- Broad arm slings—wrist and forearm injuries
- Broad bandages or FRAC straps® to secure the upper limb to the trunk or the lower limbs together

- Box splints—padded, solid surrounding supports short leg, long leg,or forearm for long bone fractures
- Traction splints—suitable for femoral shaft fractures
- Vacuum splints—to provide contoured splintage for limb fractures
- Spinal boards—principally designed as an extrication device but frequently used in spinal trauma.

Splintage is discussed more detail in individual topics on fractures.

Regional injuries: upper limb

Clavicular fractures

Cause

The vast majority are caused by a direct blow on the point of the shoulder. Less commonly, clavicular fracture follows a fall on an outstretched hand due to force transmitted up the arm.

Signs and symptoms

- Tenderness
- Swelling
- Visible deformity
- The patient frequently supports the weight of their arm

Treatment

Relieve the weight of the arm by providing support either manually or with a broad arm sling.

Potential problems

Very occasionally, the fracture may be compound, particularly if it is the result of a direct injury. There is a small risk of injury to the subclavian artery or the brachial plexus. Because of the close proximity of the chest wall, there may be an underlying chest injury.

Sternoclavicular dislocations

Cause

Sternoclavicular dislocations occur following a fall or a direct injury to the front of the shoulder. They are seen quite frequently in rugby scrumming injuries. The joint can sublux or dislocate both anteriorly or posteriorly.

Signs and symptoms

- Pain
- Tenderness
- Swelling
- Asymmetry at the inner end of the clavicle.

Treatment

Support in a broad arm sling.

Potential problems

Posterior sternoclavicular dislocations are occasionally associated with acute airway obstruction, producing stridor and respiratory distress. The treatment is to lever the clavicle forward using the fingers. If this is unsuccessful, the patient should be transported urgently to hospital.

Rarely, posterior dislocations are associated with damage to underlying major vessels and they can present with shock.

Acromioclavicular dislocations

Cause

Acromioclavicular dislocations are commonly seen following falls when the patient rolls onto the shoulder. This is a common injury of rugby players.

Signs and symptoms

Various degrees of injury occur, from simple sprains presenting as local tenderness and swelling, to dislocations where the dislocated outer end of the clavicle is obviously prominent.

Treatment

Support in a broad arm sling.

Potential problems

There are no specific frequent complications of acromioclavicular joint dislocation. In patients with a component of crush injury, other injuries should be excluded.

Dislocations of the shoulder: anterior

Cause

This is the most common type of shoulder dislocation occurring commonly in males aged 18–25yrs, caused by falls on the outstretched hand followed by external rotation of the shoulder. Anterior dislocations are common sports injuries, but also occur as a result of simple falls and, occasionally, road traffic collisions.

Signs and symptoms

Patients are often in severe pain and support their arm in the most comfortable position. The arm is held with the elbow flexed and the shoulder internally rotated. The normal contour of the shoulder is lost (Fig. 3.15).

Treatment

The arm should be supported. It cannot be splinted by the side and should be kept in a comfortable position. The patient is likely to have found this for themselves, but support on a pillow may help. Analgesia should be given, using Entonox, an NSAID, or opiates (titrated to need).

Occasionally, it may be appropriate to attempt reduction in the pre-hospital environment, although this should only be considered by those with appropriate experience.

Adequate analgesia or sedation should be given and gentle external rotation of the humerus should be attempted, with the elbow flexed to 90°. This may achieve reduction, or reduction may occur when the elbow is adducted across the chest. Successful relocation of the head of the humerus can usually be felt by the manipulator. Otherwise, if the hand on the affected side can reach to grasp the opposite shoulder without difficulty, successful reduction has been achieved.

Potential problems

Neurological complications are relatively common, especially damage to the axillary (circumflex) nerve tested for sensation over the regimental badge area on the side of the upper arm. The neurological deficit can be more dense and, rarely, there is an accompanying axillary artery injury.

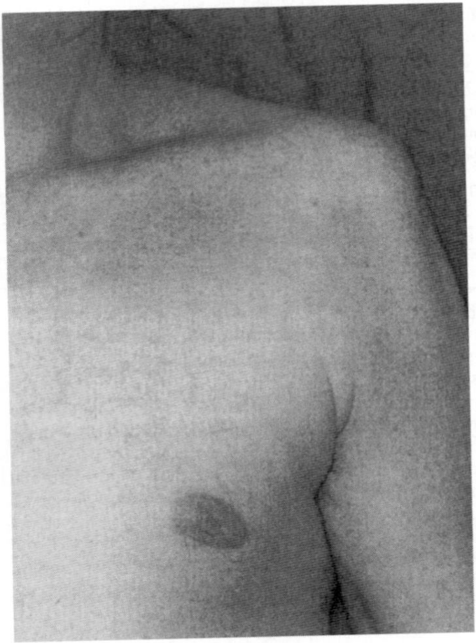

Fig. 3.15 Shoulder contour: anterior dislocation.

Dislocations of the shoulder: posterior

Cause

Posterior dislocation of the shoulder may result from a direct blow to the front of the shoulder or a fall on the outstretched hand with the arm internally rotated. Posterior dislocation classically, but rarely, complicates epileptic fits or electrocution.

Signs and symptoms

- Pain
- Deformity
- Local tenderness.

Treatment

The arm should be supported and analgesia should be given.

Potential problems

Neurological complications, whilst recognized, are rare.

Dislocations of the shoulder: inferior (luxatio erecta)

Cause

The usual cause is a superior blow with the shoulder in an abducted position. Superior dislocation of the shoulder is extremely rare.

Signs and symptoms

- Pain
- Deformity
- Loss of function.

Treatment

The arm should be supported and pain relief given.

Potential problems

Inferior dislocation may be associated with injuries to the brachial plexus or the axillary artery. There may be problems fitting the patient onto a stretcher and they may have to be transported in a sitting position.

Humeral fractures: proximal

Cause

Proximal humeral fractures may occur due to direct falls on the upper humerus or by transmitted force following a fall on the outstretched hand.

Signs and symptoms

- Pain
- Tenderness
- Deformity
- Loss of function.

Treatment

Analgesia should be considered before moving the arm. Pain may in part be relieved by immobilizing the arm. The elbow can be bent and the arm splinted in a sling with the addition of a broad bandage around the chest. Alternatively, the arm can be positioned by the patient's side and secured by a series of broad bandages around the chest and trunk. Some patients may prefer to support the arm themselves for transport to hospital.

Potential problems

If the fracture occurs as a result of significant direct violence, the possibility of other injuries (for example, chest wall injuries) should be considered.

Humeral fractures: shaft fractures

Cause

Humeral shaft fractures are usually due to direct violence (falls, road traffic collisions). They may also occur due to indirect force such as a fall onto the outstretched hand.

Signs and symptoms

- Pain
- Angulation
- Loss of function
- The patient supports the arm with the other hand
- There may be evidence of radial nerve palsy (motor and sensory).

Treatment

Analgesia should be offered and the patient allowed to support their own arm. Use of a sling or pad inside the arm and splinting to the chest with broad bandages should be considered.

Potential problems

Radial nerve palsy may occur in midshaft fractures. Very rarely, injuries to the brachial artery may occur, as can a compartmental syndrome.

There is a high incidence of associated chest injuries when humeral fracture occurs in a pedestrian hit by a vehicle.

Supracondylar fractures in adults

Cause

These commonly result from a fall directly onto the elbow. By definition, the fracture occurs in the distal third of the humerus. The fracture is invariably transverse but may have an intra-articular component.

Signs and symptoms

- Pain
- Swelling and deformity
- Loss of function
- The patient will be in pain and will usually support their own arm.

Treatment

The arm should be immobilized in the most comfortable position. If the arm is extended, it may be immobilized in a padded box splint or by padding and bandages to the trunk. If the elbow is flexed, the arm may be best supported in a broad arm sling.

Potential problems

As in children's fractures, although less frequently, there may be associated injuries to the brachial artery and the median nerve.

Supracondylar fractures in children

Cause

This is a common fracture following a fall on the outstretched hand.

Signs and symptoms

Typical features include:

- Pain
- Swelling and deformity
- Loss of function.

There is a risk of vascular compromise due to trauma to the brachial artery when the features may include pallor, coldness, parasthesae, and pulslessness in the forearm and hand. Neurological injury to the median, radial, and ulna nerves have all been recorded and clinical features will include appropriate sensory and motor signs.

Treatment

Appropriate analgesia should be given and the limb realigned, if this can be tolerated. Splintage to the trunk or a padded box splint or broad arm sling should be used to provide immobilization.

Potential problems

The main problems relate to neurological or vascular injury, particularly the latter. Regular circulatory assessment is mandatory. The late manifestations of an unrecognized ischaemic limb include compartment syndrome and the risk of developing a Volkman's ischaemic contracture.

There are other configurations of fractures about the elbow that occur particularly in children, for example, fractures of the medial and lateral condyles. The presentation is as above, although they are usually without complications, and these injuries can normally be immobilized in a broad arm sling.

Olecranon fractures

Cause

The olecranon is most commonly fractured by a fall on the point of the elbow. Following this, bony separation of the fragments occurs due to the action of the triceps muscle. Less frequently, fracture results from an unopposed forceful contraction of the triceps muscle.

Signs and symptoms

- Pain
- Inability to straighten the arm (not always found)
- Bruising and swelling.

The bone ends, particularly in the elderly, are often palpable and, in some patients, the skin is stretched and at risk of breaking down. Occasionally, these fractures are compound at the outset.

Treatment

If the fracture is compound, a sterile dressing should be applied. A broad arm sling will give adequate support in most cases. If the arm is held extended or the skin is vulnerable, it should be splinted in extension using a box splint.

Potential problems

In direct trauma, because of its close proximity, the ulna nerve may be damaged.

Radial head and neck fractures

Cause

The majority of radial head and neck fractures occur because of falls onto the outstretched hand, the fracture occurring as the force is transmitted along the radius. Rarely, the radial head may be injured by direct trauma.

Signs and symptoms

The patient complains of elbow pain, swelling, and later bruising. Forearm rotation (pronation and supination) is restricted, as is elbow extension.

Treatment

Pain may be relieved by placing the arm at 90 degrees in a broad arm sling. An ice pack may help relieve pain.

Potential complications

No significant pre-hospital complications.

Dislocations of the elbow

Cause

These commonly occur following a fall onto the outstretched hand. The majority are posterior—the ulna is displaced posterior relative to the humerus. Direct blows to the proximal forearm bones in an upwards direction may result in anterior elbow dislocation.

Signs and symptoms

- Pain
- Swelling and deformity.

There is obvious loss of the normal bony contours. The patient often supports their elbow for pain relief.

Treatment

The patient should be offered analgesia (Entonox® is effective), and the elbow should be supported or splinted in the most comfortable position. This may involve padding and splintage to the side of the body or padding and immobilization in a box splint.

Potential problems

Injuries to the brachial artery and the ulna and median nerves have been recorded.

Fractures of the shafts of the radius and ulna

There are three specific types of fracture configuration of the bones of the forearm:

1. Fractures of the shaft of the ulna, or radius, or both.
2. A fracture of the ulna with a dislocation of the radial head (Monteggia fracture).
3. Fracture of the shaft of radius with a dislocation of the distal end of the ulna (Galeazzi fracture).

Cause

Direct violence to the forearm may fracture one or both bones at the point of impact. A common self-defence injury is the so called '*night-stick fracture*' which results when the forearm is presented in self defence and is subjected to a direct blow. More commonly, fractures occur as a result of indirect violence following a fall on the outstretched hand. The applied force and angle of rotation of the forearm dictate the type of fracture pattern. Although a radiological diagnosis, isolated displaced fractures of a single bone of the forearm must be associated with an injury elsewhere, as in the Monteggia and Galeazzi fracture patterns. In children, greenstick fractures commonly occur.

Signs and symptoms

- Pain
- Swelling and deformity, including angulation and rotation
- The forearm is usually supported.

These injuries are only rarely compound.

Treatment

A broad arm sling maintaining elevation may be all that is necessary. Alternatively, the arm can be splinted in a padded boxed splint.

Potential problems

In fractures of both bones of the forearm, there is a risk that a closed injury may become compound if the arm is not immobilized.

Associated neurovascular deficit may occur. If there is delay in presentation and the history is of a high impact injury, acute compartmental syndrome is possible. The clinical features of this include:

- Extreme pain
- Marked pain on passive extension of the fingers
- Altered sensation in the hand.

The wrist

There are four main types of wrist fractures:

1. Colles' fracture
2. Smith's fracture
3. Volar Barton's fracture
4. Epiphyseal injuries in children.

Cause

The Colles' fracture is one of the most common wrist fractures and results from a fall on the outstretched hand. It usually occurs in middle-aged and elderly osteoporotic women. In displaced fractures, the appearance of the wrist is commonly described as a dinner fork deformity. The dorsal prominence is produced by the displaced distal end of the radius and carpus.

The Smith's fracture, often referred to as the 'reversed Colles' fracture,' results from a fall landing on the back of the hand (a flexed wrist). It is relatively common in motorcyclists who receive their injuries whilst still gripping the handlebars or as a consequence of landing. These fractures also occur with a dorsal wrist prominence, this time due to the volar slippage of the distal radius, carpus, and hand.

The Volar Barton's fracture occurs in a similar way to the Smith's fracture. Only the anterior portion of the distal radius is fractured and may be displaced. The differentiation from a *Smith's* fracture is made by X-ray.

Falls on the outstretched hand in children commonly produce a fracture involving the epiphyseal plate.

Signs and symptoms

- Pain
- Swelling and deformity.
- The wrist is commonly supported by the patient's other hand.

Treatment

Pain relief and the use of a broad arm sling. In more severe injuries, a padded box splint may be useful, especially in those patients with other associated injuries who require transportation in the supine position.

Potential problems

In high-energy trauma, there is a significant association between wrist fractures and fractures and injuries elsewhere in the body including the head, chest, pelvis, and other limbs. Displaced fractures may be associated with median nerve symptoms. Less frequently, the ulna nerve may be affected.

Carpal bone fractures

Cause

The most common carpal bone fracture is the scaphoid fracture commonly resulting from a fall on an outstretched hand. Traditionally, it was described as an injury complicating a 'kick-back' when using a starting handle. Scaphoid fracture is well known for its difficulty in hospital diagnosis and the typical delay in the appearance of a fracture on X-rays.

Other common carpal injuries may follow forced palmar flexion producing simple dorsal bony avulsion injuries. Isolated fractures of the other carpal bones can rarely occur, all of which will present with pain and local tenderness.

There are a variety of complex fracture dislocations of the carpus which are delineated by radiographic investigation. These usually occur in high-velocity trauma, though they should be managed in line with other wrist fractures.

Signs and symptoms

- Wrist pain
- Tenderness in the anatomical snuff box (scaphoid fracture).

Other signs of scaphoid fracture include pain in the scaphoid on axial pressure through the thumb and pain on compression of the dorsum of the scaphoid. The patient may have restricted movement in the wrist and impaired grip.

Treatment

The patient usually supports the injured wrist. Analgesia should be given and the limb should be placed in a supporting high broad arm sling.

Potential problems

Scaphoid fracture may be associated with median nerve symptoms. The differential diagnosis of tenderness in the region of the anatomical snuff box, the distal radius, and the radial styloid includes Colles' fracture, scaphoid fracture, and wrist sprain. A definitive diagnosis should be made in hospital. In pre-hospital care, they should all be treated as potential fractures.

Finger fractures

Cause

Metacarpal and phalangeal fractures are common hand injuries and follow both direct and indirect forces. Spiral fractures often occur as a result of rotational forces.

Specific fractures within the hand complex include:

- Fractures of the base of the thumb (Bennett's fracture)
- Ulnar collateral ligament of the thumb sprain or rupture
- Mallet finger
- Fracture of the fifth metacarpal (boxer's fracture)
- Finger dislocations.

Bennett's fracture is better described as a fracture dislocation at the base of the thumb metacarpal. This is an intra-articular fracture resulting in dislocation of the main component of the metacarpal.

The ulna collateral ligament of the thumb may be ruptured, often in conjunction with a bony avulsion. These injuries result from a forced abduction of the thumb, traditionally in gamekeepers but, more commonly now, as a result of falls on the dry ski slope.

Forced flexion of the extended finger may produce a bony avulsion of the extensor insertion to the distal phalanx resulting in a mallet finger deformity. These are caused by direct force (commonly a ball striking the tip of the finger) and are usually obvious clinically.

Fracture of the fifth metacarpal (often spiral in nature) commonly results from the administration of a bare knuckle punch (which is why this fracture is almost never seen in boxers). Common assailants include walls and wardrobes (allegedly).

Dislocations of the finger at the metacarpo-phalangeal joint or either interphalangeal joint (rarely both) are usually clinically obvious.

Signs and symptoms

Common signs and symptoms include pain, swelling, and deformity. When attempting to flex the finger into the palm, obvious rotation of the digit may be apparent in phalangeal or metacarpal fractures.

Treatment

The arm should be placed in a broad arm sling ensuring that the hand is supported and elevated. Light companion strapping of the injured finger, if practical, may offer some symptomatic relief, although this can usually be delayed until arrival in hospital.

Simple interphalangeal dislocations can usually be reduced in the field by longitudinal traction under analgesia (Entonox® is effective) by appropriately trained personnel.

Rings and jewellery should be removed from the injured hand as soon as possible.

Potential problems

Compartment syndrome rarely occurs following severe crush injuries to the hand.

Regional injuries: the thorax

Rib fractures

Cause

Most rib fractures result form direct force, for example, direct blows to the chest. They occur frequently in road traffic collisions, falls, sport, and assaults.

Signs and symptoms

- Pain
- Tenderness
- Shortness of breath.

The pain is usually well localized to the fracture site and is made worse by movement, including inspiration. The patient may well support the chest wall manually. Rarely, the patient will complain of clicking of the broken rib ends.

Treatment

Adequate analgesia should be provided to enable the patient to breath comfortably. Self help includes splintage of the chest wall. The patient should be allowed to position themselves in the most comfortable position, which is usually sitting up. This will also assist in making breathing easier.

Potential problems

Rib fractures on their own, occurring in fit healthy people are usually benign, albeit painful injuries. However, the elderly and those with pre-existing chest disease (for example, chronic obstructive pulmonary disease) are at serious risk of complications associated with reduced chest wall movement and underlying pulmonary contusion.

Patients suffering rib fractures may sustain intra-thoracic complications including pneumothorax, haemothorax, atelectasis, and chest infection due to alveolar hypoventilation (see pp.208–17).

There is generally a tendency to underestimate the magnitude of chest trauma.

Entonox® should not be used if there is any possibility of pneumothorax.

Flail chest

Cause

A flail chest occurs when two or more ribs are broken in two places resulting in a flail segment. This results from substantial chest trauma, for example, road traffic collision or falls from a height. As a consequence, during inspiration and the generation of negative intrathoracic pressure, the flail segment is sucked in and the lung remains underventilated. This pattern of breathing is called paradoxical movement.

Lateral flail chests are easy to see with full chest exposure. Anterior flail chests may be more difficult to visualize unless the patient is supine and the chest is viewed at trolley height from the patient's feet. The mechanism of injury should alert one to the possible presence of a flail chest: the whole of the anterior chest wall may be flail if, during an RTC, the chest has struck the steering wheel. Posterior flail chests are commonly supported by the muscle mass of the back and may only become apparent when the patient becomes exhausted.

Signs and symptoms

- Pain
- Respiratory distress.

The definitive diagnosis is made by the detection of paradoxical movements. Air entry may be decreased. The percussion note may vary depending on associated intrathoracic injuries—it will be hyper-resonant in the presence of a pneumothorax and dull due to haemothorax.

Treatment

The patient should receive high-flow oxygen at a rate of 15L per minute via a mask with a non-rebreath reservoir bag. Manual stabilization and splintage may be achieved by applying the flat of the hand to the flail segment and maintaining the indrawn position. This may also be achieved with a half litre or litre bag of saline or postural positioning over something firm to compress the flail segment. Adequate analgesia is essential.

Potential problems

These are related to associated intrathoracic injuries, in particular, pulmonary contusion. Other complications include pneumothorax, haemothorax, and, in the longer term, chest infections. Major flail chest may be associated with mechanical failure of respiration and the necessity for artificial ventilation in hospital.

Sternal fractures

Cause

The most common mechanism of injury is a direct blow to the sternum where the injury pattern may range from unicortical cracks (often seen in seatbelt injuries) to complete fractures, sometimes with overlap of the bone ends.

Sternal fractures can also occur in conjunction with thoracic wedge compression fractures due to forced flexion of the thoracic spine (for example, in falls from a motorbike).

Signs and symptoms

- Pain and tenderness at the fracture site
- The patient may hold their chest.

Other signs and symptoms may relate to associated intrathoracic injuries.

Treatment

Treatment includes analgesia, oxygen therapy, and manual support for the chest. Very rarely, in prolonged transport times, local anaesthetic can be injected into the fracture site.

Potential problems

These relate to the underlying injuries and include cardiac contusion, cardiac arrhythmias, thoracic aorta tears, and pulmonary contusion.

Regional injuries: the pelvis

Fractures of the pelvis are produced by three main mechanisms:

1. Antero-posterior compression
2. Lateral compression
3. Vertical compression.

These fractures can be classified by appreciating that the pelvis is a complete ring where instability occurs if there are two or more major areas of injury.

Type A: stable fractures

Include fractures not involving the complete pelvic ring (for example, the iliac crest, the anterior inferior iliac spine) or minimally displaced pelvic ring fractures that are stable (for example, fractures of the superior pubic rami).

Type B: rotationally unstable, vertically stable fractures

For example, open-book fractures.

Type C: rotationally and vertically unstable fractures

Involve major damage to two or more areas in the pelvic ring. These may be seen following falls from a height.

Minor pelvic fractures: pubic ramus

Cause

Fractures of the pubic rami are common, especially in elderly osteoporotic women following a fall onto the affected side. Anteroposterior (AP) compression may produce isolated ipsilateral superior and inferior pubic rami fractures and, following significant falls (for example, if rolled on following a fall from a horse), may affect both superior and inferior pubic rami ('butterfly fracture').

Signs and symptoms

The patient will complain of pain in the groin and will be tender to palpation over the fracture. Hip movements may be painful because of the close proximity of the fracture. The patient can usually manage a straight leg raise. Anterior and lateral pelvic compression is painful.

Treatment

The mainstay of pre-hospital treatment is providing pain relief, appropriate packaging, and transport to hospital. The legs should be splinted together using a pad and broad bandages and the patient should be transported in a supine position.

Potential problems

Simple falls onto the side producing pubic rami fractures are usually uncomplicated and are classified as minimally displaced or undisplaced fractures of the pelvic ring. The anteroposterior crush injuries, depending on the mechanism of injury, may be associated with significant blood loss, damage to the urethra, and, in some cases, sacroiliac injuries.

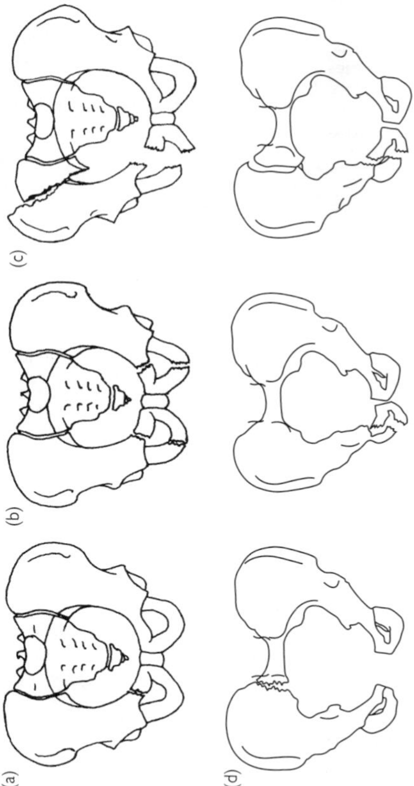

Fig. 3.16 Mechanisms of pelvic fractures: (a) stable fracture of a single pubic ramus; (b) 'butterfly fracture' (AP compression); (c) vertical shear fracture; (d) 'open book' pelvis. (a–c) reprinted with permission from McRae *Practical fracture treatment* Churchill Livingstone.

Minor pelvic fractures: avulsion fractures

Cause

These are fractures of the pelvis not involving the pelvic ring and are frequently seen in sports injuries, most commonly athletics, resulting from sudden muscle contraction. Common sites include the anterior superior iliac spine (sartorius muscle), the anterior inferior iliac spine (the rectus muscle), and the ischial tuberosity (the hamstrings).

Signs and symptoms

- Pain
- Local tenderness
- Variable loss of function.

Treatment

No specific treatment is necessary. Analgesia may be required. The patient should be transported to hospital.

Potential problems

In the pre-hospital phase of care, there are no specific potential problems.

Major pelvic fractures

Cause

Major compression fractures and the rotationally and vertically unstable injuries are most commonly the result of road traffic collisions. These fractures nearly always involve disruption of the pelvic ring although, rarely, isolated fractures of the iliac crest may occur.

Signs and symptoms

The patient will (depending on injuries elsewhere) complain of pain, tenderness, and sometimes deformity. There may be clear signs and symptoms of shock (pallor, sweating, tachycardia, tachypnoea, hypotension, and increased capillary refill time). The circulatory assessment should include a single careful examination of the pelvis (gentle controlled anteroposterior, lateral, and vertical movement of the pelvis with the hands over the iliac crest) which may demonstrate instability and pain. This examination should NOT be repeated as this may precipitate bleeding.

Depending on the pattern of injury, there may be associated urethral trauma presenting with blood per urethram and associated perineal or scrotal swelling which may or may not be recognized in the pre-hospital situation.

Treatment

The patient should be assessed following the ABCDE system. Measures to reduce blood loss include splinting the patient's legs together with the legs internally rotated, elevation of the legs, tilting the patient head down on a spinal board, the use of a commercial external pelvic splint (which has been shown convincingly to reduce the pelvic volume), or wrapping in sheet (or similar) around the pelvis and applying circumferential pressure.

Intravenous access should be obtained and fluid infused to restore or just maintain the radial pulse (non-compressible, non-controllable haemorrhage). Appropriate titrated opiate analgesia should be given.

Potential complications

The main pre-hospital complication is hypovolaemia. Patients with pelvic fractures often, as their mechanism of injury may suggest, have injuries elsewhere.

In the presence of a significant pelvic injury, a scoop stretcher should be used for the transfer to a spine board rather than a log roll.

Regional injuries: lower limb

Acetabular fractures/hip dislocations

Cause

Most fractures of the acetabulum occur as a result of force transmitted along the longitudinal axis of the femur (for example, due to impact from the dashboard in front seat car occupants) or following lateral compression injuries to the greater trochanter region (as in side impact road traffic accidents or a fall onto the side). In some instances, not only is the acetabulum fractured but the head of the femur is driven through the acetabulum producing a central fracture dislocation of the hip. Most dislocations are posterior (the head of the femur is displaced posteriorly), unless the injury is associated with excessive hip extension when the head of the femur dislocates anteriorly.

Signs and symptoms

The patient is in pain. In posterior dislocation, the hip is held flexed, internally rotated, and adducted. Attempts to straighten the leg are unsuccessful: the head is held behind the posterior aspect of the acetabulum, where in many cases there is an associated fracture of the posterior wall.

Treatment

The patient should be given high-flow oxygen and opiates titrated to achieve pain relief. The limb should be supported and splinted by opposing the good leg, insertion of padding between the legs, and the use of circumferential broad bandages or Frac straps®. Because the limbs are splinted in a flexed position, a blanket should be placed under the patient's knees.

Potential problems

Posterior dislocation of the hip is associated with sciatic nerve palsy in 10% of cases. Urgent reduction in hospital is necessary.

Anterior dislocations are associated with a risk of damage to the femoral nerve and the femoral vein and artery.

Acetabular fractures are often seen in association with more serious injury. An ABCDE approach and a secondary survey (when clinically appropriate) should be undertaken.

Fractures of the neck of the femur

The term 'fractured neck of the femur' includes intracapsular (subcapital and transcervical) and extracapsular fractures (pertrochanteric and intertrochanteric fractures).

Cause

Fractures of the neck of the femur most commonly occur in the elderly osteoporotic female population, usually following falls onto the affected side. Occasionally, the lucid and astute patient may report their leg giving way followed by a fall, suggesting a fracture due to underlying bony weakness.

Fractures in the younger age group, including children, usually follow significant violence as in road traffic collisions, falls from significant heights, or industrial accidents.

A slipped upper femoral epiphysis in children may occur after minor or insignificant trauma and present clinically like a fractured neck of femur.

Signs and symptoms

The patient will be in pain, often lying in the position that they were in immediately after the fall. Depending on the fracture pattern, which will not be known until X-rays are taken, there may be anterior hip tenderness (intracapsular fractures) or tenderness over the greater trochanter (extracapsular intertrochanteric fractures). Bruising, if seen, suggests a time delay and is usually only present in extracapsular fractures. Except in the most minor of hip fractures (undisplaced intracapsular incomplete neck fractures), the patient is unable to do a straight leg raise. In displaced fractures, the leg is classically shortened and externally rotated.

Treatment

Initially, assessment should follow the ABCDE system. The patient should receive analgesia and the leg should be repositioned and secured to the good leg using padding and broad bandages. The neurovascular status should be determined before and after any manipulation.

Potential problems

It is important to ascertain whether there was any medical reason for the fall, for example, a transient ischemic episode, epileptic fit, or collapse due to a cardiac cause. The patient's prescribed drugs should be taken to hospital.

Some patients may have been lying on the floor all night and have become hypoglycaemic and dehydrated. A blood glucose assessment is necessary. If there is a prolonged journey time to hospital, fluid replacement should be considered for correction of dehydration. Similarly, the elderly patient is at risk of developing pressure sores. Particular care should be taken to handle them carefully, especially when the patient has been lying still for any length of time, avoiding hard surfaces such as scoop stretchers or spinal boards if possible. Otherwise, the time on one of these must be kept to a minimum. A vacuum mattress, if available, should be considered in this group of vulnerable patients.

Any patient with hip pain should be transported to hospital to exclude femoral neck fracture—in those patients with no leg deformity, there may be fractures of the adjacent pubic rami.

The proximal femur is not an uncommon site of pathological femoral neck or intertrochanteric fractures due to malignancy.

Fractures of the shaft of the femur

Cause

Fractures of the shaft of the femur are common following road traffic collisions, falls from significant heights, and crush injury (for example, under falling masonry).

A fracture that occurs spontaneously or after minimal trauma suggests that it is a pathological fracture, for example, secondary to carcinoma or myeloma.

Signs and symptoms

- Extreme pain
- Deformity and swelling of the thigh
- External rotation of the leg

Palpation may reveal crepitus and mobility at the fracture site. Many high-velocity injuries are compound, some associated with extensive soft tissue injuries and blood loss.

Treatment

The initial assessment and treatment should follow the ABCDE system. High-flow oxygen should be administered. Obvious external bleeding should be controlled, usually by direct pressure using a dressing and bandage. Very rarely, control may only be achieved using the windlass technique or a tourniquet.

Vascular access should be obtained and intravenous fluid should be given if there is significant external blood loss or a delay in transportation. Intravenous morphine titrated to the patient's clinical need should be given with an antiemetic. Femoral nerve block (see pp.393–4) can be considered in entrapments or prolonged transfer times.

In patients with grossly contaminated wounds, obvious contaminating material should be wiped or washed away and a sterile moist dressing applied. Externalized bone should be relocated by traction if possible. The fracture should be realigned and approximated to the intact femur. This is achieved by a combination of longitudinal traction and rotation and should be performed in a controlled way with an assistant or bystander gripping the proximal femur. The neurovascular status of the limb should be assessed and recorded before and after any manipulation. Should the peripheral pulse be lost as a result of a manipulation, the leg should be re-positioned such that the pulse is restored. An appropriately applied traction splint will stabilize and immobilize the femur for transport.

Potential problems

With an increasing number of patients undergoing hip replacements, peri-prosthetic fractures are common. These often present with a history of fairly minor trauma. However, the physical signs are similar to uncomplicated femoral shaft fractures.

Should the distal pulses be absent both before and after realigning the femur, this should be regarded as a time-critical emergency. Rapid transfer to hospital is necessary.

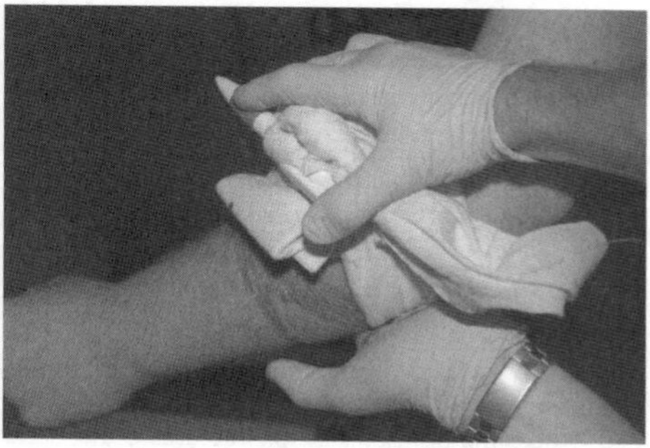

Fig. 3.17 Using the windlass technique to control bleeding. Reprinted with permission from Greaves I *et al.* (2005). *Emergency care: a textbook for paramedics,* 2nd edn. W.B. Saunders Co. Ltd.

Supracondylar fractures of the femur

Cause

Supracondylar fractures are commonly seen in the osteoporotic elderly female population, usually following a fall. The presence of a total knee replacement produces a stress interface at the proximal end, making this area particularly vulnerable to fracture.

Signs and symptoms

- Pain
- Swelling
- Tenderness and deformity just above the knee, associated with loss of function.

Treatment

Treatment should follow the same principles as for fractures of the shaft of the femur. However, the pull of the gastrocnemius muscle tends to pull the distal fragment posteriorly. Attempting to straighten the leg worsens this problem and may compromise the circulation. This fracture, which is relatively easy to recognize, should be treated by support under the knee, padding between the legs, and broad bandages to maintain the position. The distal vascular status should be assessed before and after the application of splintage. Femoral nerve block is ineffective in supracondylar fracture and traction splintage is contraindicated as it allows the distal femoral fragment to angulate posteriorly.

Potential problems

Regular circulatory assessment is necessary as this fracture is commonly associated with vascular trauma.

Patella fractures

Cause

Patellar fracture most commonly follows a direct injury, for example, on the dashboard of a car or a fall onto a hard surface. An occasional cause is crush, for example, falling masonry.

Uncommonly, patellar fracture may follow a resisted extension force, for example, when catching a shoe on the pavement whilst extending the leg, or a blocked, tackle playing football.

Signs and symptoms

- The patient is often unable to walk or stand unaided.
- The knee is swollen and after some time may become bruised.

Associated wounds make the injury compound, for example, dashboard injuries may be associated with transverse skin wounds, whereas falls to the ground are associated with abrasions, local contusions, and ragged lacerations.

Treatment

Wounds should be covered with a sterile dressing, the leg should be straightened, and position maintained in a long leg box splint.

Potential problems

In significant front end road traffic accidents producing femoral shaft fractures, there is often an associated knee injury, the differential diagnosis of which includes patella fracture.

A patient suffering a simple undisplaced patella fracture with intact medial and lateral patella retinaculae may be able to perform a straight leg raise. However, there is usually an associated extensor lag.

Resisted extension forces may also produce rupture of the quadriceps tendon at its insertion, rupture of the patella tendon, or avulsion of the tibial tubercle. In the presence of swelling, it may be difficult to differentiate these from a patella fracture.

Patella dislocations

Cause

Patellar dislocation commonly follows a muscular contraction, associated with sudden twisting or changes in direction, in 'at risk' individuals, usually women. It generally occurs when the knee is close to full extension. Predisposing causes include a narrow femoral sulcus and genu valgum (an exaggeration of the normal tibiofemoral valgus which produces a lateral vector and, therefore, a tendency to lateral subluxation or dislocation of the patella). Often, there is a history of recurrent dislocations.

Patella dislocations may also follow direct blows to the knee, with lateral dislocation being more common than medial.

Signs and symptoms

- Pain
- Reluctance to permit examination of the knee.

The misplaced patella is invariably lateral and fairly obvious on examination. The patient will not actively move their leg.

Treatment

With appropriate analgesia (for example, Entonox) , in a co-operative patient' the patella can be reduced by simply extending the knee. A click following relocation is usually followed by an expression of relief both visual and otherwise on behalf of the patient. Many patients will not tolerate this without considerable analgesia and multiple attempts, whilst the patient becomes increasingly distressed, should be avoided. Reduction can take place in hospital.

The knee should be immobilized in flexion with a blanket under the knee and FRAC Straps® or triangular bandages, and the patient transported to hospital.

Dislocations of the knee

Cause

Although associated with major trauma, for example, a dashboard injury, some dislocations occur after seemingly innocuous trauma. Patients with a grossly normal knee who say 'I dislocated my knee but it went back' have usually suffered a dislocated patella.

Signs and symptoms

Depending on the mechanism of injury, the dislocation (as described by the position of the tibia relative to the femur) can be in any direction, anterior and posterior being the most common. The dislocation produces major ligamentous disruption, meniscal displacement, and, in some cases, neurovascular injury (injuries to the popliteal vein, popliteal artery, and the common peroneal nerve being the most uaual).

Treatment

The knee should be supported and splinted in the position in which it is found. Because of the dislocation, the knee will not straighten, therefore it should be splinted to the normal leg using pads and broad triangular bandages. This is a time-critical problem requiring urgent transfer to hospital for manipulative reduction.

Potential problems

Frequent observations for distal vascular compromise should be undertaken.

Fractures of the tibial plateau

Cause

These fractures commonly occur due to significant varus or valgus forces, when the femoral condyle impacts with the tibial plateau producing a fracture of the plateau. The degree of damage depends on the force involved.

As the displacement is increased, there may be rupture of the collateral ligament (on the side of contact), cruciate ligament rupture, and meniscal damage.

These injuries are commonly seen when the bumper of a car strikes a pedestrian or when the bindings fail to release in a skiing accident.

Signs and symptoms

- Knee swelling due to the presence of a haemarthrosis
- Bruising (may take some time to develop)
- Deformity and instability depending on the extent of damage (not always present
- Inability to weight bear.

Treatment

Analgesia. The leg should be positioned as straight as possible and immobilized in a box splint. Some supplementary padding may be necessary. The neurovascular status should be checked before and after splinting.

Potential problems

Injuries to the medial tibial plateau following varus force may be associated with a common peroneal nerve injury.

Tibial and fibula shaft fractures

Cause

Tibial and fibula shaft fractures commonly follow direct and indirect trauma. Direct injury produces transverse fractures, for example, following a blow to the shin as in a kick in football or from a heavy weight falling on the leg. Isolated single bone fractures may occur.

Fractures following indirect force produce tortional/rotatory injuries with oblique or spiral fractures usually affecting both bones. This pattern of injury is commonly seen in association with sporting injuries, falls from a height, and road traffic collision.

Signs and symptoms

- Pain
- Swelling
- Deformity
- Loss of function.

In displaced fractures, there may be obvious shortening and deformity producing angulation and rotation due to the pull of the non-opposed intact muscles.

The fracture may be compound, particularly when due to direct trauma or in relation to the subcutaneous border of the tibia where there is very little soft tissue coverage.

Neurovascular damage is more common in open fractures, particularly where there has been a penetrating injury. Less commonly, vascular injury may follow proximal tibial fractures in close proximity to the popliteal artery trifurcation.

Treatment

Following appropriate analgesia, any gross contamination should be removed from the compound wound and exposed bone should be relocated beneath the skin and the limb realigned. A clean sterile dressing should be applied to any wounds present. If possible, a polaroid picture should be taken to accompany the patient to hospital. A long leg box splint, to immobilize the joint above and below the fracture, should be applied.

The neurovascular status should be assessed before and after any manipulative procedure.

Potential problems

It is not uncommon for fractures of the tibia and fibula to be accompanied by an ipsilateral femoral shaft fracture. Immobilization using a traction splint, with supporting padding and broad bandages above and below the respective fractures, is one way of managing this injury.

An acute compartmental syndrome may complicate closed tibial and fibular fractures, particularly following moderate to severe energy transfer. It occurs because of swelling within a closed fascial space and is characterized by increasing pain beyond normal, excruciating pain on passively extending the toes (stretching ischaemic muscle), and, later, pallor, parasthesia, and, ultimately, pulselesness.

Acute compartment syndrome commonly takes several hours to develop but due to delay in access to the patient, protracted entrapment, or journey times, this could become a problem for the pre-hospital carer. Treatment is by surgical decompression, and this should be regarded as a time-critical emergency. It is important to remember that the presence of a distal pulse does not guarantee that the limb is adequately perfused. In the unconscious patient, vascular compromise may initially go unnoticed.

Ankle fractures

Cause

Ankle fractures commonly occur due to rotatory forces. The talus is normally sited between the fibula and tibia (like a mortis and tenon joint) and is stabilized by the medial (deltoid) ligament, the lateral ligament complex, and the tibio-fibular ligament (syndesmotic ligament). Depending on the forces involved, trauma will produce ligamentous injuries and fractures of the malleoli (medial, lateral, and posterior) which may progress to a clinical picture of fracture dislocation.

Direct injuries may occur at the site of contact, due to compression as in falls from a height, or following forced dorsiflexion as in brake pedal injuries. These high-energy injuries commonly produce comminuted fractures of the tibial articular surface.

Signs and symptoms

The most common ankle injury is a lateral ligament sprain (partial injury) which presents with:

- Pain
- Swelling and tenderness
- Difficulty with weight bearing.

Bony tenderness over the fibular is usually pathomnemonic of an underlying fracture. Bimalleolar swelling and tenderness is suggestive of an underlying bony injury. The differentiation between a soft tissue injury and bony fracture should be made in hospital.

Treatment

The injured ankle should be immobilized in a box splint or an appropriate alternative. Dislocations, depending on the skill base of the pre-hospital care practitioner, may be reduced by simple traction and manipulation to restore normal alignment after the administration of analgesia. The limb should then be immobilized as above.

Potential problems

Fracture dislocations may be associated with distal vascular compromise and major pressure on the skin, risking necrosis. This is a time-critical injury and if manipulation and reduction is not possible at the scene due to lack of experience or appropriate skills, urgent transfer to hospital is necessary.

Some rotational injuries result in disruption of the interosseous membrane between the tibia and fibula with a proximal fibular fracture, which will account for proximal fibular pain and tenderness in the presence of an ankle fracture (Maisonneuve fracture).

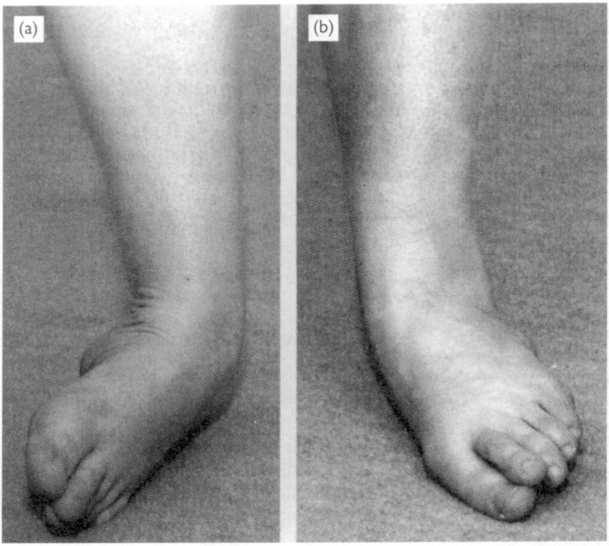

Fig. 3.18 (a) Inversion and (b) eversion of the ankle. Reprinted with permission from Greaves I *et al.* (2005). *Emergency care: a textbook for paramedics,* 2nd edn. W.B. Saunders Co. Ltd.

Fractures of the talus and calcaneum

Cause

Talar fractures commonly follow forced dorsiflexion such as may occur in road traffic collisions, where the break pedal forces the talar neck onto the front of the tibia. This injury was first described as 'aviator's astragalus' from violent dorsiflexion due to impact with the rudder pedals at the time of an aircraft crash. This injury may also occur following falls from a height.

Calcaneal fractures commonly follow falls from a height, landing on the heel. They can be bilateral, depending on the first point of contact with the ground.

Signs and symptoms

- Pain
- Inability to weight bear
- The heel will appear swollen, broader, and, in some cases, displaced into a valgus position
- Characteristic bruising tracking to the sole of the foot will occur (late).

Treatment

The limb should be immobilized in a below-knee padded box splint and the patient transported to hospital.

Potential problems

Patients sustaining injuries following falls from a height not uncommonly have other injuries including tibial plateau injuries, hip and pelvis injuries, and fractures to the thoracolumbar spine.

Injuries to the various processes of the talus and calcaneum can occur as well as more major peritalar dislocations. These injuries should be treated as above.

Midtarsal injuries

Cause

Midtarsal dislocations (between the talus and the calcaneus proximally and the navicular and cuboid distally) commonly result from forced abduction or adduction.

Signs and symptoms

- Pain
- Deformity may be masked by considerable swelling except in the early period following injury.

Treatment

The foot and ankle should be immobilized in an appropriate box splint.

Potential problems

The distal neurovascular status should be assessed and reassessed because of the risk of associated vascular injury or compartment syndrome. Lesser injuries in this region also occur, for example, navicular avulsions. All of these injuries should be treated in a similar way in the pre-hospital environment.

Tarsometatarsal dislocations

Cause

These injuries may follow a fall on the plantar-flexed foot or complicate road traffic collisions.

Signs and symptoms

- Pain
- Swelling
- Inability to weight bear.

Treatment

The treatment is simple splintage, analgesia, and transfer to hospital.

Potential problems

Occasionally, there may be vascular compromise due to a compartmental syndrome, particularly where there has been significant trauma, for example, when the foot has been run over.

Metatarsal fractures

Cause

These commonly follow direct injuries (for example, when a weight falls onto the foot) or are indirect, as part of a forced inversion or eversion to the fore foot.

Signs and symptoms

Pain, swelling, local tenderness, and an inability to weight bear are suggestive of an underlying bony injury.

Treatment

No specific treatment may be necessary at the pre-hospital scene.

Potential problems

Metatarsal fractures may occur as part of more significant foot fractures, In particular, it is imperative not to miss the Lisfranc injury which commonly involves an anterior subluxation/dislocation of the second metatarsal in association with other metatarsal injuries.

Inversion injuries to the ankle may also be associated with fractures to the proximal shaft or base of the fifth metatarsal. Stress fractures (most often affecting the second metatarsal) are common and can present with acute pain.

Phalangeal fractures

Cause

These commonly follow crush injuries, (for example as a result of a heavy weight falling on the foot) but they may also result from kicking a solid object or catching the little toe on a static object whilst walking bare foot.

Signs and symptoms

- Pain
- Tenderness
- Swelling
- Deformity (sometimes).

Very occasionally, these may be compound injuries.

Treatment

Wounds should be dressed and simple realignment and companion strapping applied if the patient will tolerate it.

Potential problems

It is often impossible to distinguish between toe dislocations and fractures. If a dislocation is obvious, simple longitudinal traction may reduce it.

The complications of fractures

Actions in the pre-hospital care phase may influence the complications that occur in the immediate, early, and late phases of patient treatment.

Immediate

A closed fracture may be converted into an open fracture by inappropriate handling, thereby increasing the risk of complications, particularly infection. In addition, delays in realigning fractures may lead to undue pressure on the skin, risking subsequent necrosis, and may delay relief of pressure on nerves and arteries.

In cases of prolonged entrapment or in long transport times, a compartmental syndrome may develop, particularly in high-energy closed long bone fractures such as of the tibia and fibula.

Removal of any gross contamination from compound fractures, although no substitute for surgical toilet and debridement, may influence the early development of infection, particularly if there is a delay in surgical treatment.

Early

Delayed or inappropriate immobilization of major long bone fractures will increase the risk of the development of fat embolism syndrome particularly in patients who have uncorrected hypoxia and hypovolaemia.

As stated above, early problems include compartmental syndrome and mishandling which could convert a fracture into an open injury.

Late complications

Late complications usually relate to delays in union or to non-union, a situation which can be linked to associated sepsis in compound injuries. Unrecognized compartmental syndromes have devastating consequences. Failure to recognize and relieve pressure on nerves has a significant morbidity.

Soft tissue injuries

Types of injury

A large number of injuries, particularly sports injuries, are soft tissue injuries. They occur most commonly in the lower limbs. Many are minor and self-limiting (for example, simple bruises to the skin and underlying tissues) but they can range from this to major skin, ligament, muscle, and tendon injuries.

The immediate care practitioner must decide whether the patient requires medical intervention or, as in the case of minor bruises and sprains, can be readily treated with rest, ice, compression, and elevation (RICE). The more serious injuries may be obvious, although peripheral nerve and tendon injuries can be difficult to recognize and require a high index of suspicion based on the mechanism of injury and a safeguard referral pattern to the emergency department.

Soft tissue injuries may follow blunt or penetrating trauma. Penetrating trauma usually produces a localized anatomical injury whereas blunt trauma may produce more diffuse injuries often associated with crush.

Patient assessment

Assessment should follow the ABCDE system of the primary survey. Soft tissues injuries may, for example, be recognized under breathing assessment where there is bruising to the chest wall or under circulation where there is an obvious major wound associated with bleeding. Other injuries may be apparent when the patient is appropriately exposed, or found during the secondary survey.

In relation to the limbs, the secondary survey includes an inspection for swelling, wounds, and deformity and an assessment of motor function (M), sensation (S), and circulation (C). The latter can be summarized by the mnemonic MSC x 4:

- Motor response—test for active movements
- Sensation—response to touch
- Circulation—pulse, pallor, and skin temperature
- x 4—all four limbs.

Injuries to specific tissues

Skin

Wounds may be classified as open or closed. Open wounds include:

- Incised wounds—for example, wounds sustained with glass or knives.
- Lacerated wounds—where the skin is irregularly torn, for example, following a blow to the face.
- Puncture wounds—for example, from a needle or garden fork.
- Graze or abrasions—partial thickness injuries to the skin.
- Contused wounds—following a fall or direct blow which splits the skin and bruises the soft tissues.
- Gunshot wounds—often associated with entry and exit wounds with significant internal disruption.

Closed wounds

Closed wounds include:

- Crush injuries—where the skin integrity is not compromised.
- Bruising—swelling and later discolouration associated with contained bleeding within the underlying tissues.

Open wounds

External haemorrhage control should follow stepwise progression, noting that most external bleeding can be controlled by simple measures. Techniques include:

- Direct pressure
- Elevation
- Wound packing
- Windlass technique (See p.257)
- Indirect pressure
- Tourniquet.

In the event of blood soaking through applied dressings, further added dressings are unlikely to arrest haemorrhage. An appropriate wound dressing should be placed within the wound and effective pressure achieved by securing this firmly in place. It may be necessary to use the windlass technique (See p.257) to control the haemorrhage.

For extensive wounds, where direct pressure would be futile, haemorrhage control may be effected by indirect pressure over a proximal artery (for example, the femoral artery or the brachial artery). Alternatively, a tourniquet can be applied.

Vessels

Bleeding from major blood vessels is usually obvious if there is an external wound and control should be effected by following the guidelines above. Contained vessel damage may produce significant limb swelling, compartment syndrome, or overt signs of distal vascular insufficiency. The features of ischaemia include:

- Pain
- Pallor
- Pulselessness
- Parathesaea
- Paralysis.

} The five Ps

Muscles

Most significant muscle injuries complicate open wounds such as lacerations, incised wounds, and wounds associated with open fractures. Less frequently, closed muscle injuries, such as ruptures of the long head of the biceps or the quadriceps muscle close to its insertion into the patella, may occur.

Sportsmen may sustain a 'pulled muscle' (for example, the hamstring). These are normally small intramuscular tears.

Treatment should be symptomatic. Where there is significant loss of function (for example, a quadriceps rupture), appropriate splintage is necessary and the patient should be referred to hospital. Simple muscle sprains can be managed initially following the RICE regimen.

Tendons

Tendon injuries, particularly to the hand, are often not recognized in the pre-hospital scene. A high index of suspicion is necessary, noting the mechanism of injury (for example, a glass or knife injury) and the anatomical site of an injury (for example, the volar aspect of the wrist or the palmar aspect of a finger). There may be visible tendons within a wound or obvious loss of function but, in many cases, the only clue to a significant injury is the location of the laceration.

It is inappropriate to probe a wound to determine the presence of any tendon injury. Since any tendon injury present will be found on that part of the tendon which was under the wound at the time of injury, it may not be apparent in a position of rest.

The wound should be managed by control of haemorrhage and application of a sterile dressing and referral to hospital. In the majority of cases, careful surgical exploration under optimal conditions will be necessary to exclude tendon or nerve injury.

Rarely, spontaneous rupture of tendons occurs following trivial trauma, for example, of the patella tendon producing an inability to straighten the leg, or the extensor tendon as in a mallet finger deformity.

Nerves

Nerve injuries may be open or closed injuries, the former associated with wounds commonly due to glass or knives. As in tendon injuries, a high index of suspicion is necessary. Treatment involves the management of the wound and referral to hospital. Closed nerve injuries may be seen, for example, in supracondylar fractures of the humerus in children and sciatic nerve injuries associated with posterior hip dislocations. Neurological injuries associated with fractures and dislocations require urgent transportation to hospital to optimize the chances of neurological recovery.

Ligaments

Partial injuries to ligaments, for example, in soft tissue sprains to the ankle, are extremely painful. Complete ligament ruptures are often surprisingly pain free and, therefore, the injury may not be recognized. The mechanism of injury is the clue to diagnosis. In both instances, the pre-hospital treatment is symptomatic. It is usual to refer these patients to hospital to exclude significant ligament injury or associated bony trauma.

Regional injuries

The wrist

Soft tissue injuries to the wrist are common, although differentiation from a bony injury is difficult since both present with swelling, pain, and some loss of function. Pre-hospital management is symptomatic with ice, analgesia, and a broad arm sling. Referral to hospital is appropriate.

The knee

Common features of knee injuries include pain, swelling, difficulty in, or inability to weight bear and a loss of function. The mechanism of injury may give a clue to the likely injury.

Quadriceps tendon rupture

This may follow resisted extension or occur spontaneously. The clinical features include:

- Localized pain, tenderness, and swelling
- Inability to extend the knee
- A palpable defect above the patella
- An inability to weight bear
- Swelling of the knee due to an associated haemoarthrosis.

Pre-hospital treatment includes splinting the knee in extension and referral to hospital.

Patella tendon rupture

This may be caused by a direct blow to the front of the knee, a penetrating knee injury, or a resisted extension injury. Clinical features include:

- Infrapatellar tenderness, swelling, and pain
- A palpable defect in the tendon
- An inability to extend the knee
- An inability to weight bear.

Pre-hospital treatment includes splinting the knee in extension, analgesia, and referral to hospital.

Reduced lateral dislocation/subluxation of the patella

The patient will usually give a history of dislocation or subluxation. There will be an associated knee haemarthrosis and tenderness over the medial patella retinaculum. Weight bearing should be discouraged and the patient should be referred to hospital to exclude associated bony injuries and for ongoing management. Ice and splintage may be necessary.

Meniscal tears

Classically, these occur due to a rotational injury whilst weight bearing on a semi-flexed knee. They occur most commonly in males and as sporting injuries, in particular in football. Common clinical features include:

- Pain
- Swelling
- Locking
- Giving way of the knee.

Locking implies a mechanical obstruction within the knee due to a displaced part of the meniscus. Patients with locked knees require referral to hospital for definitive management.

Ligament injuries

These are particularly common in footballers and skiers. Injuries include partial and complete tears to the medial collateral ligament, the lateral collateral ligament, and the cruciate ligaments. As an example, a valgus force applied to the knee may produce, in sequence:

- A partial tear to the medial collateral ligament
- A complete tear of the medial collateral ligament
- A medial meniscal peripheral detachment
- A rupture of the anterior cruciate ligament.

Clinical features include pain, swelling, tenderness, decreased function, and instability. The magnitude of the injury is usually apparent from the mechanism of injury as related by the patient. Treatment should be symptomatic including ice, splintage, and referral to hospital.

The ankle

Lateral ligament inversion sprains are the most common soft tissue injury to the ankle and present with:

- Swelling
- Tenderness
- Difficulty bearing weight.

Differentiation from a fracture can be difficult. Complete absence of tenderness over both malleoli and the fifth metatarsal makes a fracture very unlikely. Bony tenderness mandates referral to hospital for an X-ray. Minor sprains can be treated by RICE.

Achilles tendon ruptures

Achilles tendon ruptures most commonly occur due to asymptomatic degeneration in the tendon or as an acute event, often on the sports field or squash court. There may be an audible snap or the patient may feel as if they have been kicked or hit in the back of the leg, although no contact has occurred.

Clinically, there is pain and tenderness in relation to the rupture with a palpable gap if examined early. Most commonly, there is an inability to bear weight and a major compromise of plantar flexion.

Absence of plantar flexion, when the patient's calf is squeezed with the patient in the kneeling position, is diagnostic of Achilles tendon rupture. (Simmonds test).

Pre-hospital treatment is symptomatic only. The patient should be taken to the emergency department for definitive management.

Spinal injuries

Spinal injuries range from simple soft tissue sprains to fractures, stable or unstable, with the potential for spinal cord injury or the presence of established spinal cord injury. In general terms, all patients with an appropriate mechanism of injury should be regarded as having a spinal injury until proven otherwise and should, therefore, be subjected to spinal immobilization. Spinal injuries commonly follow:

- Road traffic collisions
- Falls
- Gymnastics\trampolining
- Rugby/football
- Horseriding
- Skiing
- Hang-gliding
- Aquatic activities
- Weights falling onto the back.

Road traffic collisions are the most common cause of injury and are responsible for 50% of patients suffering spinal cord injuries. Compression/flexion and extension/rotation are the common forces involved. Lesser injuries include whiplash injury due to rear end shunts producing flexion followed by extension.

Whilst the majority of injuries are in the cervical spine, 10% of these patients have a second spinal injury.

Falls, in particular, are associated with thoracolumbar fractures. Scrummage injuries in rugby are commonly associated with cervical spine injury. Aquatic sports, particularly diving into a shallow pool, often produce a combination of head and cervical spine trauma. Historically, falls onto the back in coal miners produced major thoracic and thoracolumbar fractures.

Certain criteria must be fulfilled if the spine is to be cleared of any injury at scene (See box opposite).

Assessment

If there is a high index of suspicion of spinal injury based on the mechanism of injury, the spinal column should be protected, unless the patient's spine can be cleared following the criteria detailed in the box opposite. The patient should not be allowed to get up and, ideally, should be maintained in the supine neutral position. In the case of road traffic collisions, the neck should be moved to a neutral position and inline spinal stabilization maintained prior to and during extrication. An inability to achieve a neutral position suggests the possibity of a fracture dislocation, in which case the neck should be maintained in as near neutral position as possible.

No attempt should be made to forcibly restrain or fasten down an aggressive, unco-operative patient. Such patients may sometimes tolerate a cervical collar alone, which must be accepted as 'better than nothing'. Such aggression may be the result of hypoxia and, if present, this should be identified and treated.

Criteria for clearing spine of injury

- There is no altered level of consciousness
- The patient is not under the influence of alcohol or drugs
- There is no midline spinal tenderness
- There are no neurological signs or symptoms
- There are no other distracting painful injuries
- There is no history of previous spinal injury
- The patient does not suffer from an inflammatory arthropathy such as rheumatoid arthritis or ankylosing spondylitis

Segment	Representative dematomes	Representative myotomes
C5	Sensation over detoid	Deltoid muscle
C6	Sensation over thumb	Wrist extensors
C7	Sensation over middle finger	Elbow extensors
C8	Sensation over little finger	Middle finger flexors
T1	Sensation over inner aspect of elbow	Little finger abduction
T4	Sensation around nipple	–
T8	Sensation over xiphisternum	–
T10	Sensation around umbilicus	–
T12	Sensation around symphysis	–
L1	Sensation in inguinal region	–
L2	Sensation anterior upper thigh	Hip flexors
L3	Sensation anterior mid thigh	Knee exensors
L4	Sensation on medial aspect leg	Ankle dorsiflexors
L5	Sensation between 1st and 2nd toes	Long toe extensors
S1	Sensation on lateral border of foot	Ankle plantar flexors
S3	Sensation over ischial tuberosity	–
S4/5	Sensation around perineum	–

Fig. 3.19 Motor and sensory levels. Reprinted with permission from Greaves I *et al.*, (2001). *Trauma Care Manual*. Hodder Arnold.

The conscious patient may complain of motor weakness or altered sensation, the extent of which will depend on the level of injury. Important anatomical landmarks and their relevance are summarized below (and in Fig. 3.19):

- **Injuries from C1–2**—the patient is unable to breathe because of intercostal and diaphragmatic paralysis and will die unless they receive basic life support
- **Injuries at C3–C5**—depending on the extent of the injury, the diaphragm may be functional or non-functional due to paralysis of the phrenic nerves. Over a period of time, patients who may initially be able to cope are at risk of developing respiratory failure due to exhaustion or progression of diaphragmatic deficiency due to spinal cord swelling.
- **Injuries between C5 and C7**—there is complete loss of intercostal function. However, the phrenic nerve and the diaphragm are functional. The patient displays a seesaw pattern of breathing.
- **Injuries between T1 and L2**—there will be a variable loss of intercostal muscle function and, therefore, respiratory compromise depending on the level of cord injury. The higher the level of injury, the greater the deficit. Above the level of T6, there is sufficient loss of sympathetic outflow to produce neurogenic shock. This is characterized by bradycardia, a low blood pressure (usually 70–80mmHg), and distal peripheral vasodilatation. Male patients have priaprism (sustained penile erection).

The flaccid paralysis and areflexia associated with a spinal cord injury is commonly referred to as spinal shock. This is not 'shock' in the normal pathophysiological sense but a state of electrical interruption to the cord: spinal concussion. This should not be confused with neurogenic shock and the term spinal shock is best avoided.

In the unconscious patient, there will be no specific complaint of pain and no verbal communication regarding motor or sensory deficit. The physical signs detailed above may suggest spinal cord injury. A high index of suspicion and mandatory full spinal immobilization are necessary.

Management

Primary survey

Problems due to spinal injury may be detected during the primary survey. Examples include:

- Inadequate breathing and ventilation due to intercostal or phrenic nerve compromise.
- Hypotension, bradycardia, distal vasodilatation, and priaprism due to neurogenic shock.
- Motor and sensory deficit due to neurological injury.

Secondary survey

A detailed secondary survey which involves a head-to-toe examination is normally carried out in the emergency department. During the log roll, local tenderness, deformity, and palpable steps in the spinal column may be detected. A rectal examination may reveal a lax anal sphincter.

Patient positioning

Airway always take precedence over the cervical spine. Where possible, the cervical spine should be maintained with inline spinal immobilization. The supine neutral body position is ideal. In road traffic collisions, the cervical spine should be maintained in a neutral position pending full.

Immobilization

Patients should be extricated from vehicles maintaining a stable straight spine, onto a spinal board, followed by the application of securing body straps, head huggers, and their supporting straps. It is common practice in the UK for these patients to be transported to hospital whilst on a spinal board. Where there is an extended travelling time, consideration should be given to transferring the patient onto a vacuum mattress using a scoop stretcher.

In the unconscious patient, once secured to the spinal board, the cervical collar should be released to avoid compression on the external jugular vein which can lead to raised intracranial pressure.

Transport

Consideration should be given to the use of helicopter transportation for expediency, reduced transport time, and transportation to the most appropriate hospital.

Amputation

Traumatic

Traumatic amputation is fortunately rare. Re-implantation of the amputated part(s) may be possible in guillotine type injuries, but is rarely an option in crush or avulsive amputations. Nevertheless, the amputated part should always accompany the patient to hospital since it may be used as a source of tissue for reconstruction.

Surgical

Surgical amputation is rarely necessary pre-hospital. It should not be undertaken without the necessary training and equipment.

Amputated parts

When their size permits, amputated parts should be wrapped in sterile dressings dampened with saline and placed in a waterproof bag or container. This should then be surrounded by a bag or container holding a mixture of ice and water. The amputated part must not be allowed to come into direct contact with ice for any length of time.

Blast and gunshot injuries

Introduction

Trauma caused by bomb blast and guns is increasing. Gun-related violence is now commonplace on the streets of our big cities. A responsible attitude from rescuers and scene safety are critically important. Therefore:

- Do not approach the scene until it is declared safe from the risk of further shooting, secondary devices, fire, and building collapse. The police may determine a rendezvous point at a safe distance from the incident until the scene is declared safe.
- Do not touch objects or disturb the environment except to treat patients, as the incident is a forensic scene.
- Do not disturb dead bodies unless to give access to casualties or if they are at risk of further damage or destruction.

When the scene is declared safe, it may be necessary, in the case of multiple casualties, to initiate a triage sieve. If a major incident has been declared, the rescuer should work under the directions of the appropriate incident officer.

Patient assessment should follow the normal ABCDE system regardless of the nature of the injuries.

Blast injuries

Blast injuries may occur in the following situations:

- Terrorism
- Domestic incidents (for example, gas explosions)
- Industrial incidents (for example, chemical explosions).

Blast injury mechanisms

Blast (shock) wave

Following detonation, the explosive substance is instantaneously converted into a large volume of gas, producing an expanding shock or blast wave. The shock wave is similar to a sound wave (but much faster) and produces an almost instantaneous rise in pressure. The shock front spreads out from the point of detonation as a hemisphere but the pressure declines dramatically as the distance from the detonation increases. The effect of the blast wave is accentuated, however, in closed environments where reflection from surfaces occurs and summation of incident and reflected waves results in increased pressures.

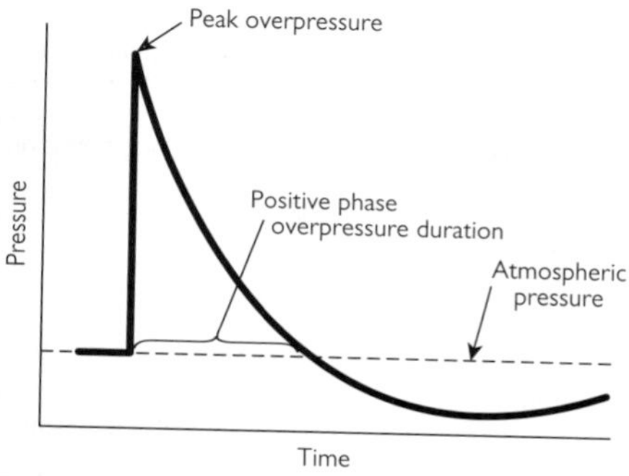

Fig. 3.20 Idealized blast overpressure waveform.

Blast wind

Behind the blast, shock wave is an area of turbulence—the dynamic overpressure or 'blast wind'. This consists of a rapidly expanding turbulent fireball of hot air and products of combustion.

Fragmentation

Most military explosives are contained in shells or cases which will fragment on detonation (grenades, mortars, and artillery shells). These weapons are designed to fragment in a way which causes the maximum possible injuring potential. These are primary fragments. Terrorist devices may use nails or ball bearings as primary fragments. Fragments of the environment such as shattered car body work, masonry, furniture, or the body parts of victims will all act as secondary fragments if sufficiently energized by the blast wind.

Thermal injury

The immense thermal output from an explosive detonation is usually associated with flash burns which, although painful, are usually of relatively minor clinical significance. Ordinary clothing usually offers a reasonable degree of protection. However, deeper, more serious burns, may occur if the environment ignites as a result of the detonation or there is an incendiary component to the explosive device. Industrial or chemical explosions are significantly more likely to be associated with serious burns and terrorists may use accelerants such as petrol in simple improvized devices.

Patterns of injury

Blast injuries are classified as follows:

- *Primary injuries*—result from the blast (shock) wave
- *Secondary injuries*—from fragments
- *Tertiary injuries*—due to the blast winds
- *Burns**
- *Crush injury**
- *Psychological effects**

* Sometimes referred to as quaternary blast injuries

Primary blast injuries

Primary injuries result from exposure of the body to the blast shockwave. The structures most at risk are those at solidfluid interfaces and those containing air such as the bowel, lung, and ear.

The most important primary effect is to the lung, producing lung contusion and haemorrhage into the alveoli.

Features of blast lung include:

- Breathlessness
- Dry cough
- Chest pain
- Restlessness
- Confusion and agitation
- Pneumothorax and haemothorax.

The incidence of blast lung is low because those near enough the detonation to suffer significant primary blast injury site usually die as a result of fragmentation or tertiary injury.

The ears are very sensitive to primary blast injury and rupture of the tympanic membrane is common. Deafness is a sign of significant blast injury. However, it only occurs if there is direct orientation of the auditory canal to the blast wave. Thus, although deafness is an indicator of significant blast exposure, its absence does not imply that the patient has escaped significant injury elsewhere.

> The patient may not be ignoring you—they may be deaf!

Injuries to gas-containing abdominal organs include immediate perforation, intestinal wall haemorrhage with delayed perforation, mesenteric tears, and retroperitineal haematomas. Although rare in explosions taking place in air, they are more commonly seen following underwater explosions.

The treatment for all scenarios follows the ABCDE system.

Secondary injuries

The majority of patients close to the explosion will have multiple injuries caused by fragments from the explosive device (bomb casing or nails) or blast wind energized debris (masonry, glass, and wood). Injuries may be blunt or penetrating, the latter invariably have significant contamination.

Tertiary injuries

Tertiary injuries are produced by the blast wind. Displacement of individuals may result in whole body disruption or disintegration, traumatic avulsion amputations, and crush injury. Other injuries may be caused by bodily impact. The amputations occur through long bones fractured by the blast wave and are avulsive, with considerable proximal damage.

Burns

Flash and flame burns occur in explosions. Flash burns are usually superficial and are related to the heat generated at the time of detonation. Flame burns may occur due to secondary ignition of the environment.

Crush injuries

Entrapment following collapse of buildings due to blast is common. Patients often sustain multiple injuries. Delay in rescue may result in a risk of crush injury progressing to crush syndrome. At scene, appropriate fluid replacement and high-flow oxygen may influence outcome. There is no role for tourniquets in crush syndrome (except for control of life-threatening bleeding from associated injuries). Vigorous fluid resuscitation and immediate evacuation is essential.

Psychological effects

Significant numbers of patients and emergency workers will suffer ongoing psychological problems following an explosion. This is undoubtedly related to the mutilating nature of the injuries and the likelihood of survivors being personally acquainted with each other and the dead.

For the majority, the outlook is good. Critical incident debriefing may be helpful and is common practice amongst emergency service personnel. All patients and personnel involved should have some arrangement for follow-up which may be in-house for the emergency services or through general practitioners for patients. Similar arrangements should be available to support hospital personnel.

Management

The essential features of management are:

- *Triage: effective rigorous triage is essential.* A triage sieve, followed by a triage sort, will identify the seriously injured amongst those with lesser injuries and will allow appropriate use of transport and hospital resources, particularly for those requiring continued resuscitation and surgery.
- The circumstances and mechanism of injury must be considered in determining transfer to hospital (for example, a non-survivable head injury).
- A high index of suspicion should be maintained for inhalation injury and impending acute lung injury, especially from explosions in confined places.
- High-flow oxygen with a non re-breather reservoir bag is mandatory if lung injury is suspected.
- Careful assessment for signs of abdominal injury—often there are very few clinical signs early on, particularly in the presence of a hollow viscous injury.
- Deafness is the hallmark of potentially significant blast injury. All such patients should be carefully assessed and transported to hospital. Absence of deafness DOES NOT imply absence of a significant blast load.
- Primary and secondary fragment injuries are very common and are almost invariably multiple. External haemorrhage should be controlled by direct pressure and wound dressings. It is not necessary to dress every wound.
- Adequate analgesia is essential for its pain-relieving and anxiolytic features.
- Avulsed limbs should be sent with patient to hospital. Re-implantation will not be possible, but they may provide tissue for reconstruction.

Gunshot injury

Wound ballistics and mechanism of injury

Wound ballistics is the study of injury caused by ballistic weapons. The degree of tissue damage caused is related to the acute energy transfer where:

$$KE = \frac{1}{2} mv^2$$

KE = kinetic energy; m = mass; v = velocity

If a bullet is stopped by tissue, all the energy is used ('transferred') causing damage to that tissue. If, however, the bullet passes through a tissue without slowing, depending on the site of impact, very little damage may occur. For example, a bullet striking the femur may be arrested in motion, shatter the femur, and produce extensive soft tissue damage whereas a bullet going front to back through the lung, without making bony contact, may cause relatively little damage. The amount of energy transferred will also be affected by the stability and shape of the missile.

Missile penetration into the body results in crushing or laceration. The results will depend on the anatomical site and the structures involved. Damage to apparently remote structures may result from missile deflection off bone or damage from secondary bony fragments.

Wounding missiles

The old concept of high-and low-velocity missiles has been replaced by the concept of energy transfer, since it is this which determines the damage produced. Wounds can therefore be described as:

- High-energy-transfer wounds
- Low-energy-transfer wounds.

The same amount of damage can have different effects depending on the anatomical site. For example, a wound to the forearm is unlikely to be fatal whereas a similar wound to the heart almost certainly will be.

The external appearance of both entry and exit wound may have little relation to the internal damage, especially if a major deflection or fragmentation of the missile has taken place. Similarly, although the exit wound is usually bigger than the entry wound, this is not invariably the case and, indeed, is clinically of no relevance in the initial management. The rescuer, therefore, should concentrate on the ABCDE assessment rather than being concerned about ballistics.

The interface of bullets with tissues

Injury severity is governed by:

- Temporary cavitation
- Bullet fragmentation
- Wound contamination.

Temporary cavitation

In low-energy wounds, tissue damage is largely confined to the tract of the missile. In high-energy transfer wounds, however, injury extends radially from the wound as a result of the formation of a temporary cavity, due to the transfer of large amounts of energy causing the tissues to accelerate away from the path of the missile. This temporary cavity results in negative pressure which sucks in dirt and debris producing gross contamination. The temporary cavity then collapses.

The amount of energy transfer is determined by the shape of the missile and the features of the tissue. Elastic tissues such as lung may stretch and remain largely intact. Solid organs such as the liver, loaded colon, or bone may suffer catastrophic injury. The maximal cavity size is often deeply placed within the wound tract, (for example, within the chest or abdomen). In the limbs, where impact on bone is a feature, the cavitation may produce an extensive large ragged wound.

Fragmentation

Energy transfer is increased if the area of the bullet striking the tissue is increased. Conventional military weapons have an outer casing or metal jacket to prevent fragmentation or deformity. However, stability may be lost on contact with human tissue. The bullet may yaw (angle from side to side) or tumble (turn over). Maximal energy transfer occurs if the long axis of the bullet is at 90 degrees to its axis of penetration, and a more extensive complex wound results.

If a bullet breaks up or deforms within body tissues, the effect may be devastating. Conventional bullets which are fully jacketed should not fragment. Bullets may be designed to fragment and deform, resulting in a maximum 'energy dump' and tissue destruction. Cavities may be large and, if affecting vital areas, often result in fatal injuries. Bullets used by the law enforcement agencies are designed to deform for maximum 'stopping' potential with minimal risk of collateral injury due to the bullet passing straight through the intended victim. Bullets can be easily altered to deform or fragment.

Wound contamination

All bullet wounds should be assumed to be contaminated. High-energy transfer wounds produce cavitation with negative pressure leading to indrawing of clothes and debris (including faecal material) into the wound.

Missile tracks

The track of a bullet cannot be predicted from the entry wound. In addition to the factors discussed above, the position of the patient at the time of wounding (which may not be known to the clinician) will materially effect the wound track.

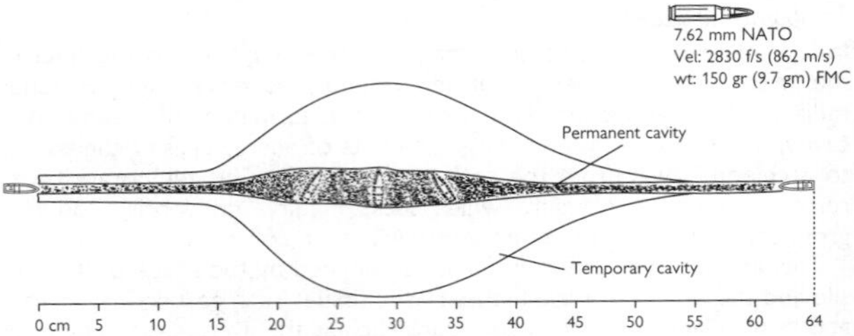

Fig. 3.21 Ballistic injury: temporary and permanent cavities. Reproduced from *Emergency War Surgery*—2nd United States revision. NATO handbook 1988. Permission requested from US Government printing office, Washington DC.

Types of missile

Bullets

Handguns generally fire jacketed lead bullets producing low-energy transfer wounds and injury along the track of the projectile. The clinical significance will depend on the tissues involved.

Police and hunting weapons are designed to produce a contained injury with a 'clean drop' and minimal risk of collateral damage. These partially jacketed bullets deform on impact and produce high-energy wounds.

Modern bullets (military and terrorist) have full metal jackets and are not intended to deform. They may fragment causing devastating energy transfer wounds.

Baton rounds

These are often incorrectly called rubber or plastic bullets. They are significantly larger than conventional ammunition and are designed to stop by inflicting severe pain from soft tissue injury. Skin penetration is very rare. UK guidelines restrict their use to impact below the victim's waist, making significant injury extremely unlikely. Fatalities in the past have usually been associated with impacts to the head or impacts in children. Basic attention to ABC, analgesia, and transfer to hospital for assessment and observation is likely to be all that is required.

Airguns

These produce single, low-energy wounds which are not normally significant, although intracranial penetration has been recorded in children and there is also a risk of significant injury to the eyes.

Shotguns

These fire multiple pellets with a range of sizes from bird shot (smallest) to buck shot. Fired at close range, they can act as a single missile causing massive tissue damage.

Management

The provision of medical care at the scene of a shooting may present certain clear risks. If the police are present, their advice MUST be followed at all times. There must be NO risk of further injury before assistance (life-saving or otherwise) is offered.

General principles

- **Make sure that it is safe to approach.**
- Follow an ABCDE protocol.
- Consider permissive hypotension in patients with penetrating chest or abdominal injuries.
- DO NOT become distracted by ballistics.
- Treat what you find, not what you expect.
- Remember that bullets behave erratically and may have penetrated several body cavities.
- Do not delay life-saving surgery by protracted on-scene times.
- Do not come to any decision on wound severity. In general, bullet entry and exit wounds give little information about the patient's condition.

- Assume serious injury in all cases and arrange rapid transfer to hospital.
- Give adequate analgesia; provide reassurance.

Management of wounds

Chest wounds should be treated conventionally using an Asherman seal®. Wounds elsewhere should simply be covered with a sterile dressing (moist if there is eviscerated bowel). Iodine should NOT be applied. Bleeding should be controlled by pressure: cavities may require packing or pressure from fingers or a fist. If necessary, a tournequet should be used. Topical haemostatic agents such as Quickclot® or Hemcon® may be used for the emergency control of life-threatening limb bleeding. The manufacturers instructions should be carefully followed.

Forensic considerations

- Never remove clothes by cutting through wound holes
- Ensure that clothes remain with individual patients and are handed to a named person (preferably a police officer)
- Do not speculate about ballistics
- Do not touch any weapons
- Do not speculate about criminal responsibility

Burn injury

Pathophysiology

A burn wound has three zones:

- Zone of coagulation—a central zone of destroyed cells producing an avascular wound area.
- Zone of stasis—an area of injured cells which may die due to associated vasoconstriction and microthrombi.
- Zone of hyperaemia—an area of minimal thermal damage with marked vasodilatation and an acute inflammatory response.

Fluid loss

Fluid loss from the burn surface occurs which is:

- Due to vasodilatation and changes in blood vessel walls
- Proportional to the extent of the burn
- Present for 36 hours after injury

In addition, all patients suffer a systemic inflammatory response and capillary leak which is related to the extent of the burn and contributes to fluid loss. In combination with cutaneous loss from the burn, this may produce hypovolaemia. Burn shock is slower in onset (greater than 1hr) than hypovolaemic shock which may be associated with other coexisting injuries (for example, a house fire and injuries sustained jumping from the building).

Infection

Super-added infection is a critical feature in burns prognosis since many burns victims ultimately die of infection. Early attention to minimizing risk is, therefore, essential. Bacterial contamination can be reduced by wearing gloves when treating or moving a burns patient.

Pain

Pain from burn injury is produced by the exposure of nerve endings in burnt skin and from inflammatory mediators. Simple covering with cool dressings will have a dramatic effect in improving patient comfort but adequate analgesia is also vital.

Hypothermia

Burns patients, especially children, are at risk of hypothermia due to over zealous cooling. **Cool the burn and warm the patient** is sound clinical practice.

Death

Early burn-related deaths are associated with airway obstruction and severe inhalation injury. Later deaths are often precipitated by sepsis with a sustained systemic inflammatory response, acute lung injury, renal impairment, and myocardial depression, leading to multiple organ failure.

Types of thermal injury

Scalds

- 40–50% of burns unit admissions are children, 85% of which are scalds in children under 3 years of age.
- Are commonly due to hot water or hot fluids from cooking, including kettles, saucepans, chip pans, cups and mugs.
- Are more common in the elderly due to an increased frequency of spilling hot liquids and slowness to react (for example, in getting out of a bath which is too hot).
- May be associated with a medical crisis such as hypoglycaemia or CVA.
- Are commonly associated with drugs and alcohol use.

Flame burns

- Are commonly associated with house fires, especially when clothes catch alight.
- Are often associated with children playing with matches or cigarette lighters.
- May result from smoking in bed (especially in the elderly).
- Occur as a result of petrol or accelerants associated with barbecue or bonfire accidents.
- May be associated with airway burns.
- Are commonly associated with drugs and alcohol use.

Explosive burns

Burns resulting directly from the detonation of explosives are usually 'flash burns' against which normal clothing offers good protection. In some cases, however, the environment catches fire, in which case conventional flame burns will predominate. Explosions involving flammable materials such as petrol or gas will be associated with extensive burning. These may be domestic or industrial incidents or associated with incendiary terrorist devices.

Contact burns

Contact burns result from skin contact with a hot object and depend on the nature and temperature of the heat source and the duration of contact.

Chemical burns

Chemical burns commonly follow domestic and industrial accidents but occasionally occur as a form of self harm. Most chemical burns require copious irrigation. Four types of chemical burns require special attention:

Cement burns

Cement is a weak alkali and causes burns on prolonged contact. It is a common source of lower leg burns in builders.

Phosphorus burns

Phosphorus ignites spontaneously even in the presence of water. Phosphorus particles should be removed using forceps. This is made easier by applying 1% copper sulphate solution which turns the particles black. Copper sulphate is in itself toxic and should not be left in prolonged contact with the skin. Copper sulphate may be available in areas where phosphate is used.

Phenol burns

Phenol is absorbed through the skin and can cause renal failure. Water or saline soaks are contraindicated. Irrigation with copious running water is of benefit.

Hydrofluoric acid burns

Hydrofluoric acid causes intensely painful, deep burns. Treatment is with copious irrigation with cold water followed by urgent transfer to hospital for calcium gluconate therapy. All rescue personnel must be protected from contact with the acid.

Electrical injury

Electrical injury may follow low or high tension current sources. Low tension characteristically produces small deep burns at entry and exit points with variable tissue damage between them. Depending on the anatomical path of conduction, there may be associated cardiac dysrhythmias. High tension burns from overhead cables may be associated with injuries due to a fall from a height.

Ionizing radiation burns

Burns from ionizing radiation are rare. They should be suspected in any patient rescued from a fire at a nuclear installation. Treatment is with copious water irrigation using soap or detergent.

It is essential that all rescue personnel avoid the possibility of contamination with radioactive materials.

Flash burns

Flash burns are caused by intense, very short exposure to severe heat, often producing superficial or partial thickness burns. They may result from flame, radiation, or explosive burn injury. Normal clothing offers good protection against flash burns which are usually confined to exposed areas.

Non-accidental injury (NAI)

Non-accidental injury is most often seen in children, but may also occur in the elderly. Characteristic injuries include cigarette burns, scalds to the feet and buttocks (from lowering into hot water), and burns with irons and other electrical appliances.

Burn depth

The anatomical depth of a burn can be divided into:

- Simple erythema—superficial burn with no skin loss. Skin is red and tender and heals within 5–10 days with no scarring (typical of sunburn).

> Erythema is NOT included when counting burn area

- Superficial partial-thickness burns—painful, with superficial blistering healing in 10–14 days.

- Deep partial-thickness burns—thick-walled blisters with a granular white skin and pinpoint red mottled areas. Associated pain may be limited because of damage to the skin adnexae.
- Deep full-thickness burns—producing white leathery charred skin with no sensation. These burns commonly follow prolonged contact with a burning agent or dry heat. Scarring is inevitable.

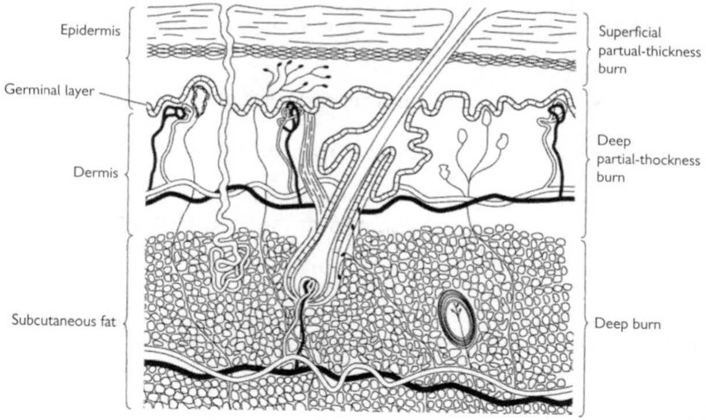

Fig. 3.22 Anatomical diagram showing burn depths. Reprinted with permission from Greaves I *et al.* (2005). *Emergency care: a textbook for paramedics*, 2nd edn. W.B. Saunders Co. Ltd.

Factors affecting the outcome of burns

Extent of burns

Surface area may be assessed using the 'rule of nines' in adults or the 'rule of fives' in children, for which standard assessment charts are available. The palm of the hand in adults (with the adducted fingers included) equates to approximately 1% body surface area. Assessment of the burns surface area is difficult in the pre-hospital environment and does not materially change management unless there is a significant transfer time to hospital. A simpler criteria is the 'rule of halves' using the following system:

- Is over half of the patient burnt?
- Is the area burnt between a quarter and a half of the patient's skin surface area?
- Is the area between an eighth and a quarter of the patient's skin surface area?
- Is the area less than an eighth of the total skin surface area?

A more detailed and accurate assessment can be carried out after arrival in hospital.

Burn site

A poorer prognosis is associated with burns to the:

- Face (often associated with smoke inhalation)
- Hands or feet
- Eyes
- Ears
- Perineum

Burns involving these areas, however small the surface area, require management in a specialist unit.

Circumferential burns to the neck may produce airway compromise, to the chest, respiratory compromise, and to the limbs may be associated with limb ischaemia. There is no role for escharotomy in normal UK pre-hospital care practice although unusual circumstances may dictate the need for local protocols.

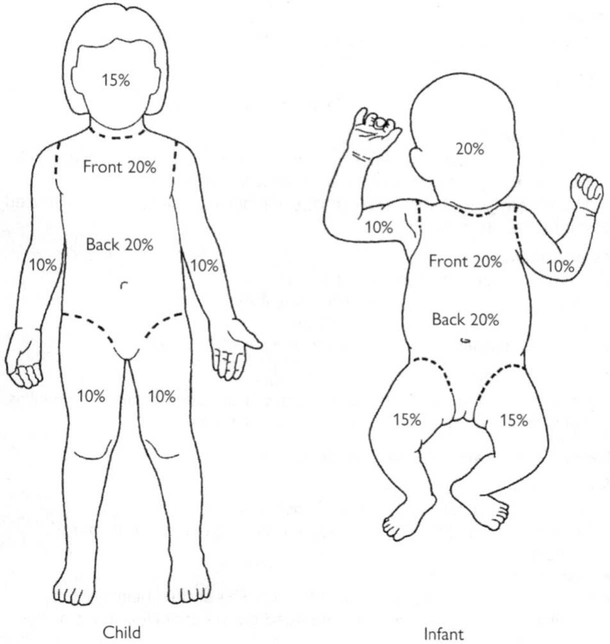

Fig. 3.23 'Rule of fives' (children and infants). The quoted percentages refer to the front *or* back of the limbs, but to the whole of the head. Reprinted with permission from Greaves *et al.* (2005). *Emergency care: a textbook for paramedics*, 2nd edn. W.B. Saunders Co. Ltd.

Inhalation injuries

Inhalation injuries are a major cause of death due to:

- Direct thermal injury by inhalation
- Inhaled toxic substances
- Systemic poisoning (for example, carbon monoxide)

Age of the patient

Mortality is increased in children under five years of age because child surface area is greater in relation to their total body size.

The elderly are at risk because of poor healing potential and reduced physiological reserve.

Associated injuries

Causes of associated injury include:

- Falls or jumps from a height in building fires
- Impact injuries in road traffic accidents
- Electrical injuries including arrythmias in electrocution

Associated medical conditions

Significant co-morbidities include ischaemic heart disease, diabetes mellitis, steroid therapy, and immunocompromised patients.

Immediate care of thermal injuries

Scene safety

- Ensure scene safety regarding avoidable risks to carers.
- Remove the patient from the heat source and extinguish flames, if necessary.
- Remove burnt and hot clothing.
- Cool the burn area for up to 20 minutes. This should begin whilst waiting for evacuation and be continued during packaging and transfer.

Primary survey

- Determine mechanism of injury.
- **A** Assess and open the airway, if necessary.
- **B** Assess breathing and ventilation and seek the signs and symptoms of smoke inhalation.

Only in extreme circumstances should intubation be attempted in the field, in which case a smaller than normal endotracheal tube should be used. Wheezing should be managed by the administration of nebulized salbutamol.

If the airway is *critically* threatened, the two options are surgical airway formation or anaesthesia and intubation. The former is safer in inexperienced hands (see page 178).

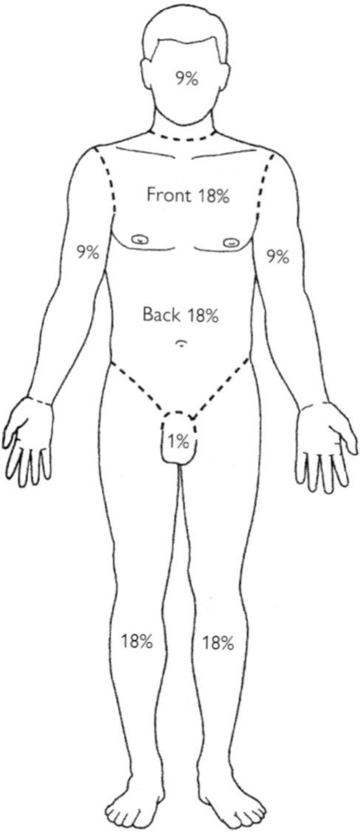

Fig. 3.24 'Rule of nines' (adults). The percentage on each limb refers to the front *or* rear aspect. A burn to the whole of the head represents 9% total body surface area (TBSA). Reprinted with permission from Greaves I *et al.* (2005). *Emergency care: a textbook for paramedics*, 2nd edn. W.B. Saunders Co. Ltd.

- **C** Assess the circulation

An accurate assessment of pulse, blood pressure, and capillary refill and subsequent monitoring is important in critical burns (greater than 15% in an adult and greater than 10% in a child). Depending on the mechanism of injury, it is important not to assume that shock is due to burn fluid loss. Intravenous cannulation, if necessary, should avoid the burn area.

Fluid replacement with normal saline or Hartmann's solution can be commenced if the patient is cannulated but must be started for burns greater than a quarter of total body surface area or if time to hospital is more than one hour from the time of injury.

A guide for fluid volume replacement is:

- Adults: 1000ml
- 10–15-year-olds: 500ml
- 5–10-year-olds: 250ml
- Under 5:20ml/kg body weight

- **D** Assess disability (neurological assessment)

As a baseline, a simple AVPU assessment is undertaken and pupillary size and response noted.

All patients are at risk of hypothermia with protracted burn cooling, especially children and the elderly. It is important to cool the burn wound but warm the patient.

Secondary survey

A detailed secondary survey is normally performed after arrival in hospital. In pre-hospital care, the following details should be ascertained, if possible:

- Time of the burn
- Burning agent
- Is the patient complaining of pain?
- Has the patient jumped or been involved in an explosion?
- Was the patient in a confined space?
- Has the patient lost consciousness at any time?
- A brief medical history; drug and allergy history

Tetanus status of the patient

Signs and symptoms of smoke inhalation

- History of being confined with the fire in a closed space
- History of unconsciousness at the time of the incident
- Exposure to smoke or gas during the incident
- Evidence of burns to the face
- Singed nasal hair
- Cough or carbonaceous sputum
- Blistering or redness in the mouth
- Evidence of laryngeal oedema (e.g. hoarseness, stridor).
- Wheezing
- Signs of airway obstruction or respiratory distress
- Full-thickness burns to the nasolabial area of the face or posterior pharyngeal swelling
- Signs of respiratory failure: the patient who is unable to speak owing to shortness of breath or exhaustion, or who is unconscious

Assessment and treatment of carbon monoxide poisoning

Most burns patients from a fire in an enclosed space have inhaled carbon monoxide.

- Signs and symptoms of mild intoxication include lethargy, muscle weakness, headache, nausea, and vomiting.
- Signs and symptoms of severe carbon monoxide poisoning are; cyanosis, coma, pulmonary oedema, and dilated pupils.

Pulse oximetry is unreliable as it will not detect the difference between carboxyhaemoglobin and oxyhaemoglobin. The classic cherry red appearance is a rare and very late feature.

Dressings

For burns of surface area less than 10%, a clean dressing soaked in cold water or normal saline should be applied. This will reduce the pain and halt or slow the burning process.

For burns over 10%, a sterile clean cloth or clingfilm® should be used. Reducing the air current over the burn will reduce pain and wound contamination. It is important to avoid circumferential dressings and clingfilm should, therefore, be gently laid over the burn wound in overlapping sheets.

Clingfilm should not be used for chemical burns as this may worsen the burn effect.

Analgesia

The ideal analgesic for burns is morphine given intravenously in aliquots according to body weight and with an antiemetic. Intramuscular and subcutaneous analgesia should be avoided in moderate or severe burns because of delayed absorption.

Patient disposal

Treatment should be given with the aim of reducing on-scene times and delivering the patient to the appropriate treatment centre. This will be the nearest appropriate A&E department unless local protocols allow direct transport to a burns facility.

Formulary

Introduction

This chapter describes the drugs most commonly used in pre-hospital care. As a result, it is restricted to indications which are likely to be encountered in the pre-hospital management of patients and only describes formulations which are used in these circumstances. For example, the use of oral amiodarone is not discussed, neither is the use of oral steroids in the management of chronic inflammatory conditions, although intravenous steroids in acute asthma and anaphylaxis are mentioned.

Only *significant acute side-effects* are listed. Details of minor and chronic side-effects can be found in the *British National Formulary*. No attempt has been made to list every recorded side-effect of each drug mentioned.

Acute allergic reactions are possible with any drug, as a result they are not specifically listed under individual entries.

Paediatric doses are given on pp.356–8.

Adrenaline

Description

Vasoconstrictor sympathomimetic catecholamine.

Presentation

- 1 in 10,000, 10ml ampoule/pre-filled syringe[1]
- 1 in 1000, 1ml ampoule/pre-filled syringe[1]
- Self-administration pens for patient's own use (Epipen®, Anapen®).

Effects

Acts on adrenergic receptors to constrict peripheral blood vessels; may also stabilize mast cell membranes.

Indications

- Cardiac arrest
- Anaphylaxis.

Dose

- Cardiac arrest—standard dose, 1mg (10ml, 1 in 10,000).
- Acute anaphylaxis—1ml, 1 in 1000 (1mg) by intramuscular or subcutaneous injection. In severe anaphylaxis with circulatory compromise, use 1 in 10,000 by slow intravenous injection, titrated to effect.

Contraindications

None.

Side-effects

Anxiety, tremor, tachycardia, headache, arrhythmias, cold peripheries, pulmonary oedema, nausea and vomiting, sweating, dizziness.

Notes

Adrenaline may also be used combined with lignocaine to reduce bleeding from peripheral vessels. If used inappropriately (for example, in fingers), this can lead to ischaemia and tissue loss. The use of lignocaine with adrenaline is NOT recommended in pre-hospital care.

Anaphylaxis patients on non-selective beta-blockers may not respond to adrenaline (but may develop severe hypertension); intravenous salbutamol may be required after arrival in hospital.

1 Other size ampoules are available but do not represent 'standard' doses; only the above should be carried.

Doses of IM adrenaline in anaphylaxis

Age	Dose	Volume of 1 in 1000 1mg/ml
Under 6 years	150μg	0.15ml
6–12 years	300μg	0.3ml
12 years and over	500μg	0.5ml

Amiodarone

Description

Class III anti-arrhythmic drug.

Effects

Inhibits the activity of peripheral vascular calcium channels and adrenergic receptors, resulting in peripheral vasodilatation, and of cardiac calcium channels, causing slowing depolarization.

Presentation

30mg/ml, 10ml ampoule for intravenous injection; also available as pre-filled syringe.

Indications

- VF or pulseless VT.
- Amiodarone should not be used for the treatment of ventricular and supraventricular arrythmias pre-hospital.

Dose

300mg by slow intravenous injection (at least 3 minutes).

Contraindications

None in cardiac arrest situations.

Side-effects

Not applicable in cardiac arrest situations.

Aspirin

Description

Irreversibly acetylates cyclo-oxygenase, the rate-limiting enzyme in the arachidonic acid cascade.

Presentation

300mg soluble tablets is recommended for use in acute coronary syndrome. Aspirin is not carried as an analgesic.

Effects

Aspirin inhibits the aggregation of platelets and platelet degranulation as well as decreasing localized vasoconstriction.

Indications

Secondary prevention of thrombotic cerebrovascular or cardiovascular disease.

Dose

300mg soluble aspirin dispersed in water.

Contraindications

- Caution in asthma
- Active peptic ulceration
- Haemophilia and other bleeding disorders
- Aspirin is contraindicated in children under 16 and during breast-feeding (Reye's syndrome).

Side-effects

Bronchospasm, gastrointestinal bleeding.

Atracurium

See pp.385–6.

Atropine

Description

A cholinergic antagonist (anticholinergic).

Presentation

- 600μg/ml, 1ml ampoules for injection (other strengths are available)
- 100μg/ml, 5ml, 10ml, 30ml pre-filled syringes
- Also available as 200μg/ml, 5ml pre-filled syringe; 300μg/ml, 10ml pre-filled syringe; and 600μg/ml, 1ml pre-filled syringe.

Effects

- Tachycardia, increased cardiac output, and increase in systemic blood pressure
- Drying of secretions
- Prevention of bradycardia in response to intubation (spinal injuries)
- Pupillary dilatation.

Indications

- Profound bradycardia with hypotension
- Organophosphate poisoning (see p.442)
- Pre-intubation prevention of bradycardia in spinal injuries.

Dose

- Bradycardia—increments of 500ug or 600ug titrated to effect (maximum dose 3mg)
- Organophosphate poisoning—(see p.442)
- Pre-medication—up to 600ug (children 20ug/kg, maximum 600ug).

Contraindications

- Other situations—angle-closure glaucoma, myasthenia gravis.

Side-effects

Constipation, bradycardia, tachycardia, arrythmias, drying of secretions and dry skin, urinary urgency and retention, pupillary dilatation with loss of visual acuity, flushing, confusion, nausea and vomiting, and dizziness (rare).

Benzyl penicillin

Description

Penicillin active against meningococcus.

Presentation

Benzyl penicillin sodium 600mg and 1.2g vials for intravenous or intramuscular injection.

Effects

Benzyl penicillin (penicillin G) is active against pneumococcus, meningococcus, and many other streptococci.

Indications

Established or suspected bacterial meningitis.

Dose

Adult 1.2g (2.4g in established disease) by intravenous injection (preferred) or intramuscular injection

Children Under 1: 300mg
1–years: 600mg
10 years and over: adult dose.

Contraindications

Penicillin allergy.

Side-effects

Allergic reactions.

Notes

Following arrival in hospital and pending sensitivity results, a cephalosporin is usually added or substituted.

Bupivacaine

See p.392.

Chlorpheniramine (chlorphenamine)

Description

Sedating antihistamine.

Presentation

- 10mg/ml, 1ml ampoule for injection
- 4mg tablets.

Effects

- Binds to H_1 receptors decreasing histamine-induced vasodilation, oedema, and secretion
- Also has anticholinergic activity.

Indications

- Symptomatic relief of allergy
- Treatment of anaphylaxis.

Dose

Oral dose—4mg

Intravenous or intramuscular dose—10mg by SLOW injection; may be repeated once

Children 1 month–1 year: 250μg/kg
1 year–6 years 2.5–5mg
6–12 years: 5–10mg

Contraindications

Urinary retention, glaucoma (due to anticholinergic effects).

Side-effects

Drowsiness, stimulation (rare), urinary retention, dry mouth, blurred vision, dizziness, confusion.

Notes

- Injection may result in transient hypotension or CNS stimulation; intravenous injection should be slow.
- Chlorpheniramine may be given sc or im, however the intravenous route is preferred when parenteral administration is necessary.

Compound analgesics

Description

Analgesics containing paracetamol and an opiate.

Presentation

There are very many proprietary compound analgesics. Immediate care practitioners should carry ONE of the following:

- Co-codamol 30/500 (codeine 30mg, paracetamol 500mg)
- Co-dydramol (dihydrocodeine10mg, paracetamol 500mg)
- Co-proxamol (dextropropoxyphene 32.5mg, paracetamol 325mg).

Effects

Combined effects of opiates and simple analgesics.

Indications

Moderate pain.

Dose

- 1–2 tablets every 4–6 hours, maximum 8 in 24 hours
- Not recommended in children.

Contraindications

Constipation and confusion may occur, so use with care in the elderly.

Notes

Compound analgesic overdoses present with the features of opiate poisoning (reversible with naloxone) and, subsequently, of paracetamol poisoning. Such overdoses are unfortunately common.

Cyclizine

Description

An antihistamine.

Presentation

50mg/ml, 1ml ampoule for intramuscular or intravenous injection.

Effects

Prevention or reduction of nausea and vomiting.

Indications

- Established nausea or vomiting
- Prophylaxis of opiate-induced nausea and vomiting.

Dose

Cyclizine 50mg iv.

Contraindications

Cyclizine is not recommended in severe heart failure and may counteract the beneficial cardiovascular effects of opiates.

Side-effects

Extrapyramidal effects.

Notes

- Cyclizine is available as a combined preparation with morphine, cyclimorph® (morphine 10mg/cyclizine 50mg in 1ml). Its use is not recommended.
- The treatment for extrapyramidal effects is benztropine 1–2mg by intravenous or intramuscular injection, or procyclidine 5–10mg by intramuscular or intravenous injection. Management of these symptoms should take place in hospital.

Dextrose

Description

Solution of anhydrous glucose.

Presentation

- 5% solution, 500ml and 1000ml bags
- 10% solution, 500ml bags

Effects

Elevation of blood glucose levels.

Indications

- Hypoglycaemia
- Fluid replacement.

Dose

- Hypoglycaemia—25–50ml 10% glucose by intravenous injection; *Children*: 10% glucose titrated to effect
- Fluid replacement—5% glucose titrated to effect.

Contraindications

None.

Side-effects

Hyperglycaemia, venous irritation, and thrombophlebitis.

Diamorphine

Description

Opiate analgesic (heroin hydrochloride).

Presentation

Powder for reconstitution; 5mg and 10mg ampoules (larger dose ampoules are available).

Effects

- Binds to opiate receptors resulting in analgesia, euphoria, and respiratory depression
- Decreases pre- and after-load (central mechanism) and increases force of ventricular contraction and ejection fraction.

Indications

- Acute pain, especially from myocardial infarction
- Acute pulmonary oedema.

Dose

Up to 5mg by slow intravenous injection (may be repeated).

Contraindications

- Acute respiratory depression
- Care in head injury.

Side-effects

Respiratory depression, nausea and vomiting, drowsiness, hypotension, tachycardia, pinpoint pupils.

Notes

Naloxone (Narcan®) must always be available if opiate analgesics are being used.

Diazepam

Description

Sedative hypnotic benzodiazepine.

Presentation

- 5mg/ml, 2ml ampoule diazepam emulsion for intravenous injection*
- 2.5mg, 5mg, and 10mg rectal tubes.

Effects

Acts through membrane GABA receptors to stabilize membranes, primarily in the CNS, and reduce depolarization.

Indications

- Cessation of epileptic fits/febrile convulsions/poisoning-induced seizures
- Sedation and amnesia for clinical procedures
- Co-administration with ketamine to reduce emergence phenomena (not required in children).

Dose

- 10–20mg by slow intravenous injection in aliquots to effect
- Rectally, 500μg/kg
- Children Status epilepticus—rectal: children over 10kg, 500μg/kg maximum 20mg; intravenous: Neonate—12 years 300–400 μg/kg; 12–18 years 10–20mg.

Contraindications

- Pregnancy or lactation (not applicable in status epilepticus)
- Respiratory depression.

Side-effects

- May cause respiratory depression and apnoea (facilities for ventilatory support must be available)
- Drowsiness, occasionally irritability, excitability and hallucinations (more common in elderly patients).

* For intravenous use, diazepam should be given as the emulsion. Benzodiazepines may also be used as muscle relaxants: use as such is not appropriate in acute pre-hospital care.

Diclofenac (Voltarol)

Description

A non-steroidal anti-inflammatory drug

Presentation

- Tablets/capsules 50mg (smaller dose tablets are available)
- Suppositories 100mg (smaller suppositories are available)
- Voltarol for intramuscular injection 25mg/ml, 3ml ampoule.

Effects

Decreases pain and inflammation by the inhibition of the prostaglandin synthesis cascade, primarily through the inhibition of cyclo-oxygenase.

Indications

Acute pain; effective in ureteric and billiary colic.

Dose

- Oral 50–100mg
- Suppository 100mg
- IM 75mg (repeated once after 30 minutes in ureteric colic).

Contraindications

- Caution in the elderly, acute renal, cardiac, or hepatic failure
- Peptic ulcer disease.

Side-effects

- No acute significant side-effects with single doses
- Caution in the elderly, acute renal, cardiac, or hepatic failure.

Etomidate

See p.381.

Fentanyl

See p.368.

Flumazenil

Description

Specific antagonist at central benzodiazepine receptors.

Presentation

100ug/ml, 5ml ampoule for intravenous injection.

Effects

Specific antagonism of benzodiazepines at central receptors.

Indications

Reversal of benzodiazepines following administration for anaesthesia or sedation.

Dose

200μg over 15 seconds followed by 100μg at one-minute intervals; usual dose 300–600μg.

Contraindications

Life-threatening condition controlled by benzodiazepine.

Side-effects

If flumazenil is administered too rapidly, agitation, fear, and anxiety may occur. Transient tachycardia, bradycardia (including complete heart block), hypertension VT and, occasionally, convulsions are possible. Acute withdrawal, including fitting, may occur in patients addicted to benzodiazepines.

Notes

Flumazenil is not licensed for use in the treatment of benzodiazepine overdose. In the majority of such cases, respiratory support is appropriate pending arrival in hospital rather than reversal at scene which may precipitate the problems described above (see side-effects) and the patient's rapid departure from the scene.

Flumazenil MUST NEVER be used in patients with a history of convulsions or who have also taken tricyclic antidepressants.

Flumazenil has a relatively short half life and repeated doses may be necessary with some longer-acting benzodiazepines.

Flumazenil IS NOT recommended for pre-hospital use.

Frusemide (furosemide)

Description

A loop diuretic.

Presentation

10mg/ml, 2ml and 5ml ampoules for intravenous injection.

Effects

Acts in the ascending limb of the loop of Henle to inhibit reabsorption of sodium and increase water loss.

Indications

Acute pulmonary oedema secondary to left ventricular failure.

Dose

Initial dose 20–50mg; larger doses may be required in severe LVF.

Contraindications

- Anuric renal failure
- Prostatic hypertrophy (may precipitate acute retention).

Side-effects

No major side-effects in the acute pre-hospital situation.

Glucagon

Description

Polypeptide hormone.

Presentation

1mg vial with pre-filled syringe (water for injections) for reconstitution.

Effects

Glucagon increases plasma glucose by mobilizing glycogen stored in the liver. (See below.)

Indications

Acute hypoglycaemia.

Dose

- 1mg by subcutaneous, intramuscular, or intravenous injection
- *Children*: under 8 years (or under 25kg) 500μg
  over 8 years (or over 25kg) 1mg.

Contraindications

None.

Side-effects

Nausea, vomiting, abdominal pain, hypotension.

Notes

Because glucagon acts by mobilizing glycogen stored in the liver, it will be ineffective in hypoglycaemia associated with starvation, chronic alcoholism, and other states in which liver glycogen stores are depleted.

Glyceryl trinitrate

Description

A vasodilator acting predominantly on the venous system.

Presentation

- 400μg metered dose sublingual spray
- 300μg, 500μg, and 600μg sublingual tablets
- slow-release preparations (including Suscard® and Sustac®), various sizes up to 10mg.

Effects

Coronary vasodilatation, reduction of venous return and left ventricular work, inhibition of platelet function (antithrombotic effect) via cGMP.

Indications

- Angina
- Left ventricular failure.

Dose

- GTN
- Angina (treatment of attack)—sublingual 0.3–1mg (tablet or spray)
- Acute LVF—5mg slow release (can be repeated).

Contraindications

Hypotension, aortic or mitral stenosis.

Side-effects

Headache, flushing, dizziness, postural hypotension, tachycardia.

Hydrocortisone

Description

An adrenal glucocorticoid.

Presentation

100mg vial for intramuscular or intravenous injection, may be supplied with or without ampoule of water for injections (2ml).

Effects

Glucocorticoids:

- Decrease capillary permeability
- Decrease release of histamine by mast cells
- Inhibit macrophage phagocytosis
- Inhibit antibody production by lymphocytes

Indications

- Anaphylactic shock
- Acute severe asthma.

Dose

- 100–200mg
- *Children*: up to 1yr, 25mg; 1–5yrs, 50mg; 6–12yrs, 100mg.

Contraindications

None in anaphylaxis or acute severe asthma.

Side-effects

Nil acute.

Ibuprofen

Description

Non-steroidal anti-inflammatory drug.

Presentation

- 200mg, 400mg, and 600mg tablets
- Paediatric suspension 100mg/ml.

Effects

Decreases pain and inflammation by the inhibition of the prostaglandin synthesis cascade, primarily through the inhibition of cyclo-oxygenase.

Indications

- Acute pain
- Pyrexia in children.

Dose

- 400–600mg orally
- Fever and pain in children:

  3–6 months, 50mg*
  6 months–1 year, 50mg
  1–4 years, 100mg
  4–7 years, 150mg
  7–10 years, 200mg
  10–12 years, 300mg
  (all doses three times daily)

Contraindications

- Caution in the elderly, acute renal, cardiac, or hepatic failure
- Contraindicated in peptic ulcer disease.

Side-effects

No acute significant side-effects with single doses.

Notes

Various slow-release preparations are also available.

* Body weight over 5kg.

Ketamine

Description

A dissociative anaesthetic/analgesic.

Presentation

10mg/ml, 20ml vial for injection*
100mg/ml, 10ml vial for injection

Effects

Ketamine has the following features:

- It is powerfully analgesic in subanaesthetic doses
- Protective glottal reflexes are relatively preserved
- It does not normally cause respiratory depression at conventional doses
- It has a long shelf life
- It does not cause hypotension, but ketamine-induced hypertension makes it *relatively* contraindicated in head injury
- It is *relatively* safe in patients with a full stomach.

Indications

- Pre-hospital anaesthesia for extrication or short procedures
- Analgesia.

Dose

- *Anaesthesia*: intramuscular—5–10mg/kg (provides 12–25 minutes of surgical anaesthesia, effective after 4–15 minutes)
- Intravenous—1–2mg/kg (provides 5–10 minutes of surgical anaesthesia, effective after 2–7 minutes)
- *Analgesia*; ketamine is an effective analgesic when used in subanaesthetic doses by either the intramuscular or intravenous route
- Repeat doses may be given as 10–20mg intravenously or 20–50mg intramuscularly.
- *Children*: as above

Contraindications

- Hypertension
- Head injury (relative, but consider clinical priorities).

Side-effects

A significant proportion of patients suffer emergence hallucinations which can be very distressing. As a consequence, a benzodiazepine should also be administered to oblate these symptoms.

* 50mg/ml is also available but NOT RECOMMENDED for pre-hospital use.

Lignocaine (lidocaine)

Description

Class Ib anti-arrhythmic.

Presentation

Anti-arrythmic

- Lignocaine hydrochloride 1% (10mg/ml), 10ml pre-filled syringe
- Lignocaine hydrochloride 2% (20mg/ml), 5ml pre-filled syringe

Local anaesthesia

- Lignocaine hydrochloride 1% (10mg/ml), 2ml, 5ml, and 10ml ampoules for injection
- Lignocaine hydrochloride 2% (20mg/ml), 2ml and 5ml ampoules for injection.

Effects

Lignocaine blocks sodium channels, reducing the conduction rate and amplitude of nerve electrical impulses.

Indications

- Ventricular arrhythmias
- Painful localized pathology
- Local anaesthesia for painful procedures.

Dose

- Ventricular arrhythmias: 100mg by slow intravenous bolus (dose may be reduced in smaller patients)
- Local anaesthesia: see notes below
- Children (local anaesthesia): 3mg/kg.

Contraindications

- Anti-arrhythmic therapy: sino-atrial disorders, atrio-ventricular block.
- Local analgesia: hypovolaemia, complete heart block.
- Solutions with adrenaline: see notes below.

Side-effects

- These are rare with single applications of topical lignocaine.
- Inebriation and lightheadedness followed by sedation, circumoral paraesthesia, and twitching; convulsions in severe cases.
- Convulsions and cardiovascular collapse on intravenous administration.

Notes

0.5% lignocaine is available for local anaesthetic use. It is NOT recommended in the pre-hospital environment.

A MAXIMUM safe lignocaine dose for an average adult is 20ml of 1% (200mg) or equivalent volume of higher concentration solution. This dose can be increased if lignocaine is given with a vasoconstrictor such as adrenaline. Use of lignocaine with adrenaline may cause gangrene if injected into digits or appendages and is NOT RECOMMENDED in pre-hospital care.

Magnesium

Description

Administered as magnesium sulphate.

Presentation

Magnesium sulphate 50%*, 2ml (1g) and 10ml (5g) ampoules, 10ml pre-filled syringe.

Effects

Precise mechanism not known; effective in acute severe asthma.

Indications

- Acute severe asthma
- Ventricular tachycardia
- Torsade de pointes.

Dose

- Asthma: 1.2–2g iv over 20 minutes
- VT, torsade de pointes, and refractory VF: 8mmoles (4ml or 2g) over 30 minutes (followed by infusion after arrival in hospital).

Contraindications

None.

Side-effects

Symptoms of hypermagnesaemia: nausea, vomiting, flushing, hypotension, arrhythmias, respiratory depression, drowsiness, and confusion.

Notes

The dose of magnesium given above for the treatment of asthma should only be given ONCE to avoid symptomatic hypermagnesaemia.

* 1ml of 50% magnesium contains 2mmol magnesium. 20% magnesium sulphate is also available (0.8mmol/ml).

Methionine

Description

Paracetamol antidote.

Presentation

250mg tablets.

Indications

The first-line treatment for paracetamol overdose is N-acetylcysteine after arrival in hospital and within four hours of the overdose. Methionine is only indicated (and need only be carried) in areas in which prompt evacuation is likely to be impossible.

Dose

- *Adult and child over 6*: 2.5g initially followed by three further doses of 2.5g every 4 hours orally.
- *Child under 6*: 1g initially followed by three further doses of 1g orally.

Contraindications

Since it is given orally, methionine is ineffective in patients who are vomiting.

Side-effects

Nausea, vomiting, drowsiness, irritability.

Metoclopramide

Description

Prokinetic antiemetic.

Presentation

5mg/ml, 2ml (10mg) ampoule for injection.

Effects

Antiemesis by central antagonism of dopamine. Cholinergic effects on the gut include increased gastric emptying, pyloric sphincter relaxation, increased lower oesophageal sphincter tone, and stimulation of peristalsis.

Indications

- Nausea and vomiting
- Adjunct treatment with opiate analgesics.

Dose

10mg by iv injection (may also be given im).

Contraindications

Not to be used in patients UNDER 20 YEARS OLD due to an increased risk of acute dystonic reactions.

Side-effects

Extrapyramidal effects (dystonia). Other side-effects are rare.

Notes

The treatment for extrapyramidal effects is benztropine 1–2mg by iv or im injection or procyclidine 5–10mg by im or iv injection. Management of these symptoms should take place in hospital.

Midazolam

Description

Sedative hypnotic benzodiazepine.

Presentation

- (Midazolam hydrochloride 1mg/ml, 50ml vial)
- Midazolam hydrochloride 2mg/ml, 2ml and 5ml ampoules
- Midazolam hydrochloride 5mg/ml, 2ml, 5ml, 10ml, and 18ml ampoules.

Effects

Acts through membrane GABA receptors to stabilize membranes, primarily in the CNS, and reduce depolarization.

Indications

- Sedation and amnesia for clinical procedures
- Co-administration with ketamine to reduce emergence phenomena (not required in children).

Dose

- 2–2.5mg (0.5–1mg in the elderly) by slow iv injection, increasing in increments of 1mg (0.5–1mg in elderly).
- *Children*: (by SLOW iv injection) 6 months–5 yrs, initially 50–100ug/kg; 6–12 yrs, 25–50ug/kg. Further increments are given to effect.

Contraindications

Severe respiratory depression, acute pulmonary insufficiency, myasthenia gravis.

Side-effects

- Respiratory depression and arrest (overdosage or too rapid administration)
- Drowsiness, confusion, ataxia, amnesia, headache, vertigo.
- Excitement and aggression (more common in children and the elderly).

Notes

Midazolam can also be given by im or rectal routes.

Morphine

Description

An opiate analgesic.

Presentation

- Morphine sulphate 10mg/ml, 15mg/ml, 20mg/ml, and 30mg/ml—1 and 2ml ampoules
- Morphine sulphate 10mg/ml—1ml pre-filled syringe
- Morphine sulphate 1mg/ml—10ml pre-filled syringe
- Larger-volume vials are available but are intended for iv infusion preparation.

Effects

Binds to opiate receptors resulting in analgesia, euphoria, and respiratory depression.

Indications

Acute severe pain

Dose

- Morphine should be given by iv injection in small aliquots titrated to effect. An initial dose of 5mg is appropriate for an adult male, 2mg for smaller or older patients. Doses of up to 30mg may be required in fit young men with severe pain.
- *Children*: neonate, 40–100μg/kg; 1–6 months, 100–200μg/kg; 6 months–12 years, 100–200μg/kg.

Contraindications

Acute respiratory depression.

Side-effects

Nausea and vomiting, drowsiness, respiratory depression, hypotension, hallucinations. Acute allergic reactions.

Notes

The labelling on ampoules of proprietary morphine is identical except for the concentration. It is imperative that this is carefully checked if dosing errors are to be avoided. Morphine should always be administered in a concentration of 1mg in 1ml (10mg in 10ml).

An antiemetic should be administered with any iv opiate, however the use of Cyclimorph® (morphine/cyclizine) is not recommended .

Naloxone and equipment for mechanical ventilatory support MUST be available when morphine (or any other opiate) is administered.

Morphine has a duration of action of about 2 hours.

Naloxone

Description

A competitive opiate antagonist.

Presentation

- 400ug/ml, 1ml ampoule
- 400ug/ml 1ml, 2ml, and 5ml pre-filled syringe
- 1mg/ml, 2ml pre-filled syringe.

Effects

Reversal of opioid effects.

Indications

- Reversal of therapeutic overdose of opiates
- Treatment of opiate poisoning (recreational overdose)
- Treatment of unexplained loss/reduction of consciousness.

Dose

- 0.4mg(400ug)–2mg repeated at intervals, as required, to a maximum of 10mg
- If naloxone is given to exclude opiates as a cause of loss of consciousness, a dose of 10mg should be given
- *Children*: intravenous 5–10μg/kg, subsequent dose of 100ug/kg if no response.

Contraindications

Caution in patients who are physically dependent on opiates; will precipitate pain in patients given opiate for analgesia.

Side-effects

Nausea and vomiting, tachycardia.

Notes

Naloxone is short-acting. As a result, when long-acting opiates are being reversed, repeated doses may be needed. Drug abusers may leave the scene after a first dose only to collapse as the naloxone wears off. In order to reduce the likelihood off this, either the opiate can be reversed only enough to ensure adequacy of respiration before arrival in hospital, or a similar dose to the intravenous one given above may be given INTRAMUSCULARLY, in addition.

Nitrous oxide/oxygen 50:50 (Entonox)

Description

50:50 mixture of oxygen and nitrous oxide (N_2O).

Presentation

Various sizes of blue cylinder with a white and blue mantle. Self administered with override valve.

Effects

Analgesia without loss of consciousness.

Indications

- Analgesia for moderate pain in fully conscious individuals
- Analgesia for short, painful procedures

Dose

Titrate to effect. Usually self administered using a demand valve. May be overridden by medical staff.

Contraindications

Contraindicated in patients in whom an air-filled cavity exists into which nitrous oxide can diffuse. These conditions include pneumothorax (so contraindicated in significant chest injury), the 'bends' (so contraindicated in patients following diving), and open head injuries.

Side-effects

See above

Notes

At temperatures less than –7°C, nitrous oxide/oxygen mixtures will separate. This may lead to inhalation of pure oxygen with no analgesic effect, followed by pure nitrous oxide leading to hypoxia. A few shakes of the cylinder will have no effect on this separation. Entonox MUST be kept above–7°C, even if this means transferring it to your vehicle immediately before departure.

Ondansetron

Description

Specific $5HT_3$ antagonist.

Presentation

- 4mg and 8mg tablets
- Ondansetron hydrochloride 2mg/ml, 2ml and 4ml ampoules for slow iv injection.

Effects

Blocks $5HT_3$ receptors in the gastrointestinal tract and CNS.

Indications

Nausea and vomiting.

Dose

- 4mg orally
- 4–8mg by slow iv injection
- *Children*: 100ug/kg by slow iv injection.

Contraindications

Caution in pregnancy and breastfeeding.

Side-effects

Sensation of warmth or flushing, transient visual disturbance and dizziness. (Rarely, fits, chest pain arrhythmias, hypotension, and bradycardia.)

Notes

May also be given orally or by im injection.

Oxygen

Description

Invisible odourless gaseous element.

Presentation

Black cylinders with a white collar and neck.

Effects

Increases alveolar oxygen tension, decreases work of breathing, and improves arterial oxygen tension.

Indications

Hypoxia (for example, due to trauma, chronic obstructive pulmonary disease (COPD), asthma, or pulmonary embolism).

Dose

High flow (12–15l/min) by Hudson mask with rebreathing bag for trauma and other causes except COPD, (in which case, low flow 24–28% by fixed or variable rate mask).

Contraindications

High-flow oxygen is contraindicated in patients with COPD and oxygen, in patients with paraquat poisoning.

Side-effects

Exacerbation or precipitation of respiratory failure if given in high dose to patients with elevated $PaCO_2$ dependent on hypoxic drive.

Sizes and capacities of conventional oxygen cylinders

Size	Capacity (litres)	Duration at 15l/min
C	170	11
D	340	22
E	680	45
F	1360	90
G	3400	225

Ambulance services are increasingly carrying the CD size lightweight cylinder which contains 460 litres of oxygen, and lasts 30min with a delivery rate of 15 litres/min.

Pancuronium

See pp.385–6.

Paracetamol

Description

A simple analgesic with weak anti-inflammatory properties.

Presentation

- Tablets: 500mg (also as dispersible paracetamol)
- Paediatric suspension: 120mg/5ml*
- Suppositories: 60mg, 125mg, 250mg, and 500mg.

Effects

Inhibits brain prostaglandin synthesis.

Indications

- Mild to moderate pain, especially in children (aspirin contraindicated)
- Pyrexia

Dose

Adults: 500mg–1g orally, maximum 4g in 24 hours orally or by suppository
Children:

- Orally:
  - 3 months–1 year—60–120mg
  - 1–5 years—120–250mg
  - 6–12 years—250–500mg.

These doses may be repeated every 4–6 hours, maximum 4 doses in 24 hours

- By suppository:
  - 3 months–1 year—60–125mg
  - 1–5 years—125–250mg
  - 6–12 years—250–500mg
  - Over 12 years—500mg–1g.

Contraindications

None for single dose in acute situation, but check with regard to patient's 24-hour total dose, especially with respect to compound analgesics containing paracetamol.

Side-effects

No significant acute side-effects.

Notes

Paracetamol is extremely toxic in overdose.

* Paediatric tablets and adult suspension (250mg/ml) are also available.

Pethidine

Description

Synthetic opioid with a shorter duration of action than morphine.

Presentation

- 50mg/ml in 1ml and 2ml ampoules for injection
- 10mg/ml in 5ml and 10ml ampoules
- Oral pethidine is not suitable for pre-hospital use.

Effects

- Analgesia
- Obstetric analgesia (pethidine does not delay labour)
- Atropine-like effects—blurred vision, dry mouth.

Indications

- Moderate pain
- Obstetric pain.

Dose

- 20–50mg by slow iv injection
- 50–100mg sc or im for obstetric analgesia.

Contraindications

- Patients taking monoamine oxidase inhibitors
- Acute respiratory depression
- Care in head injury.

Side-effects

- See morphine
- There is no evidence to suggest that pethidine has less effect than morphine on the sphincter of Oddi.

Notes

- Onset within 10 minutes, duration of action 1–2 hours
- Pethidine is associated with a greater risk of hypotension because of its alpha blockade, it is NOT RECOMMENDED for pre-hospital use.

Prilocaine

See p.392.

Propofol

See p.382.

Rocuronium

See p.385.

Salbutamol

Description

B_2 adrenergic receptor agonist.

Presentation

- Nebulizer solution 1mg/ml 2.5ml (2.5mg) nebules, 2mg/ml 2.5 ml (5mg) nebules
- Metered dose inhaler 100μg per puff.

Effects

Relaxation of smooth muscle resulting in bronchodilatation.

Indications

Acute asthma.

Dose

- 5mg as nebulized solution
- Child over 18 months—2.5mg as nebulized solution (under 18 months, 1.25–2.5 mg as nebulized solution).
- Doses may be repeated if necessary.

Contraindications

None in acute use for severe asthma.

Side-effects

Tachycardia, fine tremor, headache, peripheral dilatation, palpitation, and arrhythmias.

Notes

If a nebulizer is not available, salbutamol may be given by metered dose inhaler (MDI) via a spacer device.

Suxamethonium

See p.384.

Syntocinon (oxytocin)

Description

An oxytocic.

Presentation

- 5 units/ml, 1ml ampoule
- 10 units/ml, 1ml ampoule.

Effects

Contracts uterine muscle.

Indications

Control of excessive uterine bleeding following delivery.

Dose

5–10 units by intravenous injection.

Contraindications

Caution in patients with predisposition to uterine rupture.

Side-effects

- Rapid IV injection may cause transient hypotension
- Nausea, vomiting, arrhythmias.

Tenecteplase

Description

Fibrinolytic.

Presentation

Powder for reconstitution, 40mg (8000 units), 50mg (10,000 units) Both with pre-filled syringe of water for injections.

Effects

Acts as a thrombolytic by activating plasminogen to form plasmin which degrades fibrin and breaks up thrombi.

Indications

Acute myocardial infarction.

Dose

500–600mcg/kg (maximum 50mg) by iv injection over 10 seconds.

Contraindications

- Recent haemorrhage, trauma, or surgery (including dental extraction)
- Coagulation defects
- History of cerebrovascular disease
- Recent symptoms of peptic ulceration
- Heavy vaginal bleeding
- Severe hypertension
- Active pulmonary disease with cavitation
- Acute pancreatitis/severe liver disease
- Oesophageal varices.

Side-effects

- Nausea and vomiting
- Bleeding
- Reperfusion arrhythmias
- Hypotension.

Thiopentone

See p.383.

Tramadol

Description

A synthetic opiate with additional actions (see below). It is a non-selective OP1 and OP3 receptor agonist, acting mainly at the OP1 receptor.

Presentation

Tramadol hydrochloride 50mg/ml, 2ml ampoule.

Effects

Tramadol has opioid and non-opioid mechanisms of pain relief. It inhibits reuptake of 5HT and noradrenaline. It inhibits noradrenaline uptake and enhances serotonin release.

Indications

Moderate to severe pain.

Dose

50–100mg IV every 4–6 hours.

Contraindications

See morphine, also epilepsy (p.146)

Side-effects

- Tramadol is claimed to be less likely to cause constipation and respiratory depression than other opioids
- Confusion, fits, and anaphylaxis
- Nausea.

Pre-hospital use of tramadol is not recommended.

Vecuronium

See pp.385–6.

Paediatric doses

Adrenaline INTRAMUSCULAR for anaphylaxis

- Under 6 years: 150μg, 0.15ml
- 6–12 years: 300μg, 0.3ml
- 12 years and over: 500μg, 0.5ml

Atropine

20μg/kg, maximum 600 μg

Benzyl penicillin

- Under 1: 300mg
- 1–9 years: 600mg
- 10 years and over: adult dose

Chlorpheniramine

- 1 month–1 year: 250 μg/kg
- 1–12 years: 200 μg/kg

  or

- 1–5 years: 2.5–5mg
- 6–12 years: 5mg

Diazepam

- Rectal—children over 10kg, 500μg/kg, maximum 20mg
- Intravenous
  - Neonate—12 years 300–400 μg/kg
  - 12–18 years 10–20mg

Glucagon

- Under 8 years (or under 25kg): 500μg
- Over 8 years (or over 25kg): 1mg

Hydrocortisone

- Up to 1 year: 25mg
- 1–5 years: 50mg
- 6–12 years: 100mg

Ibuprofen

- 3–6 months: 50mg (body weight over 5kg)
- 6 months–1 year: 50mg
- 1–4 years: 100mg
- 4–7 years: 150mg
- 7–10 years: 200mg
- 10–12 years: 300mg

Ketamine

As adult doses, by weight (See p.331)

Lignocaine

Local anaesthesia, 3mg/kg

Methionine

Child over six: 2.5g initially, followed by 3 further doses of 2.5g every 4 hours

Child under six: 1g initially, followed by 3 further doses of 1g every 4 hours

Midazolam (iv)

- 6 months–5 years: 50–100μg/kg initially
- 6–12 years: 25–50μg/kg, further increments as required

Morphine

- Up to 1 month: 37.5–75μg/kg
- 1–12 months: 50–100μg/kg
- 1–5 years: 1–2mg
- 6–12 years: 2–5mg

Naloxone

10μg/kg, subsequent dose of 100μg/kg if no response

Paracetamol

Orally

- 3 months–1 year: 60–120mg
- 1–5 years: 120–250mg
- 6–12 years: 250–500mg

These doses may be repeated every 4–6 hours, maximum 4 doses in 24 hours

Suppository

- 1–5 years: 125–250mg
- 6–12 years: 250–500mg
- Over 12 years: repeat dosing as above

Salbutamol

(Over 18 months: 2.5mg as nebulized solution) under 18 months: 1.25–2.5mg as nebulized solution

Chapter 5

Analgesia and anaesthesia

Overview

Pain management is an essential part of effective pre-hospital care, particularly in traumatic injury and acute myocardial infarction. In road traffic collisions, analgesia helps facilitate extrication as well as realignment and splintage of fractures. The provision of analgesia should be regarded as normal practice that requires careful patient assessment, appropriate analgesic selection, and careful monitoring of the patient for both clinical effectiveness and adverse reactions. The method and choice of analgesia will vary depending on the skills of the practitioner.

The International Association for the Study of Pain defines pain as '*an unpleasant sensory and emotional experience associated with actual or potential tissue damage or described in terms of such damage*'. Physical trauma results in the patient experiencing both physiological and psychological discomfort which is subject to individual variation and manifestations. The sequence of both physiological and psychological events may result in an increase in morbidity. Inadequate pain relief will result in a reactionary stress response which may include hyperglycaemia, increased levels of ADH and catecholamines, enhanced coagulation, and immunosuppression. The clinical manifestations may include tachycardia, hypoxia, hypertension, deep venous thrombosis and pulmonary embolism, fluid retention, and infection.

Routes of administration

Effective analgesia should be given as quickly and safely as possible. Known drug allergies and current medication should, if possible, be identified and any potential side-effects considered prior to drug administration. The routes available for analgesic administration are:

- Oral
- Nasal
- Sublingual
- Rectal
- Topical
- Subcutaneous
- Intramuscular
- Intravenous
- Intraosseous
- Inhalation.

Oral

The oral route has no use for the relief of pain following significant trauma where the onset is slow, nausea and vomiting common, and gastrointestinal motility decreased. In addition, some patients will have an altered level of consciousness. Simple oral analgesics may be prescribed for lesser trauma such as minor soft tissue injuries.

Nasal

Some lipid soluble opioids, including Fentanyl, may be given via the intranasal route with fairly rapid systemic effects. This route is currently used by some emergency departments and its pre-hospital use is being evaluated.

Sublingual

In sublingual administration, absorption bypasses the portal system leading to a rapid response and a more predictable efficacy. This route is being currently being evaluated (for example, fentanyl lollipops.)

Rectal

Unpredictable absorption, slow drug metabolism, and practical issues make this route unsuitable for the trauma patient and reduce its relevance in pre-hospital care.

Topical

This is not a route used in acute pain management. Analgesic patches are used for chronic pain relief.

Subcutaneous

An unpredictable response, especially in the shocked patient where cutaneous vasoconstriction will reduce absorption, makes this route unsuitable for acute use in pre-hospital care.

Intramuscular

As for the subcutaneous route, slow absorption and an unpredictable response makes the intramuscular route dangerous, especially if, due to poor response, additional analgesia is subsequently given, risking a depot effect. Once the circulation is restored, rapid absorption may lead to overdosage with catastrophic consequences. Intramuscular injections should also be avoided in patients who are taking anticoagulants.

Intravenous

The ability to gain intravenous access is a prerequisite and not an option for all pre-hospital personnel. It allows delivery of analgesia promptly, predictably, and in a controlled way, and is the preferred route for the patient with significant trauma.

Intraosseous

This is an effective route for drug and fluid administration in children, commonly using the tibial metaphysis. Adult intraosseous access using selected long bone metaphyseal sites or the sternum is becoming established in cases in which intravenous access cannot be obtained. Absorption is almost as quick as the intravenous route. Infusion is facilitated by bolus injection using a syringe and three-way tap.

Inhalation

Entonox is a potent analgesic gas consisting of a 50/50 mixture of nitrous oxide and oxygen. Administration relies on the co-operation and physical capability of the patient to inhale from a well-fitting facemask or mouthpiece. It provides effective short-term analgesia.

Being more soluble than nitrogen in plasma, it diffuses into air-filled cavities and will result in deterioration in patients with air in the cranial vault, pneumothorax, and bowel obstruction. Decompression sickness is an absolute contraindication for its use.

Route of choice

For most medical and paramedical personnel working in pre-hospital care, morphine given by the intravenous route is the gold standard. Ten milligrams of morphine made up with sterile water to ten millilitres and titrated to effect is a safe and effective way of providing pre-hospital analgesia. It must be remembered that the dose of opiate required to achieve comparable levels of analgesia may vary as much as ten times between individual patients.

Useful analgesics: opioids

An opioid is a naturally occurring or synthetic drug which will bind to and stimulate an opioid receptor. An opiate is a naturally occurring drug structurally related to opium alkaloids. There are several different types of opioid receptors—OP1 (formerly μ mμ), OP2 (formerly κ kappa), and OP3 (formerly δ delta). Opioids may function as receptor agonists, partial agonists, and antagonists.

- **Agonists**
  - Have affinity and intrinsic activity
  - Bind and stimulate opioid receptors
  - Produce a dose-related effect
  - Have differing efficacy.
- **Partial agonists**
  - Bind and stimulate opioid receptors
  - Are limited by a ceiling action (beyond a certain dose, further administration has no additional effect).
- **Antagonists**
  - Bind to opioid receptors and produce no clinical effect.

Examples of specific drug actions and their receptor activity include:

- **Morphine**
  - Pure agonist
  - Acts at OP1 receptor—stimulant
  - High efficacy.
- **Naloxone**
  - Antagonist
  - Acts at OP1 and OP2 receptors
  - Reverses respiratory depression and analgesic affects
  - Short half life compared with morphine/diamorphine.

Table 5.1 Opioid receptor activity in relation to drug administration

	OP1	OP2	OP3
Effects at receptor site	Analgesia Respiratory depression Miosis Nausea Bradycardia	Analgesia Miosis Dysphoria	Anti-analgesic Dysphoria Mydriasis Respiratory stimulation Tachycardia
Agonist	Morphine Diamorphine Pethidine		
Partial agonist		Nalbuphine	
Antagonists	Naloxone Nalbuphine		

Side-effects and contraindications

Opioids acting at the OP1 opioid receptors have similar side-effects in equianalgesic dosage. In all cases, hypovolaemia increases the risk of adverse events.

Potential problems include:

- Respiratory depression
- Decreased central ventilatory response to hypercapnia and hypoxia
- Depression of the cough reflex
- Bronchospasm
- Reduction of pain-driven sympathetic activity with improved cardiovascular stability
- Bradycardia and hypotension (in overdosage)
- Sedation, euphoria, and anxiolysis
- Miosis
- Decreased gut motility
- Nausea and vomiting.

Contraindications

Opioids are contraindicated in the following circumstances:

- Pre-existing respiratory depression (rate less than 10 breaths per minute).
- Raised intracranial pressure in non-ventilated patients where respiratory depression may lead to hypercapnia and worsening cerebral oedema.
- Status asthmaticus in non-ventilated patients.
- Where appropriate drugs and equipment for the management of overdosage are not available.

Opioids should be administered with caution in the presence of hypovolaema, altered level of consciousness, and liver and renal disease.

Carefully titrated opiate analgesia may improve respiratory function in patients with rib fractures or chronic obstructive pulmonary disease complicated by trauma. Analgesia should not be withheld in head-injured patients. However, care must be taken to avoid CO_2 retention which can occur with respiratory depression.

Individual opioids with the same mode of receptor activity will produce similar side-effects in equianalgesic doses. With each and every opioid, the drug should be administered slowly whilst observing the clinical response.

Diamorphine

Description

Opiate analgesic (heroin hydrochloride).

Presentation

Powder for reconstitution, 5mg and 10mg ampoules (larger dose ampoules are available) Onset is more rapid than morphine.

Effects

- Binds to opiate receptors resulting in analgesia, euphoria, and respiratory depression.
- Decreases pre- and after-load (central mechanism) and increases force of ventricular contraction and ejection fraction

Indications

- Acute pain, especially from myocardial infarction
- Acute pulmonary oedema.

Dose

Up to 5mg by slow iv injection (may be repeated).

Contraindications

- Acute respiratory depression
- Care in head injury.

Side-effects

Respiratory depression, nausea and vomiting, drowsiness, hypotension, tachycardia, pinpoint pupils

Notes

- Naloxone (Narcan®) must always be available if opiate analgesics are being used
- Duration of action 1–2 hours
- Nausea and vomiting is less troublesome than with morphine.

Fentanyl

Description

Extremely lipid-soluble, prompt-acting, potent synthetic opioid which is more potent than morphine. 100μg fentanyl and 10mg of morphine are equipotent.

Presentation

- 50μg/ml—2ml and 10ml ampoules for intravenous injection
- Also available as cutaneous patches for intractable cancer pain.

Effects

Rapid onset analgesia (within as little as 2 minutes).

Indications

Severe acute pain.

Dose

- By iv injection 50–200μg, then 50μg as required
- *Child*: 1–5μg/kg, then 1μg/kg as required.

Contraindications

See morphine.

Side-effects

- See morphine
- May produce bradycardia of vagal origin, but maintaining blood pressure and cardiac output.

Notes

- Duration of action 30–60 minutes
- May be given nasally in the same dose.

Morphine

Description

An opiate analgesic.

Presentation

- Morphine sulphate 10mg/ml, 15mg/ml, 20mg/ml, and 30mg/ml—1ml and 2ml ampoules
- Morphine sulphate 10mg/ml—1ml pre-filled syringe
- Morphine sulphate 1mg/ml—10ml pre-filled syringe
- Larger-volume vials are available but are intended for intravenous infusion preparation.

Effects

Binds to opiate receptors resulting in analgesia, euphoria, and respiratory depression.

Indications

Acute severe pain.

Dose

Morphine should be given by intravenous injection in small aliquots titrated to effect. An initial dose of 5mg is appropriate for an adult male, 2mg for smaller or older patients. Doses of up to 30mg may be required in fit young men with severe pain.
Children: Child 100 μg/kg; 12–18 years 2.5 mg

Contraindications

Acute respiratory depression.

Side-effects

Nausea and vomiting, drowsiness, respiratory depression, hypotension, hallucinations. Acute allergic reactions.

Notes

The labelling on ampoules of proprietary morphine is identical except for the concentration. It is imperative that this is carefully checked if dosing errors are to be avoided. Morphine should always be administered in a concentration of 1mg in 1ml (10mg in 10ml).

An antiemetic should be administered with any intravenous opiate. However, the use of Cyclimorph® (morphine/cyclizine) is not recommended.

Naloxone and equipment for mechanical ventilatory support MUST be available when morphine (or any other opiate) is administered.

Morphine has a duration of action of about 2 hours.

Pethidine

Description

Synthetic opioid with a shorter duration of action than morphine.

Presentation

- 50mg/ml in 1ml and 2ml ampoules for injection
- 10mg/ml in 5ml and 10ml ampoules
- Oral pethidine is not suitable for pre-hospital use.

Effects

- Analgesia
- Obstetric analgesia (pethidine does not delay labour)
- Atropine like effects—blurred vision, dry mouth.

Indications

- Moderate pain
- Obstetric pain.

Dose

- 20–50mg by slow iv injection
- 50–100mg sc or im for obstetric analgesia.

Contraindications

- Patients taking monoamine oxidase inhibitors
- Acute respiratory depression
- Care in head injury

Side-effects

- See morphine
- There is no evidence to suggest that pethidine has less effect than morphine on the sphincter of Oddi

Notes

- Onset within 10 minutes; duration of action 1–2 hours
- Pethidine is associated with a greater risk of hypotension because of its alpha blockade, it is NOT RECOMMENDED for pre-hospital use.

Tramadol

Description

A synthetic opiate with additional actions (see below). It is a non-selective OP1 and OP3 receptor agonist, acting mainly at the OP1 receptor.

Presentation

Tramadol hydrochloride 50mg/ml—2ml ampoule.

Effects

Tramadol has opioid and non-opioid mechanisms of pain relief. It inhibits reuptake of 5HT and noradrenaline. It inhibits noradrenaline uptake and enhances serotonin release.

Indications

Moderate to severe pain.

Dose

50–100mg iv every 4–6 hours.

Contraindications

See morphine, also epilepsy.

Side-effects

- Tramadol is claimed to be less likely to cause constipation and respiratory depression than other opioids
- Confusion, fits, and anaphylaxis
- Nausea

Pre-hospital use of tramadol is not recommended.

Naloxone

Description

A competitive opiate antagonist. Time to onset 2–3 minutes. Duration of action 20 minutes.

Presentation

- 400μg/ml—1ml ampoule
- 400μg/ml—1ml, 2ml, and 5ml pre-filled syringe
- 1mg/ml—2ml pre-filled syringe

Effects

Reversal of opioid effects.

Indications

- Reversal of therapeutic overdose of opiates
- Treatment of opiate poisoning (recreational overdose)
- Treatment of unexplained loss/reduction of consciousness.

Dose

- 0.4mg (400μg)–2mg repeated at intervals, as required, to a maximum of 10mg
- If naloxone is given to exclude opiates as a cause of loss of consciousness, a dose of 10mg should be given
- *Children:* iv 10μg/kg, subsequent dose of 100μg/kg if no response.

Contraindications

Caution in patients who are physically dependant on opiates; will precipitate pain in patients given opiate for analgesia.

Side-effects

Nausea and vomiting, tachycardia.

Notes

Naloxone is short acting. As a result, when long-acting opiates are being reversed, repeated doses may be needed. Drug abusers may leave the scene after a first dose only to collapse as the naloxone wears off. In order to reduce the likelihood off this, either the opiate can be reversed only enough to ensure adequacy of respiration before arrival in hospital, or a similar dose to the intravenous one given above may be given INTRAMUSCULARLY in addition.

Sudden reversal of opioid overdosage in opioid-dependant patients can produce cardiac arrhythmias, hypotension, and convulsions.

Treatment of opiate overdosage

Opioid overdosage may be absolute (excessive administration) or relative (normal dosage given to compromised patients, commonly hypovolaemic producing excessive plasma levels). The clinical features are:

- Sedation
- Respiratory depression
- Miosis

Untreated, overdosage may lead to:

- Respiratory arrest
- Cardiac arrest

Treatments include standard ABC management:

- Securing the airway
- Supplementary oxygen
- Supporting ventilation
- Intravenous access
- Reversal with Naloxone.

Antiemetics

Nausea and vomiting are common following opioid administration. Most practitioners give an antiemetic proceeding opioid administration. Symptoms are due to stimulation of the chemoreceptor trigger zone in the fourth ventricle or direct stimulation of the vomiting centre in the medulla oblongata or the vestibule.

For more details, see Chapter 4 (Formulary):

- Cyclizine, p.319
- Metoclopramide, p.335
- Ondansetron, p.341.

Other analgesics

Mild to moderate pain may be managed by paracetamol and non-steroidal anti-inflammatory drugs (NSAID). Pre-hospital usage may be limited by the route of administration and the adequacy of pain relief.

Aspirin, see p.312
Paracetamol, see p.345
Ibuprofen, see p.330
Voltarol, see p.323
Compound analgesics, see p.318

Nitrous oxide/oxygen 50:50 (Entonox)

Description

Entonox is a 50:50 mixture of oxygen and nitrous oxide (N_2O). Nitrous oxide is a colourless, sweet-smelling, non-irritant, non-inflammable gas. It is insoluble in blood, hence its rapid clinical effect, and 15 times more soluble than nitrogen in plasma.

Presentation

Various sizes of blue cylinder with a white and blue mantle. Self administered with override valve.

Effects

Analgesia without loss of consciousness.

Indications

- Analgesia for moderate pain in fully conscious individuals
- Analgesia for short painful procedures
- Rapid onset within 60 seconds, analgesic effect for 3–4 minutes.

Dose

Titrate to effect. Usually self administered using a demand valve. May be overridden by medical staff. Overdosage does not occur with self admin istration.

Contraindications

Contraindicated in patients in whom an air-filled cavity exists into which nitrous oxide can diffuse. These conditions include pneumothorax (so contraindicated in significant chest injury), the 'bends' (so contraindicated in patients following diving), and open head injuries.

Side-effects

See above.

Notes

At temperatures less than –7°C, nitrous oxide/oxygen mixtures will separate. This may lead to inhalation of pure oxygen, with no analgesic effect, followed by pure nitrous oxide leading to hypoxia. A few shakes of the cylinder will have no effect, on this separation. Entonox MUST be kept above –7°C, even if this means transferring it to your vehicle immediately before departure.

Ketamine

Description

A dissociative anaesthetic/analgesic in the form of a white crystalloid powder

Presentation

- 10mg/ml—20ml vial for injection
- 100mg/ml—10ml vial for injection.

Effects

Ketamine has the following features:

- It is powerfully analgesic in subanaesthetic doses
- Protective glottal reflexes are relatively preserved
- It does not normally cause respiratory depression at conventional doses
- It has a long shelf life
- It does not cause hypotension, but ketamine-induced hypertension makes it relatively contraindicated in head injury
- It is relatively safe in patients with a full stomach.

Indications

- Pre-hospital anaesthesia for extrication or short procedures
- Analgesia.

Dose

Anaesthesia: im 5–10mg/kg (provides 12–25 min of surgical anaesthesia, effective after 4–15 min)

Iv 1–2mg/kg (provides 5–10 min of surgical anaesthesia, effective after 2–7 min)

Analgesia: ketamine is an effective analgesic when used in subanaesthetic doses by either the intramuscular or iv route

Repeat doses may be given as 10–20mg iv or 20–50mg im

Children: as above

Contraindications

- Hypertension (including pre-eclampsia)
- Head injury (relative, but consider clinical priorities)

Side-effects

- A significant proportion of patients suffer emergence hallucinations which can be very distressing. As a consequence, a benzodiazepine should also be administered to oblate these symptoms.
- Tachycardia and hypertension (sympathomimetic effects)
- Mild respiratory stimulation and bronchodilatation
- Cerebral blood flow and intracranial pressure may both be increased
- Increased salivation in children

Note

Analgesia may also be achieved using other routes for ketamine administration including:

- Intramuscular 1–4mg/kg
- Orally 5–10mg/kg
- Intranasally 6–8mg/kg

Oral or intranasal administration is not recommended.

The authors prefer to use the preparation 10mg/kg. Carrying three preparations of different strengths risks confusion, particularly if used in a dark, badly lit environment.

Anaesthesia

Introduction

The administration of drugs to facilitate intubation (rapid sequence induction—RSI) should only be undertaken by skilled emergency care practitioners (usually doctors in the UK) who have undergone the necessary training, have the clinical competency, have access to practice the skill, and appropriate clinical indemnity. This procedure should not be undertaken by anybody who does not fulfil these criteria.

The administration and maintenance of a general anaesthetic requires three groups of drugs:

- Intravenous anaesthetic agents to achieve unconsciousness
- Opioid analgesics for the provision of pain relief and to modify the stress response to intubation
- Muscle relaxants or neuromuscular blocking agents which decrease or abolish muscle tone

Before considering sedation or anaesthesia, especially in a combative or restless patient, it is essential to seek and correct:

- Hypoxia
- Hypovolaemia
- Hypoglycaemia

Drug abuse, alcohol, and head injury additionally make the management of these patients hazardous.

Intravenous anaesthetic agents

Unconsciousness is usually achieved rapidly and by one arm to brain circulation time. Consciousness will be regained after bolus injection, unless maintenance anaesthetic agents are administered. Drug dosage should be reduced in the hypovolaemic patient and the elderly.

Etomidate is probably the safest induction agent for use in pre-hospital care since it is more cardiovascularly stable. In addition, it reduces cerebral oxygen requirement which may have benefit in patients with raised intracranial pressure. The drug profiles of other potent anaesthetic agents are detailed below. Ketamine may be the drug of choice in hypovolaemic/hypotensive patients who are combative or difficult to assess since ketamine administration is associated with an increase in blood pressure alone of all the intravenous induction agents.

Etomidate

Description

A carboxylated imidazole anaesthetic induction agent.

Presentation

2mg/ml—10ml ampoule for intravenous injection.

Effects

Induction of anaesthesia

Indications

Anaesthesia for:

- Intubation
- Analgesia
- Extrication
- Surgical procedures

Etomidate causes less hypotension than other commonly used induction agents and is, therefore, probably the drug of choice in trauma.

Dose

Adults and children, 150–300μg/kg

Contraindications

None.

Side-effects

- Pain on injection (use a large vein, lessened by simultaneous administration of an opiate)
- Involuntary movements (lessened by simultaneous administration of an opiate or benzodiazepine)
- Nausea and vomiting (20% of cases).

Notes

The major benefit of etomidate is its cardiovascular stability. It is not suitable for continuous infusion due to its potential to induce adrenocortical function.

Propofol

Description

A general anaesthetic induction agent.

Presentation

- Propofol is presented as an emulsion.
- 1% propofol (10mg/ml)—20ml ampoule for IV injection/infusion (1% propofol is also available in 50ml bottles, 50ml pre-filled syringes, and 100ml bottles. 2% propofol (20mg/ml) is available in 50ml vials for IV infusion.)
- Only one concentration of propofol should be carried and the 1% is recommended.

Effects

- Induction and maintenance of anaesthesia
- Anticonvulsant activity.

Indications

Anaesthesia for:
- Intubation
- Analgesia
- Extrication
- Surgical procedures

Control of status epilepticus (after other methods have failed)

Dose

Induction of anaesthesia

1.5–2.5mg/kg (reduce dose in the over 55s)

Child: administer slowly until anaesthesia achieved—over 8 years, usually 2.5mg/kg; under 8 years may need as much as 4mg/kg

Maintenance of anaesthesia

Intermittent doses of 25–50mg or by iv infusion 4–12mg/kg/hr

Child: (over 3 years) 9–15mg/kg/hr

Contraindications

Hypotension.

Side-effects

- Hypotension
- Nausea and vomiting (less common than with etomidate)
- Pain on injection (may be avoided by adding 20mg of lignocaine to the propofol ampoule)
- Transient apnoea on induction if injection is too rapid.

Notes

Induction of anaesthesia occurs within 30 seconds of injection.

Thiopentone

Description

A short-acting barbiturate anaesthetic agent.

Presentation

Powder for reconstitution, 500mg vial.

Effects

- Induction and maintenance of anaesthesia
- Anticonvulsant activity.

Indications

Anaesthesia for:

- Intubation
- Analgesia
- Extrication
- Surgical procedures.

Control of status epilepticus (after other methods have failed).

Dose

Induction of anaesthesia

25mg/ml solution, 100–150mg over 10–15 seconds (reduce dose and slower injection in elderly or debilitated); further bolus as necessary, after 30–60 seconds or up to 4mg/kg

Child: up to 4mg/kg then 1mg/kg as required

Raised intracranial pressure, 1.5–3mg/kg repeated as required

Contraindications

Porphyria

Side-effects

- Hypotension
- Reduced respiratory rate and tidal volume
- Reduced cerebral blood flow and intracranial pressure
- Local tissue damage secondary to extravasation.

Notes

Induction of anaesthesia is rapid but a long half life means that effects may persist for up to 24 hours

Ketamine

See p.331

Muscle relaxants (neuromuscular blocking agents)

These drugs facilitate endotracheal intubation by abolishing muscle tone and protective laryngeal reflexes. They can be divided into two types, depolarizing and non-depolarizing agents.

Depolarizing muscle relaxants: suxamethonium (succinylcholine)

Description
A depolarizing neuromuscular blocker.

Presentation
Suxamethonium chloride 50mg/ml—2ml ampoule for iv injection.

Effects
Neuromuscular blockade.

Indications
Endotracheal intubation, especially in rapid sequence induction.

Dose

- *Intravenous*
  - Initial dose 1mg/kg
  - Subsequent doses 0.5–1mg/kg at 5–10 minute intervals
  - Neonate and infant 2mg/kg, child 1mg/kg
- *Intramuscular*
  - Infant up to 4–5 mg/kg, child up to 4mg/kg, maximum 150mg
  - Suxamethonium is the most rapidly acting neuromuscular blocker (30–45 seconds), its effectiveness manifest by twitching or fasciculation. Recovery occurs in 3–5 minutes. Total paralysis lasts approximately 4 minutes.

Contraindications

- Family history of malignant hyperthermia
- Low cholinesterase activity (1 in 3000 Europeans have a reduced ability to break down suxamethonium)
- Suxemethonium may precipitate potassium release and fatal cardiac arrest with delayed administration post injury in patients with spinal cord or brain injury or in any other patient with pre-existing muscular dystrophy. Use immediately after injury is not associated with these problems.

Side-effects

- Bradycardia with repeated use
- Raised intracranial pressure
- Malignant hyperpyrexia
- Muscle pain after use.

Notes
Suxamethonium is the muscle relaxant of choice in the trauma patient. It does not cross the placenta.

Non-depolarizing muscle relaxants

Description

Non-depolarizing neuromuscular blockers which compete with acetylcholine for receptor sites at the neuromuscular junction

Presentation

Atracurium

Atracurium besylate 10mg/ml–2.5, 5ml and 25ml, ampoules for injection

Rocuronium

Rocuronium bromide 10mg/ml—5ml and 10ml ampoules for injection

Vecuronium

Vecuronium bromide powder for reconstitution—10mg vial for injection with water

Pancuronium

Pancuronium bromide 2mg/ml—2ml ampoule for injections

Effects

Neuromuscular blockade

Indications

Paralysis at induction and during maintenance of anaesthesia
Rocuronium is more suitable for intubation cover (see durations of action, below); atracurium is appropriate for maintenance of paralysis

Dose

Atracurium (adult and child)
Intubation: 300–600μg/kg by iv injection
Maintenance: 100–200μg/kg iv as required

Rocuronium (adult and child over 1 month)
Intubation: 600μg/kg by iv injection
Maintenance: 150μg/kg iv (elderly 75–100μg/kg iv) as required

Vecuronium
Intubation: 80–100μg/kg by iv injection
Maintenance: 20–30μg/kg iv as required
Child: up to 4 months 10–20μg with further doses as required to achieve effect; over 5 months, as adult, reduced dose may be needed for intubation

Pancuronium
Intubation: 50–100μg/kg by iv injection
Maintenance: 10–20μg iv as required
Child: intubation 60–100μg/kg iv, maintenance 10–20μg/kg iv as required
Neonate: 30–40μg/kg then 10–20μg/kg

Contraindications
Use will be more prolonged in patients with myasthenia gravis and in hypothermia. Lower doses should, therefore, be used.

Side-effects
- Histamine release (atracurium, pancuronium)
- Tachycardia and hypertension (pancuronium).

Notes
Atracurium is the most commonly used competitive neuromuscular blocker in the UK

Durations of action
- *Atracurium*: effective within 90–120 seconds, duration 30–40 minutes
- *Rocuronium*: effective after approximately 60–120 seconds, duration 30–45 minutes
- *Vecuronium:* effective after approximately 3 minutes, duration 25–40 minutes
- *Pancuronium:* effective after 2–3 minutes, duration 65–100 minutes

Non-depolarizing muscle relaxants can be reversed with anticholinesterases such as neostigmine. Because anticholinesterases act at para-sympathetic endings as well as neuromuscular junctions, a parasympatholytic drug, such as atropine, shoud be administered to prevent bradycardia and increased bronchial secretions.

Rapid sequence induction (RSI)

The decision to undertake RSI depends on the clinical competencies of the attending team. In most patients, the airway can be managed in a stepwise fashion and adequate ventilation achieved using a two-person bag-valve-mask technique until arrival in hospital.

The indications for RSI in the pre-hospital arena are:

- Airway protection in acute or impending airway obstruction (for example, unconsciousness, facial burns)
- Failure to oxygenate the patient by any other measures (for example massive flail chest.
- To control and optimize ventilation in head injury patients. It is desirable to aim for low normal pCO_2 though this is not routinely measured in the pre-hospital environment.
- To control the aggressive or agitated patient
- To control status epilepticus when other measures have failed

RSI involves securing the airway by the use of therapeutic agents and endotracheal intubation. Many trauma patients have a full stomach or decreased gastric emptying. RSI is designed to minimize the risks of pulmonary aspiration. Ideally, full RSI requires four operators:

- One person to intubate
- One person to provide in-line stabilization of the neck
- One person to provide cricoid pressure
- One person to administer drugs and intravenous fluids

The stages of RSI can be summarized as:

- Preparation
- Pre-oxygenation
- Induction and cricoid pressure
- Intubation
- Confirmation of endotracheal placement
- Failed intubation drills.

Preparation

- All appropriate kit should be tested and immediately to hand, laid out in a systematic way.
- Alternative equipment (for example, LMA, needle or surgical airways) should be available in the event of failure to intubate.
- All drugs should be drawn up and labelled ready for use.

Pre-oxygenation

- 12–15 litres of oxygen using a non-rebreathe mask with reservoir bag should be administered.
- If ventilation is inadequate, the patient should receive pre-oxygenation using the two-person bag-valve-mask technique.
- Simple airway adjuncts such as the oropharyngeal or nasopharyngeal airway may help facilitate pre-oxygenation.

Induction

- Induction of anaesthesia is achieved using an intravenous induction agent given rapidly without titration.
- As the induction agent is given, cricoid pressure is applied (see below).
- A neuromuscular blocker (usually suxamethonium 100mg) is given immediately after the induction agent.

In hypovolaemic/hypotensive patients, the use of ketamine or suxamethonium in isolation should be considered, adding drugs for sedation later.

Cricoid pressure (Sellicks manoeuvre)

- Cricoid pressure is applied as soon as the induction agent is given to reduce the risk of regurgitation and aspiration.
- Cricoid pressure should only be released when directed to do so by the intubator once the cuff is inflated.

Intubation

- Manual in-line stabilization of the cervical spine replaces cervical collars and supporting head blocks and straps.
- Intubation is performed as soon as the muscle relaxant has worked (following muscular twitching if suxamethonium is used).
- Prolonged attempts at intubation must be avoided, returning to bag-valve-mask ventilation.
- Longer-acting non-depolarizing drugs should be drawn up and given after successful intubation.

A McCoy laryngoscope (straight blade) is preferred by many practitioners. Unless there is a complete view of the whole laryngeal inlet, intubation should be facilitated using a gum elastic bougie.

Confirmation of endotracheal placement

Placement should be confirmed by:

- Auscultation over both axillae and stomach
- End tidal CO_2
- Observation of the patient's chest

Failed intubation

- If there is any doubt about tube placement, it should be withdrawn and the patient ventilated using a two-person bag-valve-mask technique.
- Following re-oxygenation, further attempts can be undertaken.
- If unsuccessful, alternative techniques include the use of the laryngeal mask airway (LMA) or intubating laryngeal mask airway (ILMA).
- As a last resort, a needle or surgical cricothyroidotomy (cannot intubate, cannot ventilate) should be undertaken.

Those practitioners with RSI competence must be able to undertake a surgical airway.

Local anaesthesia

An effective local anaesthetic block can produce quality analgesia without sedation, nausea and vomiting, or depression of respiration. In excess, or used inappropriately, their use can have a fatal outcome.

Pharmacology

Local anaesthetic drugs reversibly interrupt axonal conduction by blocking sodium channels. Their potency is related to lipid solubility and the speed of action is inversely proportional to their degree of ionization. The duration of action is related to protein binding and the degree of local vasoconstriction. Many local anaesthetics act as vasodilators and efficacy can be enhanced by the addition of adrenaline as a vasoconstrictor. Adrenaline must be avoided near any end artery. The periphery of a nerve is blocked before its centre part. Therefore, the time to anaesthesia is significantly shorter for small nerves such as digital nerves than larger nerves (for example, the femoral nerve).

Complications of local anaesthesia: toxicity

Toxicity may be absolute, when too much is administered, or relative, when the correct amount has been injected intravascularly or into a highly vascular area leading to systemic absorption. Toxicity can be avoided by ensuring there is no aspiration of blood prior to injection and by careful dosage calculation.

The features of local anaesthetic toxicity are:

- Perioral numbness with a metallic taste
- Light headedness
- Tinnitis
- Visual disturbances
- Slurring of speech
- Muscle twitching and convulsions
- Coma
- Hypotension and bradycardia
- Ventricular arrythmias
- Apnoea
- Cardiac arrest.

The speed of onset will depend on the mechanism of the toxicity—clinical features of toxicity will occur within two minutes of intravenous injection whereas it may take 30 minutes for the clinical features to develop following an absolute overdosage.

Treatment

- Stop injecting the local anaesthetic
- Assess and manage the airway
- Assess and ensure adequate ventilation
- Administer 12–15 litres of oxygen via a non-rebreathe mask and oxygen reservoir
- Obtain vascular access (if not already in place)
- Obtain baseline observations and monitor frequently
- Treat convulsions with diazemuls (see p.146)
- Treat hypotension by leg elevation and bolus fluid therapy.

- Treat life-threatening symptomatic cardiac arrhythmias (cardiac pacing may be required)
- Consider bretylium for refractory ventricular fibrillation.

Hypersensitivity reactions

Anaphylactic and anaphylactoid reactions are rare. Treatment follows conventional guidelines.

Nerve damage

Nerves may be traumatized by sharp needles. In conscious patients, injections must be stopped if the patient complains of local severe pain or pain in the distribution of the relevant nerve. As there is no feedback in the unconscious patient, nerve blocks should be avoided.

Altered clinical assessments

An effective local block will compromise patient assessment. It is essential to complete neurological assessment and assessment for compartment syndrome in the relevant areas prior to local block administration.

Local anaesthetic agents

Lignocaine (lidocaine)

See also p.332.

Description

Class Ib anti-arrhythmic and local anaesthetic.

Presentation for local anaesthesia

- Lignocaine hydrochloride 1% (10mg/ml)—2ml, 5ml, and 10ml ampoules for injection
- Lignocaine hydrochloride 2% (20mg/ml)—2ml and 5ml ampoules for injection.

Effects

Lignocaine blocks sodium channels, reducing the conduction rate and amplitude of nerve electrical impulses.

Indications

Local anaesthesia for painful procedures.

Dose

A MAXIMUM safe lignocaine dose for an average adult is 20ml of 1% (200mg) or equivalent volume of higher concentration solution. This dose can be increased if lignocaine is given with a vasoconstrictor such as adrenaline. Use of lignocaine with adrenaline may cause gangrene if injected into digits or appendages and is NOT RECOMMENDED in pre-hospital care.

Children (local anaesthesia): 3mg/kg

Contraindications

- Local analgesia: hypovolaemia, complete heart block
- Solutions with adrenaline: see notes below.

Side-effects

- Light headedness followed by sedation, circumoral paraesthesia, and twitching; convulsions in severe cases
- Convulsions and cardiovascular collapse on intravenous administration.

Notes

0.5% lignocaine is available for local anaesthetic use. It is not recommended in the pre-hospital environment.

Prilocaine

Prilocaine has a similar profile to lignocaine but is slightly less toxic.

Dose (adult)

- Infiltration: 0.5% up to 80ml
- Nerve block: 1% up to 40ml, 2% up to 20ml.

Duration of effect

1.5–3 hours.

Bupivicaine

A longer-acting local anaesthetic usually used for nerve blocks. Bupivacaine is more toxic than lignocaine.

Dose (adult)

- Infiltration: 0.25% up to 60ml
- Nerve block: 0.25% up to 60ml, 0.5% up to 30ml.

Duration of effect

3–4 hours.

Local anaesthetic blocks

Wound blockade

Faced with a painful wound, restricted analgesics, and a long transfer time to hospital, local anaesthetics can be instilled into the wound or injected into the sides of the wound for symptomatic relief.

Specific blocks

Before performing a specific block, the procedure should be explained to the patient and consent obtained. Monitoring and intravenous access must be in place.

Axillary blocks, *wrist blocks* (ulnar, median, and superficial branches of the radial nerve), *triple blocks* (femoral sciatic and obturator nerves), and *foot* and *ankle blocks* (saphenous, tibial, deep peroneal, superficial peroneal, and sural nerve) are all specialist blocks and are not commonly practised in pre-hospital care unless by experienced trained personnel in special circumstances.

Two blocks in common use, however, are the femoral nerve block and the metacarpal block.

Femoral nerve block

The femoral nerve block produces analgesia and anaesthesia in the anterior thigh, femur, and hip region.

- Place the patient supine with the hip abducted and slightly externally rotated (hip flexion risks inadvertent vascular puncture)
- The key landmark is the femoral artery as it emerges below the inguinal ligament
- From medial to lateral, the essential anatomy is vein, artery, nerve
- Insert a needle approximately 1cm lateral to the artery aiming in a cranial direction at a depth of 2–3.5cm
- Aspirate to exclude vascular puncture and inject at this point
- Instil 10–15ml of 1% lignocaine or prilocaine

The time to onset of a femoral nerve block is 15–30minutes with a duration of effect of 4–6 hours.

Metacarpal digital nerve blocks

The digital nerves lie parallel to the long axis of the metacarpal bones at the level of the distal palmar crease at a depth of 0.5–1.0cm.

- Insert a 23g needle at the appropriate site and depth
- Exclude vascular puncture
- Instil 3–5ml of 1% lignocaine or prilocaine

The time to onset of action is 3–5minutes with a duration of action of 45–60 minutes. Vasoconstrictors should NEVER be used at this site.

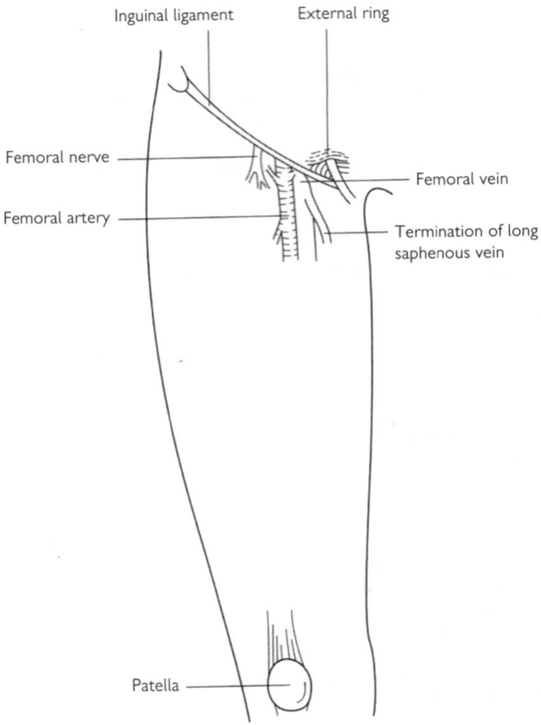

Fig. 5.1 The femoral nerve block. Reprinted with permission from Greaves I *et al.* (2000). *Trauma care*. Hodder Arnold.

Poisoning and substance abuse

Approach to the poisoned patient

In many cases, the toxic agent will not be known and when it is, options for specific treatment are usually limited. Only a very few antidotes are available for pre-hospital use (see pp.406–7). As a consequence, a generic approach to the poisoned patient is essential. This will follow the ABCDE sequence:

- **A**irway (with C spine control if there is any possibility of significant trauma)
- **B**reathing—with high-flow oxygenation
- **C**irculation
  - Establish intravenous access
  - Monitor pulse, BP, SaO_2, and ECG
- **D**isability—establish and record the conscious level using AVPU and **DON'T FORGET TO CHECK THE PUPILS!**
- **E**xposure—as required to exclude other significant injury

Airway

A patent airway should be established and maintained at all tines. The technique used will vary according to the patient's level of consciousness. **If the conscious level is reduced, an oral or nasopharyngeal airway can be inserted.** Intubation may be necessary. Many patients will also have taken alcohol and will, therefore, be prone to vomit. Appropriate use should be made of the recovery position and working suction MUST be available.

Breathing

High-flow oxygen should be administered and respiration supported as required.

Circulation

Intravenous access should be obtained in all but the most trivial of poisonings. This must not delay transfer of the critical patient. Inadequate circulation may result from a wide range of mechanisms. Wherever possible, arrythmias should be treated in hospital and rapid evacuation is essential. The arrythmias associated with tricyclic antidepressants respond to alkalinization with sodium bicarbonate. If there is no sign of arrythmia or heart failure, judicious administration of intravenous fluids can be used to raise the blood pressure. Pulse oximetry, ECG monitoring, and blood pressure monitoring should be routine.

Disability

Check AVPU (p.187) and pupils.

Assessment of the pupils may provide vital information. Pin point pupils are characteristic of opiate poisoning but also occur in organophosphate poisoning (the context may aid in diagnosis). Dilated pupils occur in the anticholinergic syndrome associated with overdose of atropine, tricyclic antidepressants and other agents. Assessment of the AVPU response will determine the depth of reduction of conscious level.

Dilated pupils

- Atropine
- Tricyclic antidepressants
- Phenothiazines.

Constricted pupils

- Opiates
- Organophosphates.

Exposure

Exclude or identify injuries due to the overdose or alcohol.

Complete exposure of the patient should be avoided in the pre-hospital environment and an exhaustive (and probably fruitless) search for clues should not delay transfer to hospital as long as appropriate attention has been paid to airway and breathing. Nevertheless, some clues such as needle marks from intravenous injection, sores around the mouth (from inhalation of chemicals) or burns from caustic substances may be identified.

Further information

In most cases, time need not be wasted seeking specialist advice. This can be done after arrival in hospital. If transfer is likely to be prolonged or delayed, or the poisoning appears trivial, advice can be sought from the UK National Poisons Advice Centre (see box).

DON'T EVER FORGET GLUCOSE

UK National Poisons Advice Centre
0870 600 6266
They will direct the call to the relevant local centre

Differential diagnosis of the poisoned patient

In many cases, it will be obvious that a patient has been poisoned, and questioning the patient or witnesses, or scene assessment will rapidly confirm this. However, patients with serious suicidal intentions may go to considerable lengths to hide what they have done, or if the patient is unconscious, the clues may be more subtle. A high index of suspicion is therefore essential. In addition, in some cases, the poison may be unknown or more than one substance may be involved. Mixed overdoses are far from uncommon, and industrial poisonings more often than not involve multiple chemicals which may further react with each other to complicate the clinical picture.

Poisoning should be suspected if:

- The patient's conscious level is altered
- Symptoms occur in an unusual age group
- The context suggests prevalence of drug abuse
- Bizarre symptom complexes or signs are present
- There is obvious reluctance to provide information.

Because the symptoms and signs of poisoning are so varied, and in the majority of cases non-specific, it is equally important not to jump to the conclusion that a patient has been poisoned and to exclude other potentially treatable causes.

Diagnoses which should be excluded include:

Metabolic

- Hypoxia
- Hypoglycaemia
- Electrolyte abnormality.

Traumatic

- Head injury
- Hypotension due to haemorrhage.

Neurological

- Stroke
- Subarachnoid haemorrhage
- Post-ictal state.

CHECK FOR

- Pill bottles and medicine containers (take them to hospital)
- Signs of alcohol consumption
- Medic-Alert® bracelet
- Injection marks
- Paraphernalia of drug abuse
- Signs of previous self harm
- Suicide note (rare).

Symptom complexes in poisoning

There are a number of symptoms or groups of symptoms which together provide useful clues to the likely causative agent.

A list of drugs and common recognizable presentations is given below and in Table 6.1:

Coma with stable vital signs

- Benzodiazepines

Hyperthermia

- Anticholinergics
- Neuroleptics (major tranquillizers/antipsychotics)
- Sympathomimetics
- Phencyclidine and hallucinogens
- Aspirin.

Hypothermia

- Sedatives, opiates, alcohol (reduce CNS activity)
- Insulin and oral hypoglycaemics.

Hypotension with normal mental state

- Calcium channel blockers.

Tachypnoea

- CNS stimulants
- Aspirin
- β agonists
- Agents causing pulmonary oedema—including organophosphates, chlorine
- Agents causing hypoxia—including cyanide, carbon monoxide
- Agents causing metabolic acidosis—including methanol, ethylene glycol.

Dilated pupils

- Tricyclic antidepressants
- Amphetamines (see p.463)
- Phenothiazines.

Constricted pupils

- Opiates
- Organophosphates.

In many cases it will not be possible to identify the agent precisely, so:

TREAT THE PATIENT, NOT THE DRUG

Table 6.1 Common recognizable presentations

Syndrome	Causes	Symptoms	Signs	Comments
Opioid	Opiates	Confusion	Reduced conscious level Pinpoint pupils Respiratory depression Hypotension	Responds to naloxone
Cholinergic	Organophosphates	Sweating, salivation, blurred vision, vomiting, wheeze, diarrhoea, muscle cramp	Tachycardia, hypo/hypertension, fasciculation, paralysis, respiratory failure, ataxia, fits, coma	
Anticholinergic	Atropine Tricyclic antidepressants Phenothiazines	Lethargy, confusion, hallucinations, fits, blurred vision, urinary retention, dry mouth, flushing	Ataxia, cardiac failure, respiratory failure, dry skin, dilated pupils, abdominal distension	
Sympathomimetic	Aminophylline Cocaine Amphetamine, Caffeine Phencyclidine	Excitation	Fits Tachycardia Hypertension	
Benzo diazepine	Diazepam Temazepam	Coma	Vital signs normally stable Hypotension and respiratory depression can occur	

Decontamination

Decontamination is only very rarely necessary in the pre-hospital environment but the following steps should always be followed:

- Remove the patient from the contaminated area (or seek fire brigade assistance)
- Remove contaminated clothing
- Use copious lavage to remove skin or eye contamination
- Keep the patient warm
- Provide necessary resuscitation
- DO NOT DELAY removal to hospital.

Gastric lavage should never be attempted pre-hospital. Similarly, there is no role for routine use of emetics (ipecacuanha) either in children or adults. Where there is concern because of very prolonged transfer times or unavoidable delays, advice should be sought on a case-specific basis from the nearest poisons unit, A&E or receiving department.

Activated charcoal (50g in an adult po) is appropriate in some overdoses or poisonings, as indicated in the text. It is recognized, however, that many immediate care practitioners will not carry activated charcoal and that many patients will not tolerate drinking it. Needless to say, charcoal can only be given if the patient is able to protect their own airway.

Antidotes

The majority of specific antidotes are only available in hospital and, in some cases, from specialist centres. There are, however, a number which have a valuable pre-hospital role.

Flumazenil

Flumazenil is a highly effective competitive antagonist to benzodiazepines. However, its use has been associated with serious complications including fits in those who have also taken drugs which cause fits (in whom the benzodiazepine is controlling epileptic activity). Flumazenil may also precipitate acute withdrawal in chronic benzodiazepine users. **It cannot therefore be recommended for pre-hospital use.** If respiratory depression occurs as a result of benzodiazepine overdose, the airway should be protected and ventilation supported (with monitoring) and the patient transferred rapidly to hospital.

Glucagon

Glucagon is used in beta blocker overdose for those patients who do not respond to atropine. The initial dose is up to 5mg iv followed, if necessary, by an intravenous infusion in hospital. It also has a role in insulin overdose.

Calcium

Calcium chloride (or gluconate) is used in the management of calcium channel blocker overdose.

Dextrose

10% dextrose is used in the management of hypoglycaemia in adults and children.

Naloxone

Naloxone (Narcan®) is a highly effective pure opiate antagonist. The initial dose is 400–800μg/kg iv in adults (5–10μg/kg in children). Considerably higher doses may be needed and can be given safely. If naloxone is being given to exclude opiate overdose as a cause of loss of consciousness, a dose of 2mg should be given. Failure to respond to this dose effectively excludes opiate overdose.

If abruptly reversed, many intravenous drug abusers will become verbally (and physically) aggressive and leave the scene. Since naloxone has a shorter half life than many opiates, recurrence of symptoms may then occur unwitnessed. As a consequence, opiate-induced coma is best not reversed unless there is significant respiratory compromise. Even then, an alternative is to support respiration until arrival in hospital. Administration of a similar dose of naloxone (400–800mcg) intramuscularly may reduce the chances of further problems if non-cooperation seems likely, since it has a significantly slower onset.

Atropine

Atropine is used in the management of organophosphate poisoning and drug-related symptomatic bradycardia.

Sodium bicarbonate

Sodium bicarbonate is the antidote for tricyclic antidepressant (TCA) overdose and is effective against TCA-induced arrhythmias. Most pre-hospital care personnel do not carry it, however, and critical patients are probably best transferred, as rapidly as possible, to hospital for further assessment and management.

Table 6.2 Commonly available antidotes

Poison	Antidote	Initial adult dose
Benzodiazepines	Flumazenil (Anexate®)	NOT RECOMMENDED
Beta blockers	Glucagon	2–5mg
Calcium channel blockers	Calcium, glucagon	10ml 10ml
Insulin/oral hypoglycaemics	Dextrose	50ml 50%
Opiates	Naloxone (Narcan®)	400–800mcg
Organophosphates	Atropine	2mg
Tricyclic antidepressants	Sodium bicarbonate	1–3mmol/kg

Poisons

Angiotensin converting enzyme (ACE) inhibitors

Examples

Captopril, cilazapril, enalapril, fosinopril, imidapril, lisinopril, perindopril, ramipril.

Clinical features

- Drowsiness
- Hypotension
- Tachycardia.

Management

- Pre-hospital treatment is not usually required
- Cautious fluid administration should be considered if the patient is hypotensive
- Activated charcoal 50g (if available)
- Transfer to A&E.

Adder bite (see also snake bite)

The adder (Vipera berus) is the only native poisonous snake in the UK.

General features

Adder bites are usually a feature of the summer since the adder hibernates during the winter. Only about 50% of bites are associated with envenomation (painful swelling at the bite is indicative of venom injection, but systemic envenomation may occur without it). Two puncture marks about one centimetre apart are usually found on the distal part of a limb. There is usually immediate pain.

Clinical features

Local

- Painful local swelling (within one hour) with bruising
- Regional (tender) lymphadenopathy.

Systemic (may occur without local signs)

- Vomiting, abdominal pain, and diarrhoea (may be of very rapid onset)
- Hypotension
- Loss of consciousness
- Oedema of the trunk face and lips
- Non-specific ECG changes may occur in severe poisonings.

Management

- Reassurance
- Clean the area of the bite and apply a sterile dressing
- If the hospital is more than 30 minutes away, place a bandage around the limb proximal to the bite, tight enough to impede venous return but not tight enough to obstruct arterial flow.
- Where possible, avoid use of the bitten limb
- Keep the bitten limb dependent
- Warn the hospital about the patient
- If the snake is dead, take it to hospital with the patient
- DO NOT waste time (and risk being bitten) trying to capture the snake
- DO NOT incise or suck the wound.

Alcohol (see ethanol or methanol)

Antibiotics

General features

Deliberate overdoses of antibiotics are rare, presumably because they are known to be relatively safe.

Clinical features

There are usually no ill effects. Nausea, vomiting, and diarrhoea may occur.

Management

- No pre-hospital treatment is required
- Transfer to hospital is appropriate for symptomatic management and psychiatric assessment.

Anticholinergic drugs and agents

Examples

- Atropine (and related drugs)
- Antihistamines
- Antipsychotics
- Tricyclic antidepressants
- Anti-Parkinsonian medications
- Plants.

Clinical features

- Hallucinations
- Confusion
- Lethargy, coma
- Fits
- Cardiac and respiratory failure
- Ataxia
- Dry skin and mouth
- Dilated pupils, blurred vision
- Tachycardia
- Flushing
- Urinary retention.

Management

- Cardiac monitoring
- Fits are usually transient and may be prevented by avoidance of stimulation. They may also, however, suggest progression to cardiac arrest. Immediate treatment is not usually necessary but, if required, the drug of choice is diazemuls.
- Sinus tachycardia
- Dysrhythmias should not be treated unless VT is present and the hospital transfer time prolonged, in which case lignocaine should be used.
- Urgent transfer to hospital is essential.

Anticoagulants

Examples

- Warfarin (acenocoumarol, phenindione).

Warfarin and related compounds (super warfarins) are the active ingredients in a range of proprietary rodent killers, although consumption of sufficient to cause serious symptoms is rare.

Clinical features

- Spontaneous bleeding
  - Nose, gums, GI tract, and urinary
  - Haemoptysis
  - Skin (rare)
  - Brain (rare).

The duration of onset of bleeding is sufficiently long that symptomatic presentations are very rare. Most patients present before symptoms develop.

Management

The management will depend on whether the patient is on long-term anticoagulation or not. Patients should be referred to hospital for assessment and fresh frozen plasma treatment, if required. Most accidental ingestions will not require treatment other than observation and serial clotting studies. Rapid complete reversal is clearly not appropriate in those who are normally therapeutically anticoagulated.

Antifreeze (see ethylene glycol)

Antihistamines

Examples

Astemizole, terfenadine, loratadine, chlorpheniramine, promethazine

Clinical features

- Flushing
- Increased temperature
- Anxiety/agitation
- Dry mouth and mucous membranes
- Dilated pupils
- Fits (rare)
- Cardiac arrhythmias (rare)
- Delerium/coma (rare).

These are the features of acute anticholinergic syndrome. Severe anticholinergic syndrome is more common with older antihistamines such as chlorpheniramine and promethazine than with newer ones such as astemizole.

Antihistamines are also found in a range of proprietary cough medications.

Management

- Maintain and establish a patent airway
- Monitor pulse, BP, ECG, and SpO_2
- Diazemuls for persistent or repeated seizures
- Bicarbonate 1–3mmol/kg (if available) for life-threatening arrhythmias
- Urgent transfer to hospital.

Barbiturates

Examples

Amylobarbitone, butobarbitone, quinalbarbitone, phenobarbitone

General features

Barbiturate overdoses were once very common. With prescriptions now restricted to long-term barbiturate users, they are rare.

Clinical features

- Drowsiness
- Dizziness
- Ataxia
- Coma
- Respiratory depression
- Hypotension
- Hypothermia
- Skin blistering occurs in a minority of patients.

Management

- Establish and maintain a clear airway (the gag reflex is lost in severe overdoses)
- Support respiration
- Activated charcoal 50g (if available) with airway protection
- Urgent transfer to hospital.

Batteries

General features

Small children are at risk of swallowing 'button' type batteries of the kind found in toys, watches, and a wide variety of everyday items.

Clinical features

The majority of swallowers will not show any symptoms. When these are present, they include:

- Retrosternal discomfort
- Nausea and vomiting
- Cough
- Difficulty in swallowing.

Later symptoms (which may be life-threatening) relate to erosion of the battery through the oesophageal wall, internal electrical burns, and the local and systemic effects of leaking chemicals. As a result, these ingestions must be taken seriously.

Management

ALL patients who are known or suspected to have swallowed a button type battery should be directed or taken to hospital for X-ray and further management. Where possible, a sample of the type of battery should accompany the patient.

Benzodiazepines

Examples

Nitrazepam, loprazolam, temazepam, diazepam.

Clinical features

- CNS depression (drowsiness to coma)
- Respiratory depression
- Hypotension (rare)
- Ataxia (in children, rare)
- Dysarthria.

Management

- Establish and maintain a secure airway (use the recovery position if necessary)
- Support respiration
- Evacuate to hospital.

FLUMAZENIL should **NOT** be used in the pre-hospital environment. Its use can be complicated by convulsions, arrhythmias, and anxiety. Fatal reactions are recorded. In addition, its use may precipitate fitting in epileptics or those who have taken a mixed overdose which also includes epileptogenic substances.

Beta blockers

Examples

Propranolol, acebutolol, atenolol, metoprolol, oxprenolol, sotalol

Clinical features

Beta blocker overdoses may be severe and regular fatalities occur.

Cardiovascular

- Bradycardia
- Hypotension and circulatory failure
- AV block/conduction abnormalities
- Ventricular arrythmias
- Cardiac arrest.

Other

- Airway constriction
- Respiratory depression
- Hypoglycaemia
- Sedation or coma
- Fits.

Depending on the beta blocker, symptoms may take up to two hours to develop.

Management

- Careful management of airway and breathing
- ECG monitoring
- URGENT transfer to hospital
- Give activated charcoal if transfer to hospital is likely to be delayed or prolonged
- For bradycardia: atropine 500μg iv (repeated if necessary)
- Glucagon 2–5mg iv stat for significantly symptomatic patients. Larger doses than those conventionally carried are often required, including continuous intravenous infusion after hospital arrival.

Bleach

General comments

The active constituent of most household bleaches is sodium hypochlorite in varying concentration. Bleaches are corrosive and give off chlorine when they react with gastric acid.

Clinical features

The majority of patients are young children, who rarely take enough to cause serious problems, presumably because of the unpleasant taste and smell. Symptoms include:

- Nausea and vomiting
- Soreness in the mouth
- Abdominal pain (rare).

Late symptoms include oesophageal perforation, haemorrhage, and shock.

Management

- Ensure a patent protected airway
- Give milk
- Transfer to A&E for assessment and monitoring.

Calcium channel blockers

Examples

- Verapamil
- Amlodipine, nifedipine, nimodipine, nicardipine
- Diltiazem.

Clinical features

Symptoms are normally apparent within 1–6 hours, but may be very delayed in overdose of sustained release preparations. Children are particularly at risk from ingestion of calcium channel blockers and deaths have been reported following ingestion of very small quantities.

- Brady/tachycardias, sinus arrest, heart block
- Cardiac arrest
- Heart failure, cardiogenic shock
- CNS depression/coma
- Fits (rare—more common in children)
- Hyperglycaemia (rare).

Management

- Establish and maintain a patent airway (use recovery position if necessary)
- Give high-flow oxygen
- ECG monitoring, oxygen saturation monitoring
- Atropine (500μg aliquots) for bradycardia
- Calcium iv (gluconate or chloride 10%, 10–20ml slowly)
- URGENT transfer to hospital.

Intravenous fluid boluses may be used with care for hypotension, and external pacing may occasionally be necessary.

Carbamazepine

Clinical features

- Drowsiness
- Confusion
- Ataxia, loss of co-ordination
- Dizziness
- Nystagmus, pupillary dilatation (not always), strabismus
- Fits
- Coma
- AV block
- Ventricular arrhythmias.

Management

Carbamazepine overdose is similar to tricyclic antidepressant overdose, although the complications are usually less severe. Supportive measures are usually all that are required. Significant arrythmias are treated with sodium bicarbonate by intravenous bolus usually after arrival in hospital.

Carbon monoxide

General comments

Carbon monoxide is a colourless, odourless gas which is the product of incomplete combustion of carbon-containing compounds. Sources include:

- Car exhaust fumes
- Methane, coal, propane, butane, oil, kerosene, wood, and other fuels
- Paint stripper
- Smoke from burning organic substances.

In many cases, poisoning results from CO accumulation in a confined space where there is inadequate ventilation, ventilation has been blocked, or heating appliances are faulty.

Mechanism of action

CO binds to haemoglobin to form carboxyhaemoglobin, reducing its oxygen-carrying ability. The affinity of haemoglobin for CO is approximately 250 times that for oxygen.

Clinical features

A high index of suspicion is essential. CO poisoning is more common in cold weather and in the circumstances listed above.

Early

- Headache
- Dizziness
- Nausea
- Vomiting (may be bloodstained).

Later

- Confusion
- Lethargy
- Nystagmus
- Ataxia
- Syncope
- Shivering.

Severe poisoning

- Coma
- Pulmonary oedema
- Hypotension
- Increased muscle tone, hyperreflexia, clonus, abnormal plantar responses
- Myocardial infarction
- Cardiac arrest.

The classical 'cherry pink' skin colour of CO poisoning is rare.

Management

- Remove the patient AND YOURSELF from the toxic atmosphere
- Establish and maintain a patent airway
- ADMINISTER HIGH-FLOW OXYGEN
- Rapid transfer to hospital with intensive care facilities.

CAUTION: pulse oximetry gives falsely high readings in CO poisoning and should not be used (see pp.80–1).

Chlorine

General comments

Chlorine is widely used in industrial processes, including the manufacture of plastics, bleaches, and hydrochloric acid. It is also used in water purification and may result from the mixing of bleach and other household cleaners. Chlorine produces patchy necrosis of respiratory mucosa and acute pulmonary oedema.

It is a greenish yellow gas which is heavier than air and may accumulate in low or enclosed areas.

Mechanism of action

Reacts with water to form hydrochloric acid, resulting in tissue irritation and pain.

Clinical features

- Mucous membrane irritation
- Coughing, choking, dyspnoea, bronchospasm, chest pain, hypoxia, and pulmonary oedema
- Respiratory arrest
- Respiratory symptoms which are likely to be worse in those with pre-existing lung disease (for example, asthma)
- Nausea and vomiting.

Management

- Remove from further exposure and give high-flow oxygen
- Check peak flow
- Salbutamol for bronchospasm
- Artificial ventilation, if required
- Copious lavage of exposed skin with water
- Eye exposure: copious lavage with water or N.saline followed by fluorescein staining or ophthalmology referral for assessment.

Corrosive substances—acids and alkalis

Uses

Widely used in the chemical industry; also used in some domestic cleaning products.

Clinical features

Skin

- Burns, often to hands and face.

Ingestion

- Burning pain in lips, throat, chest, and epigastrium
- Vomiting.

Inhalation

- Pulmonary oedema.

Eyes

- Corneal ulceration.

Management

- Establish and maintain a patent airway; administer high-flow oxygen
- Give milk (to help neutralize the corrosive)
- Analgesia as required
- Prolonged irrigation with water for skin contamination
- Immediate lavage of contaminated eyes with water (tap water is fine) at scene
- Transfer to hospital.

Attempts to neutralize an acid with alkali or vice versa are CONTRA-INDICATED.

CS gas

General comments

CS gas is used for riot control, control of violent or aggressive personages by the police, and in exercises by the Armed Forces.

Clinical features

- Burning eyes with blepharospasm
- Upper respiratory burning
- Bronchospasm and dyspnoea
- Panic.

Management

- Remove from contaminated area
- Remove clothing
- Irrigate the eyes
- Showering
- Transfer to hospital for management and assessment of associated injuries.

CS gas 'clings' to clothing and 'off-gassing' may continue for some time, causing distress to rescue personnel, especially in enclosed spaces such as the back of an ambulance.

Patients who refuse to attend hospital should be advised to shower on arrival at home and to leave their clothes outside.

Cyanide

General comments

Cyanide is widely used in industry in processes including metal extraction, laboratory analysis, electroplating, and photography. It may also result from the burning of a wide range of synthetic products such as plastics. There are also natural sources including apricot and cherry kernels and some nuts. Cyanide inhibits a wide range of enzymes, most importantly, cytochrome oxidase.

Clinical features

Early neurological symptoms include:

- Headache
- Anxiety
- Confusion
- Dizziness
- Weakness
- Patients may subsequently develop coma and convulsions.

Cardio-respiratory symptoms include:

- Dyspnoea
- Tachypnoea
- Pulmonary oedema
- Tachy bradycardia
- Respiratory and cardiac arrest
- Death may not occur for several hours.

Management

- Ensure the patient is removed from the toxic environment—DO NOT ENTER HAZARDOUS AREAS
- Remove contaminated clothing—DO NOT GET CONTAMINATED
- Wash contaminated skin thoroughly.

There are a number of cyanide antidotes including dicobalt edetate (600mg iv followed, if the response is unsatisfactory, by 300mg) or sodium nitrite and sodium thiosulphate. Both these regimes are potentially toxic in the absence of cyanide poisoning and the diagnosis should be reasonably likely before they are used. In some cases, transfer to hospital (with the kit) may be the most reasonable option. One or other antidote should be available at sites where there is a risk of cyanide poisoning.

Detergents and related substances

Examples

Soaps, detergents, fabric conditioners.

General comments

Usually consumed by toddlers and small children.

Clinical features

- Nausea, vomiting, and diarrhoea
- Other symptoms are rare but substances containing benzalkonium chloride are more toxic and may cause coma, convulsions, and respiratory failure.

Management

- Encourage fluids
- Administer milk
- Discuss with poisons advice centre (see p.399) in mild cases
- Transfer to hospital in potentially serious cases.

Digoxin and related drugs (cardiac glycosides)

Examples

Digoxin, digitoxin.

Clinical features

Overdoses of cardiac glycosides are rare, the symptoms are:

- Nausea, vomiting, diarrhoea
- Fatigue, confusion, lethargy, delirium (rarer)
- Hyperkalaemia leading to arrhythmias
- Sinus arrest, sinus bradycardia, AV block
- Ventricular arrythmias (rarer).

Management

- Cardiac monitoring
- Consider activated charcoal if transfer is delayed or likely to be prolonged
- Atropine for symptomatic bradycardia
- Conventional management for other arrhythmias (isolated ventricular ectopics do not need treatment)
- Transfer to hospital for further therapy, potentially including digoxin–specific antibodies
- Calcium is contraindicated as it may worsen arrhythmias.

Disinfectants

Clinical features

- Burns of lips, mouth, and upper GI tract
- Hoarseness, stridor, airway obstruction
- Ataxia, CNS depression, coma (pine oil-containing disinfectants)
- Shock, hypothermia, respiratory failure, myocardial damage, shock (phenol-containing disinfectants).

Management

- Establish and maintain a patent airway
- Give milk (in conscious patients)
- Transfer urgently to hospital.

These overdoses should be taken seriously as a number of detergents still contain toxic substances such as phenol. Evacuation to hospital is, therefore, appropriate.

Ethanol

General comments

Although drunkenness is extremely common, severe alcohol poisoning is, fortunately, extremely rare. It occurs more commonly in young adults unused to habitual alcohol excess. Probably the most common cause of alcohol-related death (apart from trauma) is airway obstruction, often secondary to vomiting.

It should be remembered that ethanol potentiates the CNS depressant actions of a wide range of drugs. In addition, patients under the influence of alcohol fall, get assaulted, and often neglect themselves. The possibility of associated injuries and medical conditions should not be forgotten.

Clinical features

- Confusion, aggression, disinhibition
- CNS depression leading to coma
- Hypotension
- Hypothermia
- Respiratory failure
- Hypoglycaemia in children.

There is usually the characteristic smell of alcohol on the breath. Hypoglycaemia is rare in adults but much more common in children.

Management

- Establish and maintain a patent airway (use the recovery position if there is no possibility of cervical spine injury); ensure working suction is available
- Assist ventilation (where necessary) and administer high-flow oxygen
- Check a BM stix®
- In mild cases, the patient may be left in the care of a responsible adult
- In serious cases (for example, where the airway is threatened), the patient should be admitted to hospital for observation.

NOTE

High concentrations of ethanol are also found in perfumes, aftershaves, mouthwashes, and over-the-counter cough and cold remedies.

Ethylene glycol

General comments

Ethylene glycol is the active ingredient in antifreeze and motor coolant fluids. Cases of ethylene glycol poisoning have also resulted from deliberate contamination of alcoholic drinks such as wine.

Clinical features

- Ataxia
- Slurred speech
- Nausea and vomiting
- Convulsions
- Drowsiness and coma.

Later symptoms (after 12 hours) are predominantly cardiorespiratory, including arrhythmias, bronchopneumonia, and cerebral oedema. These are unlikely to be encountered in the pre-hospital environment.

Management

- Establish and maintain a patent airway
- Treat complications symptomatically
- Transfer to hospital URGENTLY for investigation and management.

The diagnosis of ethylene glycol poisoning is often far from obvious. If it can be established with reasonable certainty that the patient has taken ethylene glycol, and they are capable of taking it, ethanol (as whisky, gin, or vodka containing 40g/l ethanol) can be given my mouth. Ethanol 'mops up' alcohol dehydrogenase, reducing the metabolism of ethylene glycol into toxic metabolites.

Fungi—poisonous

Examples

- Amanita phalloides ('death cap' mushroom)—the most common cause of fatalities from eating mushrooms
- *Gyrometra spp*
- *Psilocybe spp.*

Clinical features

A wide range of symptoms is possible. Early nausea, vomiting, and diarrhoea may occur. Other symptoms include profuse sweating, salivation, abdominal pain, hallucinations, headache, flushing, and blurred vision.

Management

Early management is supportive, with urgent evacuation to hospital. Wherever possible, a sample of the ingested fungus (fungi) should accompany the patient to hospital. Intravenous fluids may be commenced and an antiemetic given.

Hypoglycaemic agents

Examples

Tolbutamide, chlorpropramide, gliclazide, glipizide, tolazamide, glibenclamide. These are sulphonylureas; metformin (a biguanide) does not cause hypoglycaemia in overdose.

Clinical features

- Reduced conscious level or coma
- Pupillary dilatation (not always present)
- Neurological abnormalities including upgoing plantars and hyper-reflexia
- Fits.

Hypoglycaemia due to sulphonylurea overdose can be extremely prolonged and recurrent, even after treatment. Careful monitoring and repeated BM stix readings are, therefore, essential.

Management

- Establish and maintain a secure airway
- 10% dextrose by slow IV injection (IV glucagon is an alternative, initial dose 1mg)
- Fits may respond to correction of hypolycaemia; otherwise use diazemuls 2.5mg every 30 seconds until control is achieved
- Urgent transfer to hospital.

NOTE: glucagon is ineffective in patients with inadequate glycogen stores such as alcoholics.

Insulin

Clinical features

- Reduced conscious level or coma
- Pupillary dilatation (not always present)
- Neurological abnormalities including upgoing plantars and hyper-reflexia
- Fits.

Management

- Establish and maintain a secure airway
- 50% dextrose (50ml initially) by slow iv injection (iv glucagon is an alternative, initial dose 1mg)
- Fits may respond to correction of hypoglycaemia; otherwise use diazemuls 2.5mg every 30 seconds until control is achieved
- Urgent transfer to hospital.

Depending on the insulin injected, repeated doses of glucose or a dextrose infusion may be necessary to prevent recurrence of symptoms.

Regular monitoring of BM stix is essential

Iron

Clinical features

For such a widely prescribed (and self-prescribed) medication, iron can be remarkably toxic in overdose or poisoning. Accidental ingestion of iron supplements is not uncommon in children.

- Vomiting (or haematemesis) and diarrhoea (may be black or grey)
- Abdominal pain
- Lethargy, drowsiness, coma
- Fits
- Shock
- Later symptoms (after about 12 hours) include shock, acidosis, jaundice, and renal failure.

Management

- Establishment and maintenance of a patent airway
- Symptomatic treatment of complications
- URGENT referral to hospital.

Where possible, the remaining medication or its container should accompany the patient to hospital so that an estimate of the amount of elemental iron ingested can be made.

Lithium

Clinical features

- Nausea, vomiting, and diarrhoea
- Tremor, hyperreflexia, agitation
- Fits
- Coma.

Non-specific ST depression and T wave inversion may be found on the ECG. Malignant arrhythmias are rare.

Management

Pre-hospital management is supportive. A patent airway should be established and maintained. If transfer to hospital is likely to be delayed or prolonged, an intravenous infusion should be commenced. ECG monitoring is essential.

Mefenamic acid

Mechanism of action

Mefenamic acid is a non-steroidal anti-inflammatory drug.

General features

Prescribed for menorrhagia and dysmenorrhoea, as well as arthritides and related conditions, mefenamic acid (Ponstan®) is relatively commonly taken in overdose.

Clinical features

- Muscle twitching
- Fits
- Diarrhoea and vomiting.

Management

- Establish and maintain a protected airway
- Diazemuls for prolonged or recurrent seizures
- Urgent evacuation to hospital
- Give activated charcoal if transfer is likely to be delayed or prolonged.

Methanol

General comments

Methanol is used in windscreen washer fluids, as a component of methylated spirits (not in significant levels), as a fuel antifreeze additive, and as an industrial solvent. Methanol poisoning may result from the consumption of contaminated or adulterated wines.

Clinical features

- Nausea, vomiting
- Abdominal pain and diarrhoea, rigid abdomen
- Visual abnormalities (including blurred vision, flashing lights, and decreased visual acuity). May progress to blindness.
- Photophobia
- Headache
- Dizziness
- Breathlessness
- Sweating
- Convulsions (rare)
- Cardiorespiratory failure.

Management

- Establish and maintain a patent airway (use the recovery position if there is no possibility of cervical spine injury)
- Assist ventilation (where necessary) and administer high-flow oxygen
- Diazemuls for fitting
- If the patient is well enough and hospital transfer is likely to be prolonged or delayed, oral ethanol can be given in the form of whisky, gin, or vodka (40% proof).
- Urgent transfer to hospital.

Metoclopramide

Clinical features

Overdosage or poisoning with metoclopramide does not appear to be a problem. A minority of patients, however, suffer acute dystonic reactions. These include chewing movements, spasms of torticollis, and oculogyric crisis. These movements cannot be controlled by the patient, who remains fully conscious throughout.

Management

The treatment of acute dystonia is procyclidine 5–10mg im (adult dose) or benztropine 1–2mg im or iv (adult dose). If one of these is not available, the patient should be reassured and transferred to A&E for treatment.

Monoamine oxidase inhibitors (MAOIs)

Examples

- Phenelzine, tranylcypromine, isocarboxazid, moclobemide
- The anti-parkinsonian agent, selegiline, and the chemotherapeutic agent, procarbazine, are also MAO inhibitors.

Clinical features

- Headache
- Agitation
- Hallucinations
- Flushing
- Sweating
- Muscular rigidity
- Tachycardia
- Tachypnoea
- Hypotension, bradycardia, and asystole
- Abnormal muscular movements (writhing, grimacing)
- Coma
- Nystagmus
- Hyperpyrexia
- Hypertension.

Symptoms may initially be entirely absent, even in very serious overdoses.

Management

- Scrupulous attention to ABC
- Diazemuls for seizures, rigidity, and agitation
- Conventional ALS protocols for dysrhythmias (bretylium is contra-indicated and atropine and beta blockers should be avoided)
- Fluids iv for hypotension
- Passive cooling measures for hyperpyrexia
- Urgent transfer to hospital
- Consider activated charcoal if transfer is likely to be delayed or prolonged

Opiates

See drugs of abuse, p.478.

Organophosphate insecticides (including carbamates)

Examples

There are many insecticides in these two groups. They are used extensively and are relatively common causes of poisoning, either deliberate or accidental.

Uses

Agricultural and horticultural.

Clinical features

Mild poisoning

- Anxiety and restlessness
- Skin redness and erythema
- Nausea, vomiting
- Abdominal pain and diarrhoea
- Sweating
- Hypersalivation
- Bronchospasm/bronchorrhoea
- Miosis (not present in every case)
- Dizziness
- Headache.

Moderate/severe poisoning

- Reduced level of consciousness
- Muscle fasciculation and weakness
- Pulmonary oedema
- Fitting
- Cardiac dysrhythmias.

Management

- Remove patient from contaminated area
- Remove contaminated clothing
- Wash contaminated skin with soap and water
- Establish and maintain a patent airway (suction for increased secretions)
- High-flow oxygen
- ECG and pulse oximetry
- Atropine 2mg iv every 10 minutes (approximately) until the patient feels better or tachycardia, dry flushed skin, dry mouth, and dilated pupils are evident
- Diazemuls for anxiety and fitting
- URGENT evacuation to hospital.

Rescuers must at all times ensure that they do not themselves become poisoned.

Paracetamol

General features

In normal individuals, the minimum toxic dose of paracetamol is in the region of 150mg/kg (90mg/kg in children). This level is considerably lower in chronic alcohol abusers, malnourished patients, those on anticonvulsants, and HIV patients.

Clinical features

There are no immediate features of paracetamol overdose. Nausea and vomiting may occur within a few hours. The diagnosis is based on information from the patient or witnesses and the presence of circumstantial evidence such as empty pill bottles.

Late complications include cerebral oedema, encephalopathy, hepatorenal failure, serum electrolyte abnormalities, and rashes.

The presence of a reduced conscious level or coma in the early stages of paracetamol overdose suggests that a CNS depressant has also been taken. Compound analgesics such as co-codamol (codeine and paracetamol), co-dydramol (dihydrocodeine and paracetamol), and co-proxamol (codeine and dextropropoxyphene) are possible causes of this, although two entirely separate medications may have been taken.

Management

The patient should be transferred to hospital for assessment of paracetamol levels and further management, including N-acetyl cysteine where appropriate.

In extremely remote areas where transfer is likely to be very prolonged or delayed, each case should be discussed with the receiving hospital and consideration given to the administration of oral methionine (adult dose 2.5g 4hrly to a total of 10g).

Paraquat

Examples

Paraquat is a bipyridylium herbicide present in a wide range of commercial weed control products of which the most frequently encountered is probably Weedol®. Many proprietary herbicides are mixtures of herbicidal compounds and other substances such as petroleum distillates.

Clinical features

The clinical features depend on the portal of entry:

Oral ingestion

- Mucous membrane irritation
- Nausea and vomiting
- Abdominal pain and diarrhoea.

With increasing dose:

- Shock (fluid loss and direct myocardial effect)
- Pulmonary oedema
- Oropharyngeal ulceration.

The later effects of paraquat poisoning include renal necrosis, haemorrhagic pulmonary oedema, ataxia, coma, and demyelination.

Inhalational exposure

- Sore throat
- Huskiness of speech
- Epistaxis.

More serious symptoms are rare.

Skin and eye contamination

Blistering may occur but thorough decontamination should prevent systemic toxicity. Splashes into the eyes result in blepharospasm, lacrimation, and corneal ulceration. Thorough lavage is essential.

Management

- Careful assessment and management of ABC
- Symptomatic treatment of complications
- Administration of activated charcoal 50g (if carried)
- URGENT evacuation to hospital.

DO NOT GIVE OXYGEN IN PARAQUAT POISONING

Pepper spray

General comments

Pepper spray is used as a personal protection system by members of the police services. The active ingredient is capsaicin, extracted from chilli peppers.

Clinical features

- Burning eyes and mucous membranes
- Burning skin.

Management

- Remove from the contaminated area
- Remove clothing
- Irrigate the eyes (local anaesthetic may be used)
- Showering
- Consider transfer to hospital.

Petroleum distillates and turpentine

Examples

Petrol, diesel, paraffin, lighter fuel, turpentine, turpentine substitute, furniture polish, kerosene, gasoline, glues, typewriter correction fluid.

Clinical features

Most patients are likely to be symptom free. However, symptoms may include:

- Vomiting
- Diarrhoea (rare)
- Cough/haemoptysis
- Wheezing/ breathlessness
- Decreased level of consciousness or coma (rare)
- Fitting (rare).

Management

- Careful attention to ABC
- High-flow oxygen
- Symptomatic treatment of complications
- Urgent evacuation to hospital.

Phenothiazines and haloperidol/droperidol

Examples

- Chlorpromazine, promazine, promethazine
- Thioridazine
- Haloperidol, droperidol
- Fluphenazine, prochlorperazine, trifluoperazine
- Flupenthixol.

General comments

Members of this group of drugs are prescribed for a wide range of conditions, the most common indication being as antipsychotics. Others are indicated in the treatment of nausea, vomiting and motion sickness, and for their antihistamine properties.

Clinical features

- CNS depression (coma rare)
- Hypotension
- Hypo-/hyperthermia
- Acute dystonic reactions
- Fitting
- Cardiac arrhythmias/non-specific ECG changes.

Management

- Careful attention to ABC
- Activated charcoal 50g (if carried) if patient is fully conscious
- Arrhythmias should be treated conventionally, but may be ineffective until hypoxia and acidosis are corrected
- Urgent transfer to hospital.

The treatment of acute dystonia is procyclidine 5–10mg im (adult dose) or benztropine 1–2mg im or iv (adult dose). If one of these is not available, the patient should be reassured and transferred to A&E for treatment.

Phenytoin

Clinical features

- Nausea and vomiting
- Dysarthria
- Ataxia
- Choreo-athetoid movements
- Dizziness and nystagmus
- Drowsiness and confusion
- Coma (rare)
- Fits.

Management

- Ensure a patent airway
- Monitor ECG
- Give activated charcoal 50g (if available)
- Commence iv fluids if transfer times prolonged or transfer delayed
- Urgent transfer to hospital.

Plant toxins

Examples

- Cotoneaster
- Dieffenbachia
- Foxglove
- Hemlock
- Hogweed
- Holly
- Honeysuckle
- Mistletoe
- Yew.

General approach to poisoning with plant toxins

- Careful attention to ABC
  - Establish and maintain a patent airway
  - iv access.
- Decontamination of dermal exposure with soap and water
- Symptomatic treatment as required (see below)
- Seek appropriate advice
- Ensure that a sample of the plant accompanies the patient to hospital.

Cotoneaster

Presentation

The red berries of this garden shrub enclose seeds which contain cyanogenic glycosides. It is extremely unusual for sufficient to be taken to cause serious problems although abdominal pain, vomiting, and diarrhoea may occur.

Management

No treatment is usually necessary. In the case of large ingestions, activated charcoal should be given. Symptomatic treatment may be required.

Dieffenbachia

Presentation

Dieffenbachia (and the related *Monstera* and *Philodendron spp*) are common house plants. Their leaves contain oxalate crystals and cause intense burning pain in the lips and mouth. Hypersalivation occurs and the tongue, lips, and oral mucosa swell, often rendering speech difficult. Airway compromise is possible but rare.

Management

Symptomatic relief is possible with ice cubes, ice cream, or milk. Analgesia should be given. Airway compromise may mandate intervention including orotracheal intubation.

Foxglove

Presentation

Foxglove, oleander, and lilly of the valley all contain cardiac glycosides. Symptoms of ingestion include nausea, vomiting, visual disturbance, changes in mental state, and cardiac arrythmias.

Management
Treatment is generally supportive. Cardiac monitoring is essential. Arrhythmias may respond to conventional therapy but digoxin-specific antibody treatment in hospital is also effective. Calcium is absolutely contraindicated.

Hemlock

Presentation
Water hemlock and related species contain a number of dangerous toxins and ingestion of small amounts can be fatal. Symptoms include nausea, vomiting, abdominal pain, and sweating. Fits occur and death is secondary to status epilepticus and cardiac arrest. Very small quantities may result in fatal poisoning.

Management
Establishment and maintenance of a patent airway, activated charcoal if available, control of fitting with diazemuls, and urgent transfer to hospital.

Hogweed

Presentation
Giant hogweed sensitizes skin to ultraviolet light causing burning.

Management
Conventional management for superficial burns: analgesia, non-adherent dressing. Hospital or GP follow-up.

Holly

Presentation
The red berries of holly are sometimes eaten by inquisitive children. Most will develop no problems with the quantities they are likely to eat. When symptoms occur, they are vomiting, abdominal pain, and diarrhoea.

Management
None, usually. Symptomatic management when required.

Honeysuckle

Presentation
The berries of this common plant are sometimes eaten by young children. Symptoms are unusual but include vomiting and abdominal pain.

Management
No treatment is usually required. Symptomatic treatment may occasionally be necessary.

Mistletoe

Presentation
Children rarely eat enough berries or leaves to cause problems. When they do, symptoms include vomiting, abdominal pain, diarrhoea, and, rarely, bradycardia and circulatory failure. Muscle weakness also occurs.

Management

Children who have eaten more than three berries or leaves require admission to hospital for observation. If there is any doubt, referral to hospital is appropriate. Activated charcoal may be given.

Yew

Presentation

All parts of the yew are poisonous. Symptoms are rare but include vomiting, abdominal pain, diarrhoea, and rarely, fits, reduced conscious level, respiratory depression, tachy- and brady-dysrhythmias, hypotension, and cardiac arrest.

Management

Immediate transfer to hospital is essential. Treatment is symptomatic, with conventional treatment for dysrhythmias.

Pulmonary irritants

Chlorine is considered separately (see p.423).

General comments

A wide range of gases act as pulmonary irritants, the majority associated with chemical processing. Examples include: acrolein, ammonia, formaldehyde, hydrogen chloride, hydrogen fluoride, hydrogen sulphide, and phosgene. In many cases, it will not be possible (at least in the early stages) to identify the agent involved.

Clinical features

Initial exposure results in rhinitis and conjunctivitis, followed by sinusitis and laryngitis. Further exposure causes inflammation of lung tissue, eventually leading to pulmonary oedema. Individual irritants will also produce a wide range of specific clinical problems.

Symptoms of respiratory irritant poisoning include:

- Cough
- Shortness of breath
- Bronchospasm
- Chest pain
- Haemoptysis
- Headache
- Cardiac arrhythmias.

Management

- Ensure that the patient is away from the contaminated area
- Remove contaminated clothing
- Decontaminate with water
- Establish and maintain a patent airway
- Look for signs of thermal airway injury
- Serial chest examinations
- Administer high-flow oxygen
- Consider salbutamol for bronchospasm
- Monitor SaO_2 and ECG
- Transfer to hospital.

Salicylates

Examples

- Aspirin
- Decongestants
- Cold, cough, and 'flu' remedies
- Musculoskeletal pain medications (including Benorylate®).

Clinical features

Salicylates stimulate the brain respiratory centre, leading to respiratory alkalosis and compensatory metabolic acidosis. Lactic acidosis follows.

- Vomiting
- Gastrointestinal irritation and haematemesis
- Tinnitus
- Hyperpnoea
- Lethargy.

Severe poisoning

- Fitting
- Coma
- Hyperthermia
- Hypoglycaemia
- Pulmonary oedema
- Cardiorespiratory failure.

Symptoms can begin within 1 to 2 hours following ingestion, but they may be significantly delayed. Symptoms of severe poisoning are unlikely to be seen in the pre-hospital environment.

Management

- Establish and maintain a patent airway
- Support respiration if necessary
- Conventional management of complications such as fitting
- Give activated charcoal (50g) if available
- Urgent transfer to hospital
- If transfer to hospital is likely to be prolonged or delayed, commence cautious iv administration of crystalloid.

Serotonin uptake inhibitors—selective serotonin inhibitors (SSRIs)

Examples

Citalopram, fluoxetine, fluvoxamine, paroxetine, sertraline.

General comments

The SSRIs were introduced as a safer alternative to the tricyclic antidepressants. Serious overdoses are, therefore, rare.

Clinical features

- Bradycardia
- Nausea and vomiting
- Tremor
- Lethargy
- Dizziness
- Depressed conscious level
- Fitting.

Management

- Careful attention to ABC
- Activated charcoal (50g) if available
- Monitor ECG
- Transfer to hospital.

Snake bite (see also adder bite)

A wide range of snakes is held in zoos and by private individuals. In such cases, the type of snake may be known. Prolonged and hazardous attempts to capture the snake should be avoided and the patient transferred rapidly to hospital. IT IS possible to be bitten by a dead snake! Advice regarding management and provision, where appropriate, of specific antivenom, can then be sought from the local poisons unit (see p.399 for telephone number) or tropical medicine unit.

Management

- Do not apply a tourniquet (a bandage may be applied proximal to the bite, which is tight enough to occlude superficial veins only)
- Do not apply ice
- Do not suck on the wound
- Apply a splint to immobilize the bitten limb
- Keep the patient calm and rested
- Urgent transfer to hospital.

Tetracyclic antidepressants

Examples

Mianserin.

Clinical features

- Drowsiness
- Hypo- or hypertension.

Management

- No specific pre-hospital management is required; attention should be paid to ABC management
- Activated charcoal 50g (if available)
- Transfer to hospital for further management and psychiatric assessment is appropriate.

Theophyllines

Examples

- Theophylline
- Aminophylline.

Theophyllines are present in a wide range of cough and decongestant preparations. The majority of preparations are slow release and, as a result, symptoms of poisoning may not be apparent until more than 12 hours after ingestion.

Clinical features

- Nausea, vomiting
- Diarrhoea (rare)
- Haematemesis
- Restlessness, anxiety, hyperactivity
- Pupillary dilatation
- Tremor
- Hyperventilation
- Tachycardia
- Supraventricular and ventricular arrhythmias including VF
- Myoclonus, increased muscle tone, involuntary limb movements
- Fitting.

Management

- Careful attention to ABC
- Establish and maintain a patent airway
- Support respiration
- Administer activated charcoal (50g adult dose) if available, repeated if transfer is delayed or prolonged
- Monitor ECG and SpO_2
- Manage fitting with diazemuls or rapid sequence initiation of anaesthesia if the skills are available
- Tachy-dysrhythmias respond to beta blockers (if available), otherwise follow conventional managment
- Urgent transfer to hospital.

Toiletries and cosmetics

General comments

Aftershaves, deodorants, make-up, perfumes, shampoos, hair lacquer and remover, shaving cream, nail varnish (and remover), bath crystals.

These preparations variously contain ethanol, other alcohols, waxes, lanolin, and an assortment of chemical compounds. They are commonly consumed by children, fortunately in small quantities.

Non-toxic substances

The following are relatively non-toxic and consumption of enough to cause serious problems is unlikely:

- Shampoo
- Skin creams and lotions
- Make-up and lipstick
- Shaving cream
- Bubble bath.

They may, however, cause nausea and vomiting.

Substances containing ethanol

Preparations containing ethanol, such as perfumes and aftershave, are not usually consumed in sufficient quantities to be of harm.

Potentially toxic substances

Nail varnish and its remover are potentially toxic.

Management

Transfer to hospital for assessment and observation in potentially serious cases.

Tricyclic antidepressants

Examples

With sedative properties

Amitriptyline, clomipramine, dothiepin, doxepin, mianserin, trimipramine

Less sedative

Imipramine, lofepramine, nortriptyline, amoxapine

Clinical features

Tricyclic antidepressant (TCA) overdose should always be considered potentially life-threatening. Deterioration may be very rapid and within 1 hour of ingestion.

- Dry flushed skin, dry mucous membranes
- Urinary retention
- Pupillary dilatation, blurred vision
- Decreased bowel sounds
- Altered mental state (including hallucinations and delirium)
- Altered conscious level, coma
- Fitting
- Arrhythmias
  - Sinus tachycardia
  - ↑ QRS duration
  - ↑ PR interval
  - Heart block
  - SVT
  - VT (including toursade de pointes)
- Hypotension.

Management

- Establish and maintain a patent airway
- Support respiration as required
- Establish intravenous access—cautious iv fluids for hypotension
- Monitor ECG and SpO_2
- Give activated charcoal (50mg) if safe to do so
- Avoid unnecessary stimulation (may precipitate fits)
- iv diazepam for prolonged fitting (brief fits may resolve spontaneously)
- Asymptomatic arrhythmias should be observed if perfusion is adequate and the BP is acceptable. Serious symptomatic arrhythmias are best treated with sodium bicarbonate (50ml, 8.4% slow iv infusion) but this is unlikely to be available pre-hospital. If necessary, these arrhythmias can be treated with lignocaine
- Transfer to hospital urgently.

Venomous bites and stings

See also: adder bite (p.409), snake bite (p.455)

Jellyfish stings

Presenting features

- Pain
- Paraesthesia
- Paralysis
- Pruritic rash
- Anaphylactic reactions (rare)
- Hypotension (rare).

Management

- Wash with salt water (or normal saline) or diluted (1:20) vinegar for 30 minutes
- Remove tentacle fragments carefully (use forceps or thick gloves—a single layer of surgical glove can be penetrated)
- Give analgesia
- Do not rub the area or wash in fresh water.

Sea urchins

Presentation

See above.

Management

- Analgesia
- Prophylactic antibiotics
- Immerse in hot water
- Carefully remove spines (can be performed in hospital; retained spines are radio-opaque).

Spider bites

Presentation

There are no toxic native spiders in the UK. Such species may occasionally escape from private collections or bite keepers in zoos. Symptoms include (depending on the species):

- Local pain
- Muscle cramp
- Sweating
- Nausea
- Diarrhoea
- Tachycardia
- Hypertension
- Anxiety.

Management

- Specific antisera may be available in specialist centres or zoos which keep toxic species
- Diazemuls will lower blood pressure, slow tachycardia, and calm the patient
- Morphine (or a similar opiate) should be given for pain
- Monitor BP, ECG, and PaO_2
- Transfer to hospital.

Substance abuse

Substance abuse is becoming increasingly common and is a problem that every pre-hospital practitioner is likely to meet sooner or later. This section deals with the presentation and management of commonly abused drugs. Some of the complications which are discussed are fortunately rare, but may be fatal if incorrectly treated. Specific management points are given, but this in no way lessens the importance of good supportive care and careful attention to ABC. It is important to remember that, in many cases, these substances will have been taken in combination, most often with alcohol.

Drug abusers are probably everybody's least favourite patients. They are frequently aggressive, demanding, and almost never grateful. It is even more important, therefore, that personal prejudices are not allowed to interfere with management which must be of the highest standard for the protection of patient and clinician. Patients who are under the influence of drugs and other substances are at particularly high risk of further injury or harm and are owed a duty of care in this regard also.

Amphetamines

Description

Amphetamines and methamphetamine stimulate the sympathetic nervous system and block reuptake of catecholamines, dopamine, and serotonin.

Methods of abuse

Oral.

Clinical features

Effects occur within 1 hour and last 4–6 hours with smaller doses, up to 48 hours after larger.

Sympathomimetic effects

- Tachycardia, cardiac arrhythmias* (usually supraventricular)
- Dilated pupils and blurred vision
- Hypertension (may result in CVA*)
- Pallor
- Sweating, dry mouth.

Central effects

- Agitation
- Talkativeness
- Drowsiness, coma*
- Paranoia
- Visual hallucinations
- Convulsions.*

A hyperpyrexial syndrome may also occur

Immediate management

- Intravenous access
- Monitor ECG
- Diazemuls for fitting, agitation, or psychosis (also reduces hypertension agitation and tachycardia)
- Activated charcoal can be given within 1 hour of oral ingestion if hospital transfer is likely to be prolonged
- If transfer is likely to be prolonged or delayed, hyperthermia should be treated with cold intravenous fluids. Damp sponging should be carried out to reduce the core temperature.
- Transfer to hospital (SVT and hypertension can be treated after arrival, unless this is likely to be delayed).

> Hallucinating patients must not be left alone!
> Their behaviour may put themselves and others at risk.

* severe poisoning.

Amyl nitrate

Description

Conventionally used in the management of cyanide poisoning.

Methods of abuse

Ingestion and inhalation.

Clinical features

- Headache
- Nausea and vomiting
- Sweating
- Flushing
- Chest tightness
- Confusion
- Fitting (rare)
- Cyanosis may occur due to methaemoglobinaemia.

Immediate management

- No specific management is required
- Monitor: pulse, BP, respiratory rate
- Maintain a patent airway and administer oxygen 15l/min
- Transfer to hospital.

Benzodiazepines

Description

Prescription drugs.

Methods of abuse

Oral ingestion.

Clinical features

- Drowsiness
- Confusion
- Mid position or dilated pupils
- Ataxia (slurred speech) and nystagmus
- Coma (rarely deep GCS <10)
- Hypotension (usually mild)
- Respiratory depression
- Cardiorespiratory arrest (after iv use).

Immediate management

Supportive care for the patient with a reduced conscious level. Particular care should be paid to airway maintenance.

Flumazenil is NOT licensed for the treatment of deliberate benzodiazepine overdose. The correct pre-hospital management is supportive care pending arrival in hospital. Rarely, flumazenil treatment may be appropriate but it should be used with caution and complete reversal should not be attempted.

Flumazenil is ABSOLUTELY contraindicated in a patient with a history of convulsions or those who have also ingested tricyclic antidepressants in whom it may precipitate fits and ventricular arrhythmias. Acute withdrawal may result from the use of flumazenil in those patients addicted to benzodiazepines

Activated charcoal is not indicated.

Cannabis

Description

Psychoactive substances derived from the plant *Cannabis sativa*. Marijuana refers to any part of the plant used for its pharmacological effects; hashish is dried resin from the flowers. Common names include: grass, pot, hash, reefer ganja, bhang, and spliff.

Methods of abuse

- Dried, then smoked or eaten
- Occasionally injected.

Clinical features

These will depend on the mood, personality of the individual, environment, and the amount consumed.

After smoking, the onset of effects is 10–30 minutes; after ingestion, 1–3 hours. Duration of effects, 4–8 hours.

Low dose

- Euphoria
- Altered perception
- Relaxation
- Drowsiness
- Hypertension, tachycardia
- Slurred speech
- Ataxia, lack of co-ordination
- Appetite stimulation
- Injected conjunctivae
- Dilated pupils.

High dose

- Acute paranoid psychosis
- Anxiety, panic attacks
- Confusion
- Hallucinations and distortions of time and space.

Intravenous abuse may result in diarrhoea, nausea, vomiting, and abdominal pain, as well as hypotension and pulmonary oedema. Management of psychotic features is discussed on p.484.

Immediate management

Supportive therapy and observation is usually all that is required. Diazemuls may be used for sedation, if required. Hypotension responds to intravenous fluids.

Cocaine/crack cocaine

Description

- Cocaine is an alkaloid from the leaves of the coca bush from South America.
- Cocaine: cocaine hydrochloride is a white crystalline powder or colourless crystals
- Crack cocaine: crack cocaine ('crack') is cocaine separated from the hydrochloride base, and usually sold as 'rocks'.

Methods of abuse

- Cocaine is 'snorted' (sniffed) or injected intravenously
- Crack is smoked.

Clinical features

When cocaine is snorted, effects occur very rapidly and may last up to 90 minutes. Smoked crack produces its maximum effect in about 10 minutes and has begun to wear off after about 15–20 minutes.

Mild/moderate intoxication

- Euphoria
- Slurred speech and ataxia
- Restlessness, tremor, agitation, and aggression
- Hallucinations
- Pupillary dilatation
- Nausea and vomiting
- Pallor, cold sweats
- Tachycardia, tachypnoea, ventricular ectopics/arrhythmias, hypertension.

Severe intoxication

- Drowsiness and coma
- Convulsions
- Incontinence
- Hyperreflexia
- Circulatory and respiratory failure—leading to hypotension, hypoxia, and arrhythmias
- Severe hypertension—leading to stroke, intracerebral haemorrhage, and infarction
- Artery spasm—leading to myocardial and intestinal ischaemia and AMI
- Hyperthermia.

A paranoid delusional state may occur with chronic usage. Psychotic reactions to individual doses may also occur. Hallucinations may also occur.

Severe depression and aggression may follow the 'high' and may result in suicide attempts or violent behaviour against others.

Pneumothorax may be found as a result of valsalva manoeuvres performed to increase the absorption of inhaled cocaine.

Immediate management

The patient should be assessed in a quiet environment.

- Monitor: ECG, pulse, BP
- Establish and maintain a patent airway; ensure intravenous access
- Diazemuls for fitting, agitation, or psychosis (also reduces hypertension agitation and tachycardia)
- Transfer to hospital.

If transfer is likely to be prolonged or delayed, hyperthermia should be treated with tepid sponging. Cold intravenous fluids may be necessary.

Activated charcoal can be given within one hour of oral ingestion if hospital transfer is likely to be prolonged.

Ecstasy

Description

Ecstasy (3,4 methylenedioxymetamphetamine, MDMA) is a derivative of amphetamine.

Methods of abuse

Oral ingestion.

Clinical features

- Euphoria and increased sensuality
- Dehydration
- Hyperthermia
- Agitation
- Convulsions
- Muscle spasm
- Abdominal pain
- Hypotension
- Coma
- Cerebral haemorrhage and infarction
- Cardiac arrhythmias.

Effects of chronic use include anorexia, palpitation, jaw stiffness, teeth grinding, sweating, and insomnia

Immediate management

- Intravenous access
- Monitor ECG
- Diazemuls for fitting, agitation, or psychosis (also reduces hypertension agitation and tachycardia)
- Activated charcoal can be given within one hour of oral ingestion if hospital transfer is likely to be prolonged. If transfer is likely to be prolonged or delayed, hyperthermia should be treated with damp sponging to reduce the core temperature. Cold intravenous fluids should be considered.
- Transfer to hospital (SVT and hypertension can be treated after arrival, unless this is likely to be delayed).

Note

The common causes of death following ecstasy use appear to be arrhythmias (early) and a hyperthermic neuroleptic malignant-like syndrome (late).

Gammahydroxybutyric acid

Description

GHB is sold (illegally) for body building and weight loss. It is also used as a psychedelic agent.

Methods of abuse

Sold as a powder, GHB is dissolved in water and taken orally.

Clinical features

Symptoms are dose dependent and include:

- Nausea
- Diarrhoea
- Drowsiness, confusion, coma
- Vertigo
- Tremor
- Extrapyramidal signs
- Agitation
- Bradycardia
- Hypotension
- Cardiorespiratory depression (severe poisoning)
- Fits.

Immediate management

- Monitor: BP, pulse, respiratory rate, and pulse oximetry
- Check: BM stix
- Diazemuls for fits
- Atropine for bradycardia
- Transfer to hospital.

Hallucinogenic fungi

Description

A wide range of fungi are ingested for their hallucinogenic properties. The most common of these is *Psilocybe semilanceata* (liberty cap).

Methods of abuse

Oral ingestion.

Clinical features

Symptoms usually begin within 30–90 minutes following ingestion and include:

- Nausea and vomiting
- Abdominal pain
- Dilated pupils
- Hallucinations (visual and auditory)
- Agitation, tremor
- Drowsiness
- Depression.

Immediate management

- Evacuation to hospital
- Diazemuls for sedation, if required.

Ketamine

Description

A dissociative anaesthetic/analgesic.

Methods of abuse

- Commercial ketamine is injected intramuscularly or intravenously
- Street ketamine is sniffed or smoked.

Clinical features

The onset of action is rapid and the psychological effects usually last less than one hour:

- Euphoria
- Psychological effects/confusion:
  - Synaesthesia (experiencing a stimulus with the 'wrong' sense)
  - Out-of-body experiences
  - Depersonalization
  - Persistent repetition of acts or words
- Agitation
- Aggression
- Vomiting
- Slurred speech
- Blurred vision
- Numbness
- Dizziness and ataxia
- Hypertension and tachycardia
- Rarely, convulsions, cardiac and respiratory arrest, raised intracranial pressure, and pulmonary oedema may occur.

Emergence reactions may be profoundly unpleasant including vivid dreams, hypersensitivity to light, and hallucinations.

Immediate management

- Monitor: pulse, BP, ECG, and pulse oximetry
- The patient should be maintained wherever possible in a quiet dark environment to reduce emergence phenomena. Diazemuls may be used for agitation and will also reduce emergence symptoms.
- Transfer to hospital.

Lysergic acid diethylamide (LSD)

Description

A synthetic hallucinogen.

Methods of abuse

Usually ingested, either impregnated onto small squares of paper or as tablets or capsules. Rarely, taken intravenously, nasally, or by smoking.

Clinical features

Effects are usually seen within an hour after oral ingestion; more rapidly after intravenous abuse.

Patients may present with a 'bad trip':

- Hallucinations (usually auditory)
- Acute anxiety state (anxiety, panic, agitation, sweating, piloerection)
- Aggression
- Confusion.

Other effects include:

- Coma
- Nausea, vomiting
- Dilated pupils
- Tachycardia, tachypnoea
- Visual disturbance
- Weakness, tremor, ataxia
- Salivation, lacrimation
- Focal neurological deficit
- Acute psychosis with behavioural change, hallucinations, paranoia, and mania may occur.

Immediate management

- Monitor: pulse, BP, pulse oximetry
- The patient should be maintained in a quiet, dark environment with minimal stimuli and gently reassured. Diazemuls should be used if sedation is necessary or to control fitting.

Methanol

Description

Commonly found in antifreeze, it is also consumed deliberately and accidentally in contaminated alcohol.

Methods of abuse

Oral.

Clinical features

Initial symptoms (under two hours) resemble ethanol intoxication:

- Drowsiness
- Confusion
- Irritability.

After a latent period of 6–30 hours or longer, dizziness, drowsiness, abdominal pain, diarrhoea, coma, and fits may follow. Hypoglycaemia may occur.

Ocular effects may also occur up to 24 hours after ingestion. These include blurred vision with opacities within the visual fields, impaired acuity, and impaired papillary response to light. Permanent blindness may follow.

The minimum fatal dose of methanol in an adult is 60ml.

Immediate management

- Monitor: ECG, pulse, BP, and pulse oximetry
- Check BM stix
- Evacuate to hospital for further management. If evacuation to hospital is likely to be prolonged or delayed, 2.5ml/kg 40% proof spirit (whisky, gin, vodka, etc) should be given orally. Further doses may be necessary after arrival in hospital. Activated charcoal does not absorb alcohols.
- Diazemuls for fitting.

Opiates

Description

Synthetic and naturally occurring narcotic analgesics. The most commonly abused opioid is heroin (diamorphine).

Methods of abuse

Oral, intravenous, smoking.

Clinical features

The classic features are:

- Pinpoint pupils
- Respiratory depression or arrest
- Reduced conscious level or coma.

Signs of intravenous drug abuse (needle track marks, thrombosed veins, skin puncture marks) may also be present.

Symptoms of severe poisoning may also include:

- Pulmonary oedema (non-cardiogenic)
- Hypotension
- Hypothermia
- Fits—more common with dextropropoxyphene.

Immediate management

- Monitor: pulse, BP, respiratory rate, pulse oximetry
- Ensure a patent protected airway and support respiration if required (bag-valve-mask is usually appropriate).

Naloxone is a specific antidote for opiates. The dose is 0.4mg (400μg)—2mg repeated at intervals as required to a maximum of 10mg. If naloxone is given to exclude opiates as a cause of loss of consciousness, a dose of 2mg should be given.

Children: intravenous 10μg/kg, subsequent dose of 100μg/kg if no response

Naloxone is short-acting. As a result, when long-acting opiates are being reversed, repeated doses may be needed. Drug abusers may leave the scene after a first dose only to collapse as the naloxone wears off. In order to reduce the likelihood off this, either the opiate can be reversed only enough to ensure adequacy of respiration before arrival in hospital, or a similar dose to the intravenous one given above may be given INTRAMUSCULARLY in addition. Complete opioid reversal may precipitate an acute withdrawal syndrome.

Activated charcoal may be given within one hour of poisoning if naloxone is not available AND transfer to hospital is likely to be delayed or prolonged.

Opiate-induced fits may respond to naloxone. If this fails, diazemuls should be used.

Phencyclidine

Description

A psychedelic agent.

Methods of abuse

Oral ingestion.

Clinical features

- Anxiety
- Paraesthesia, decreased sensitivity to pain, synaesthesia
- Nystagmus, ataxia, dysarthria
- Disorientation
- Hallucinations
- Rigidity and catatonic movements
- Fitting
- Coma
- Tachycardia, hyper/hypotension
- Respiratory impairment or arrest.

Immediate management

- The patient should be assessed in a quiet environment
- Monitor: pulse, BP, pulse oximetry, respiratory rate
- Urgent transfer to hospital.

Volatile solvents

Description

The most commonly abused solvents are toluene, butane and xylene in such fluids as cleaning fluids, adhesives, typewriter correction fluid, lighter fluid, and glues.

Methods of abuse

Inhalation, often from a soaked rag or in a plastic bag.

Clinical features

Clinical effects occur within a few minutes:

- Euphoria
- Ataxia and dizziness leading to falling and injury
- Nausea and vomiting
- Hallucinations
- Respiratory and eye irritation
- Rash around the nose
- Drowsiness
- Headache
- Double vision
- Chest tightness.

Serious side-effects include confusion, drowsiness and coma, fits, arrhythmias, and pulmonary oedema. Sudden death is most likely to be due to arrhythmia but asphyxiation (when the bag is placed over the head) or aspiration of vomit may also occur.

The acute 'high' is likely to last less than 1 hour. Drowsiness may last many hours.

Immediate management

- Monitor: pulse, BP, ECG, and pulse oximetry
- Establish and maintain a patent airway
- Evacuate to hospital for further management.

Note

Butane is inhaled from a plastic bag and produces respiratory depression, coma, hypotension, and arrythmias. Supportive treatment only is required.

Common street names for drugs of abuse

A	*Amphetamine*
Acid (blotter acid)	*LSD or ecstasy*
Angel dust	*Phencyclidine*
Bart (Simpson)	*Ecstasy*
Base	*Cocaine free base*
Bazooka	*Cocaine*
Beast	*LSD*
Bennies	*Amphetamines*
Bhang	*Cannabis*
Big O	*Opium*
Blow	*Cocaine*
Boy	*Heroin*
Brown stuff	*Opium*
Bullet	*Amyl nitrate*
Bush	*Cannabis*
C	*Cocaine*
Candy	*Cocaine*
Cake	*Cocaine*
Charlie	*Cocaine*
Chinese (rock)	*Heroin*
Coke	*Cocaine*
Crap	*Heroin*
Crystal	*Amphetamine*
Cube juice	*Morphine*
Dennis the menace	*Ecstasy*
Dexies	*Amphetamine*
Dike	*Dipipanone (opiate)*
Disco biscuits	*Ecstasy*
Doll (dollies)	*Methadone*
Dome (dome dots)	*LSD*
Dope	*Cannabis*
Dose	*Cocaine*
Dots	*LSD*
Downers	*Barbiturates*
Dreamer	*Morphine*
Dust	*Cocaine/opium*
Dynamite	*Cocaine*
E	*Ecstasy*
Embalming fluid	*Phencyclidine*
Flake	*Cocaine*
Freebase	*Cocaine free base*

Ganja	*Cannabis*
Gas	*Volatile solvents*
Ghost	*LSD*
Glass	*Amphetamines*
Glue	*Solvents*
Grass	*Cannabis*
H	*Heroin*
Hard stuff	*Cocaine*
Happy dust	*Morphine*
Harry	*Heroin*
Hash	*Cannabis resin*
Hash oil	*Cannabis oil*
Hashish	*Cannabis resin*
Hit	*Cocaine*
Hocus	*Morphine*
Homegrown	*Cannabis*
Horse(shit)	*Heroin*
Ice	*Amphetamine or cocaine*
Jam	*Cocaine*
Joint	*Cannabis*
Joy sticks	*Cannabis*
Junk	*Heroin*
Kitkat	*Ketamine*
L	*LSD*
Lady	*Cocaine*
Leaf	*Cocaine*
M	*Morphine or ecstasy (MDMA)*
Magic dust	*Hallucinogens*
Marijuana	*Cannabis*
Mary Jane	*Cannabis*
Meth	*Amphetamine*
Microdot	*LSD*
Monkey	*Morphine*
Noise	*Heroin*
Paki (black)	*Cannabis*
Poppers	*Amyl nitrate*
Pot	*Cannabis*
Purple haze	*LSD*
Reefer	*Cannabis*
Resin	*Cannabis*
Roaches	*Cannabis*
Rock	*Heroin*

Shit	*Cannabis*
Shrooms	*Hallucinogenic fungi*
Skunk	*Cannabis*
Smack	*Cocaine or heroin*
Smoke	*Cannabis*
Snort	*Cannabis*
Speed	*Amphetamines*
Spliff	*Cannabis*
Stuff	*Heroin*
Sulphate	*Amphetamine*
Tea	*Cannabis*
Uppers	*Stimulants*
Vitamin K	*Ketamine*
Weed	*Cannabis*
White dove	*Ecstasy*
White lightening	*LSD*
Whizz	*Amphetamine*
XTC	*Ecstasy*

Chapter 7

Acute psychiatric emergencies

Psychiatric emergencies

True psychiatric emergencies needing urgent resolution are relatively rare. When they do occur, they require sensitivity and the formulation of a careful management plan. Referral to hospital may not be the most appropriate option and the patient may already be known to the psychiatric services. Nevertheless, a key component of the management of psychiatric emergencies is the identification of the small number of patients who present a risk either to their own health or to the safety of those who are attempting to help them. As a result of this risk, the law which applies to psychiatric patients is different to that which applies to those who do not suffer from mental illness, and a vital part of the correct management of these patients is a knowledge and understanding of the *Mental Health Act*.

Patient assessment—mental state examination

It is obviously impossible to carry out a full mental state examination in many pre-hospital situations. It is possible, however, to gain enough information to allow sensible management decisions to be made using a simplified system of assessment.

The key features of a psychiatric history are:

- Presenting complaint
- Past psychiatric history
- Past medical history
- Medication
- Drug and alcohol use
- Social situation and family history (including psychiatric history).

The presenting complaint can be considered under the following headings:

- Appearance and behaviour
- Speech form (rate, quantity, and coherence) and content
- Mood (depressed, manic, labile, inappropriate)
- Beliefs and thoughts
  - Passivity—direction or manipulation of thought and thought content by an other agent
  - Phobias
  - Worries
  - Obsessions
  - Suicidal/homicidal thoughts
- Delusions (false fixed unshakeable beliefs)
- Hallucinations
- Cognition (orientation, concentration, memory)
- Insight.

Patient assessment—physical examination

A physical examination should be carried out wherever possible in order to exclude or confirm an underlying organic cause for the presenting complaint (see box).

Suicide risk

Assessment of suicide risk is notoriously difficult and the pre-hospital doctor must ere on the side of caution. It is important not to be misled by the comments of others who may underplay the significance of events. In addition, parasuicidal actions may have a fatal outcome due to ignorance of the consequences on the patient's part. This is particularly the case in drug ingestions. In general, the more violent the method attempted by the patient, the greater the intent to die. Suicidal risk factors are listed in the box below.

Any patient who appears to be demonstrating a significant risk of a further completed suicide attempt should be taken to the local A&E department or mental health facility, depending on local services and protocols.

When there is a perceived significant risk that a patient will take their own life, but they are not obviously detainable under the Mental Health Act, it is permissible under common law to restrain them pending formal psychiatric assessment.

More common organic causes of psychiatric illness

- Hypoglycaemia
- Infection
- Cardiac failure
- Alcohol abuse (delirium tremens)
- Substance abuse
- Subdural haematoma.

Risk factors for a successful suicide attempt

Mental health issues

- Present or previous psychiatric illness, especially depression
- Personality disorder
- Previous suicide attempt or self harm
- Suicidal thoughts
- Family history of suicide.

Physical health issues

- Chronic physical illness.

Demographic and social factors

- Male sex
- Age >40
- Single, unmarried, divorced
- Unemployed
- Problem drinking.

Other

- Recent life crisis.

Psychiatric conditions

Psychosis

Presentation

Psychotic patients demonstrate disordered thinking and behaviour. These symptoms may or may not be sufficiently characteristic to assign a diagnostic label such as schizophrenia. Psychotic symptoms may also complicate depression (depressive delusions are usually consistent with the mood of the patient; non-congruous delusions are a feature of schizophrenia).

Delusions

Delusions are firmly held, unshakeable beliefs that are not consistent with the patient's social, religious, and cultural background. Delusions may be paranoid, controlling, or persecutory, but the patient may also believe themselves to be equipped with special abilities or a particular mission. The patient may be deluded that they are being watched or bugged or that television programmes or newspapers contain messages of significance to them. Somatic delusions are those attached to the patient's bodily function or appearance.

Hallucinations

Hallucinations are false perceptions which can occur in any sensory modality. Auditory hallucinations are most common; visual hallucinations are characteristic of delirium (an organic cause) and tactile hallucinations may occur secondary to drug abuse. Delusional explanations may be formed for hallucinatory experiences and some hallucinations may lead the patient to specific courses of action. Both delusions and hallucinations (classically olfactory) may occur in temporal lobe epilepsy.

Behavioural abnormalities

Behavioural abnormalities in psychosis may vary from the threatening and aggressive to the withdrawn and uncommunicative. Speech may be unintelligible and accompanied by wild gesturing, swearing, and antisocial behaviour. The patient may be preoccupied with responding to his delusions or hallucinations. In some, relatively rare cases, the patient may be at risk of harming themselves or others.

Management

The most important aspect of the management of a psychotic patient is control of their behaviour. The best way to achieve this is by a calm empathic approach. There is no value in attempting to reason a psychotic patient out of their delusional beliefs, and this is only likely to inflame an already difficult situation.

It is essential that a risk assessment is made and that appropriate assistance is sought, if necessary. Otherwise, an approach based on inappropriate force and aggression must be avoided since it is unlikely to be helpful and may compound the delusional beliefs of the patient.

When sedation is required, the most appropriate for pre-hospital use is probably haloperidol (2–10mg intramuscularly).

Depression

Presentation

The characteristic features of depression are:

- Misery
- Lethargy and lack of motivation
- Disturbed sleep
- Disturbed appetite
- Low self esteem
- Lack of libido
- Anxiety
- Guilt
- Self neglect
- Suicidal thoughts.

Risk factors for depression are given in the box below.

Risk factors for depression

- Low social class
- Single status
- Family history
- Unemployment
- Urban environment
- Medical and psychiatric co-morbidity
- Drug and alcohol abuse
- Loss of the patient's mother before age 11
- Those who are confined to the home (women)
- Three or more young children (women)
- Lack of social support (women)

Management

The most important aspects of management are a patient approach and a sympathetic ear. An assessment of suicide risk factors should be performed (p.483) and appropriate referral made to the psychiatric services. This may involve direct referral to A&E or, rarely, detention under common law or the Mental Health Act, pending formal psychiatric assessment.

Mania

Presentation

The characteristic presenting symptoms of mania are:

- Overactivity
- Distractability
- Agitation
- Irritability
- Impulsive behaviour.

Manic behaviour may also be flamboyant, provocative, violent, or sexually disinhibited. The patient may also suffer delusions and hallucinations.

Management

The most important aspect of management is a calm rational approach. On occasion, physical restraint may be necessary but should only be used when there is no alternative. Adequate numbers of personnel must be available. If medication is necessary, haloperidol or a benzodiazepine should be used.

Anxiety disorders

Presentation

The characteristic symptoms of anxiety are:

Physical

- Tachycardia/palpitation
- Dry mouth
- Sweating
- Breathlessness
- Flushing
- Tremor
- Urinary frequency
- Nausea and diarrhoea

Psychological

- Fear
- Apprehension
- Loss of patience/irritability
- Insomnia.

Hyperventilation syndrome may occur with dyspnoea, carpopedal spasm and perioral tingling.

Management

The main treatment aim is reassurance. Hyperventilation is treated by getting the patient to breathe in and out of a paper bag until the symptoms resolve. This should be done in the sitting position whilst the patient takes *slow shallow* breaths. Referral for longer-term management is likely to be necessary.

Personality disorders

Patients with personality disorder can be extremely difficult to manage. They often appear hostile and impatient and do not easily interact with those attempting to care for them. Indeed, such patients seem to have a remarkable ability to antagonize carers, with the inevitable consequence that their management is often suboptimal.

Unfortunately, these patients are at a significantly increased risk of successful suicide despite often long histories of previous non-fatal self harm. It is vital, therefore, that an objective approach is taken and a formal assessment carried out. Any suicidal ideation must be taken seriously and appropriate referral to the psychiatric services made.

Legal and ethical issues

The Mental Health Act 1983

The Mental Health Act 1983 states the law governing the management of patients with mental illness. The sections that are most likely to be used by pre-hospital care practitioners are sections 2,3,4, 135, and 136.

Section 2 Admission for assessment

Section 2 concerns admission for assessment and is usually applied when there is no previous history of diagnosed mental disorder or the patient is not known to the local psychiatric services. Admission must be necessary for assessment of the patient's condition, in their best interests, and required for the safety of others.

Section 2 is valid for 28 days. Application is made by an approved social worker or (less commonly) the nearest relative and recommendation for admission is by two doctors, one of whom must be approved under the Mental Health Act (Section 12) and is usually a consultant psychiatrist. An approved social worker can be contacted via the local social services department.

At the end of the 28-day period, the patient must be discharged or converted to Section 3. Patients admitted under Section 2 may request a mental health tribunal review after 14 days.

Section 3 Admission for treatment

Section 3 is intended to provide for compulsory admission for the treatment of a mental illness. Application is by an approved social worker and recommendation must be made by two doctors, of whom one must be approved under the Act (as for Section 2). Admission is for 60 days.

To be eligible for Section 3, the patient must suffer from mental illness, mental impairment or severe mental impairment, or psychopathic disorder which is sufficiently serious to require treatment in hospital. Alternatively, detention in hospital must be necessary for the safety of others.

Once an application has been made, it is considered to be in force.

Section 4 Emergency admission for assessment

Section 4 covers emergency admission, which can be recommended by any doctor (who does not have to be approved under the Act). Application is made by an approved social worker or nearest relative. Section 4 can only be used in an emergency when Section 2 cannot be used due to the unavailability of staff. The duration of admission permitted under section 4 is 72 hours (before conversion to Section 2 is necessary).

Section 135 Removal to a place of safety (via a magistrate)

Under Section 135, a social worker may apply to a magistrate for a warrant to remove a patient to a place of safety if he believes that the patient's mental illness means that the patient is unable to care for himself or he considers that the patient is being neglected or mistreated. Section 135 allows entry into the patient's home. The maximum duration for which the patient can be held under Section 135 is 72 hours.

Section 136 Removal to a place of safety (by the police)

Section 136 allows the removal of a mentally ill person to a place of safety by a police officer in an emergency situation when it is not possible to involve a social worker or approved doctor. The patient must be in need of care or control in their own best interests or in the interests of others. The place of safety is usually the nearest hospital or police station. The patient can be detained for a maximum of 72 hours pending assessment and transfer to a more appropriate section of the Act.

Table 7.1 Relevant sections of the Mental Health Act 1983

Grounds	*Application by*	*Medical recommendation*	*Maximum duration*
Mental disorder,	Approved social worker or nearest relative	Two doctors, one approved under the Act	28 days
Mental illness, psychopathic disorder, mental impairment, severe mental impairment	As above	As above	6 months
Mental disorder (urgent need to admit)	As above	Any doctor	72 hours
Mental disorder	Magistrate	N/A	72 hours
Mental disorder	Police officer	N/A	72 hours

Managing the violent patient

The key to the successful management of the violent or potentially violent patient is risk assessment. Some important risk factors for violent behaviour are shown in the box. An awareness of these allows preparation *before* a crisis occurs.

The following management points may be helpful:

DO

- Keep a sideways posture relative to the patient; avoid 'aggressive' eye contact
- Keep your hands visible
- Talk calmly and allow the patient to speak
- Try to identify the cause of the aggression and deal with it
- Have an escape plan.

DO NOT

- Interview the patient alone
- Interview the patient in an environment in which you could be trapped
- Fidget or look at your watch
- Make promises that cannot be kept
- Be critical.

Risk factors for violent behaviour

Psychiatric
- Psychopathic personality
- 'Command' hallucinations (to harm others)
- Delusional beliefs of persecution
- Mania
- Dementia.

Psychological
- Anxiety or fear about personal safety
- Anger or conflict (with inability to manage it)
- Inability to cope.

Organic
- Learning disability
- Drugs or alcohol
- Delirium
- Brain injury or disease.*

Demographic
- Young male
- Previous history of violence
- Group pressure/tolerance of violent behaviour.

* Including head injury, frontal lobe damage, meningitis, epilepsy, and encephalitis

Chapter 8
Paediatrics

Taking a paediatric history

The essential components of a paediatric history are:

- History of the presenting complaint
- Previous medical history
- Social and family history.

Immediate assessment and attention to life-threatening problems precedes a full history. However, even in a crisis, obtaining an AMPLE history takes only a short time and can provide vital information:

A Allergies
M Medicines
P Past medical history
L Last food and drink
E Events leading to current problem

Allergies

Allergic reactions to medicines and food in children are becoming increasingly common, especially allergy to nuts. Parents of children with known severe allergies often carry an adrenaline self-administration device (Epipen®).

Medicines

Regularly prescribed medication gives vital information about the child's active medical problems and underlying health issues.

Past medical history

The past medical history may provide crucial information, such as the presence of congenital cardiovascular or neurological problems and recurrent illnesses including asthma or diabetes.

Last food and drink

Recent food and drink is a risk for regurgitation, especially for children with an altered level of consciousness. Vomiting occurs quite frequently in children with minor injuries and febrile illnesses.

Events leading up to the current problem

The mechanism of injury or details of current medical problems help in predicting patterns of injury or determining the medical diagnosis. Aspects of the history should include:

Information from the scene

The position of vehicles, vehicle deformity, and the position in which the child was found all provide vital clues to potential injuries. In the case of medical illnesses or domestic accidents, the state of the home and the well-being of siblings may give useful clues to the current problem. The pre-hospital carer is in the unique position to know the home environment and the possibility of physical abuse.

Information from carers

Children are usually accompanied by a parent, relative, family friend, or teacher. Carers, nursery nurses, and school teachers will often know about a child's medical illnesses, medication, and social circumstances.

Information from witnesses

Information from witnesses may provide valuable details regarding the mechanism of injury. Was the child run over? Were they projected over the bonnet? Were they hit by another vehicle? Were they unconscious?

The child's own history

Communicating with a child can be difficult. Questions should be pitched appropriately for the child's age. Language and intellect may be barriers to understanding. Equally, a child may respond more appropriately to its parent or carer rather than to a stranger.

ABCDE

Direct questioning logically follows an ABCDE sequence:

Airway

- How long has the child had problems?
- Could the child have inhaled a foreign body?
- Has the child been distressed?
- Has the child been drooling? (consider epiglottitis)
- Has the child been eating/drinking normally?

Breathing

Has the child:

- Had the problem before?
- Been responding normally?
- Been distressed?

If there is a known respiratory problem, has the child:

- Ever required steroids?
- Ever been admitted to hospital with a similar problem before?
- Ever been admitted to an intensive care unit with breathing problems?
- Had a cough, cold, ear infection, or sore throat?

Circulation

- When did the problem start?
- Does the child have any heart problems?
- Does the child have a rash?
- Has the child had diarrhoea or vomiting?
- Has the child been responding normally?

Disability

- When did the problem start?
- Has the child been responding normally?
- Does the child have a rash?
- Has the parent or carer noted any agitation or drowsiness?
- Has the child had a head injury?

The following questions may be helpful in particular circumstances:

In the case of fitting:
- Has the child ever had fits before?
- Was the child unwell before the fit?
- Has the child had a raised temperature?
- Did the child have a tonic/clonic reaction?
- How long did it last?

In all cases of unconsciousness/diabetes:
- Is the child known to be diabetic? (check a BM stix®)
- If so, has the child had their normal insulin?
- Has the child been eating and drinking normally?
- Has the child been behaving normally?

Environment
- In what position is the child most comfortable?
- Is the child too hot or too cold?

Important questions in neonates and infants:
- Has the child had a raised temperature or been shivering?
- Has the child had a reduction or increased urine output (dry or wet nappies)?
- Is the child sleepy?

Are there any symptoms of child abuse?
- Non-accidental injury
- Emotional neglect
- Neglect
- Sexual abuse
- Organized or ritual abuse.

Features suggestive of non-accidental injury include:
- Inappropriate delay in seeking help after significant injury
- Previous history of frequent injuries
- Mechanism of injury not appropriate
- Vague or no history of trauma
- Different explanations for cause of injury
- Different history from the child
- Inconsistent history for the child's chronological age
- Inappropriate response to carers and parents.

Patient handover

The child should be handed over to medical staff using the Mechanisms, Injuries, Symptoms, Treatment (MIST) system.

Identification and management of the seriously ill or injured child

The optimal management of the critically injured or ill child requires the accurate assessment, recognition, and treatment of immediately life-threatening and urgent problems. The approach to the ill or injured child follows the ABCDE system. Diagnosis is of secondary importance to the life-saving procedures. Assessment of the child demands a full understanding of the important anatomical and physical differences between children and adults.

Weight

Weight varies with age. The most rapid growth occurs within the first year (average birth weight 3.5kg, average weight at age 1, 10kg). The rate of growth then slows prior to the pubertal growth spurt and finishes when the epiphyseal growth plates fuse.

Weight can be estimated between 1–10 years of age using the formula:

Weight (kg) = (Age in years + 4) x 2

Drug dosage calculation is related to the child's body weight. Appropriate *aide memoires* in the form of tables or tapes are available to assist in calculating weight, equipment sizes, and drug dosage and should be checked prior to any paediatric drug administration.

Vital signs

Heart rate

Heart rate varies with age from 120–140 beats per minute in the newborn to that of 60–70 beats per minute in a healthy adolescent.

Age (years)	Respiratory rate (breaths/minute)	Pulse rate (beats/minute)
Under 1	30–40	110–160
1–5	25–30	95–140
6–12	20–25	80–120

Fig. 8.1 Normal paediatric vital signs.

The most common cause of bradycardia in children is hypoxia. Tachycardia may be due to pain, anxiety, or physiological compensation to maintain vital organ perfusion.

Blood pressure

Blood pressure varies with age and can be calculated using the formula:

Systolic blood pressure (mmHg) = 80 + (age in years × 2)

Blood pressure can be difficult to measure in pre-hospital care. Children have very robust compensation mechanisms and only become hypotensive as a pre-terminal event. A hypotensive child is at serious risk of cardiovascular collapse as the compensatory mechanisms fail rapidly once hypotension is established.

Respiratory rate

Respiratory rate varies with age. It should be noted that infants are obligatory nasal breathers. Conditions such as acute bronchiolitis risk airway blockade. Infants use the diaphragm as the main muscle of ventilation. The child may exhaust easily. In addition, large amounts of air can be trapped in the stomach restricting movement of the diaphragm. The use of accessory muscles of ventilation, intercostal recession, and tracheal tug are all features of respiratory distress.

Recognition of ABC problems

The child responds to trauma and acute illness by physiological compensation. When this is exhausted, decompensation follows, which if untreated will lead to death. Ventricular fibrillation is uncommon in children, the most frequent arrest rhythm being asystole precipitated by hypoxia and acidosis. The prognosis for cardiac arrest is appalling. Therefore, the emphasis must be on its prevention.

Airway

- The airway should be checked for obstruction from foreign objects and vomit. Blind finger sweeps *should not* be undertaken.
- Upper airway obstruction may produce choking due to foreign bodies or airway narrowing due to croup, epiglotitis, or thermal injury.
- The child may exhibit stridor or a barking cough due to airway narrowing.

Breathing

- An increased respiratory rate in the child at rest may be due to an airway or circulation problem as well as a breathing problem.
- Increased use of the muscles of ventilation and accessory muscles is a sign of ventilatory distress.
- Effective breathing is demonstrated by adequate symmetrical chest movements and equal breath sounds on auscultation.
- Wheeze or grunting respiration may be apparent. A silent chest (for example, in asthma) is a bad prognostic sign indicating inadequate ventilation and impending respiratory arrest.

Circulatory assessment

A systematic assessment of the heart rate, skin colour, temperature, capillary refill, and central and peripheral pulses should be performed.

- Tachycardia may be due to many factors including pain and anxiety. It is also seen as part of the cardiovascular response to infection and hypovolaemia.
- Bradycardia is a sign of cardiovascular decompensation.
- Comparative volumes of the central and peripheral pulses will give an indication of peripheral circulatory shut down.
- Capillary refill is assessed by pressing the skin for 5 seconds, then counting the time for the skin colour to return on the release of the pressure. A figure less than 2 seconds is normal. Prolongation in the absence of a limb injury with circulatory compromise or hypothermia indicates circulatory compromise.
- Altered mental state leads to confusion, aggression, and obtundation.
- Respiratory rate increases due to hypoxia and progressive metabolic acidosis.
- Pre-terminal features include skin mottling and cyanosis.

Signs of respiratory illness

- Tachypnoea
- Use of accessory muscles
- Wheezing or grunting respiration
- Silent chest
- Tachycardia
- Bardycardia (pre-terminal event)
- Skin pallor
- Cyanosis
- Decreasing level of consciousness.

Disability

The level of consciousness should be assessed using the AVPU system:

A		**A**lert
V	response to	**V**oice
P	response to	**P**ain only
U		**U**nresponsive

A central painful stimulus such as pressing over the supra-orbital ridge is preferred. Peripheral stimulation may not produce a response in the presence of a spinal cord injury. A child who is a P or U responder is at risk of airway compromise due to the loss of protective airway reflexes.

The child's posture should be recorded, for example, decerebrate (arms extended) or decorticate (arms flexed). Abnormal stiffness and floppiness should be recorded. Pupils should be observed for size, shape, and reactivity. Unilateral dilatation in the presence of a head injury suggests an intracranial collection. Sinus bradycardia and an elevated blood pressure suggest raised intracranial pressure.

Monitoring

Vital signs must be observed including:

- Pulse rate
- Respiratory rate
- Glasgow Coma Scale (GCS)
- Oxygen saturation
- ECG trace
- BM stix®
- End tidal CO_2 (if intubated).

In the event of any deterioration, the primary survey should be repeated. All children with significant ABC problems should be regarded as having a time-critical emergency.

The Glasgow Coma Scale voice component requires adaptation in younger children (see Fig. 8.2)

Response elicited	Score
BEST EYE OPENING RESPONSE	
Open spontaneously	4
React to speech	3
React to pain	2
No response	1
BEST MOTOR RESPONSE	
Moves normally and spontaneously or obeys commands	6
Localizes pain	5
Withdraws in response to pain	4
Flexes abnormally to pain (decorticate movements)	3
Extends abnormally to pain (decerebrate movements)	2
No response	1
BEST "VERBAL" RESPONSE	
Smiles, follows sounds and objects, interacts	5
Cries consolably or interacts inappropriately	4
Cries with inconsistent relief or moans	3
Cries inconsolably or is irritable	2
No response	1

Fig. 8.2 Paediatric Glasgow Coma Scale.

Management of ABC emergencies

Airway

- Manual manoeuvres including chin lift or jaw thrust. The head should be maintained in the neutral position in neonates and the 'sniffing the morning air' position in older children. (see Figs 8.3 and 8.4).
- Inline stabilization of the cervical spine is necessary in trauma.
- Aspiration of any vomit or secretion.
- Removal of foreign bodies under direct vision—DO NOT perform a finger sweep.
- Oropharyngeal airway insertion if there is no gag reflex present.
- Consideration of Bag–Value–Mask (BVM) venlilatory support.
- Consideration of endotracheal intubation or needle cricothyroidotomy as appropriate (consider surgical cricothyroidotomy if child over 12 years of age).

Notes

An *oropharyngeal airway*, if used, must be inserted following the contour of the tongue and is best inserted using a tongue depressor (unlike in the adult where the airway is inserted upside down and then rotated). In a child, this procedure may damage the soft tissues. The airway may induce wretching and vomiting.

An appropriately sized *nasopharyngeal airway* may be used to support the airway and must be inserted carefully, following lubrication, to avoid damage to the nostrils and the adenoids.

Endotracheal intubation should only be undertaken by trained, competent practitioners. All except completely unresponsive children will require drug-assisted rapid sequence induction to facilitate intubation. In the majority of cases, the airway can be opened as above and ventilation achieved using a 1- or 2- person bag-valve-mask technique until arrival at hospital.

When all attempts to open the airway are unsuccessful, a *needle cricothyroidotomy* may be performed. This will usually maintain life for a short period of time. The patient requires rapid transport to hospital for a definitive airway.

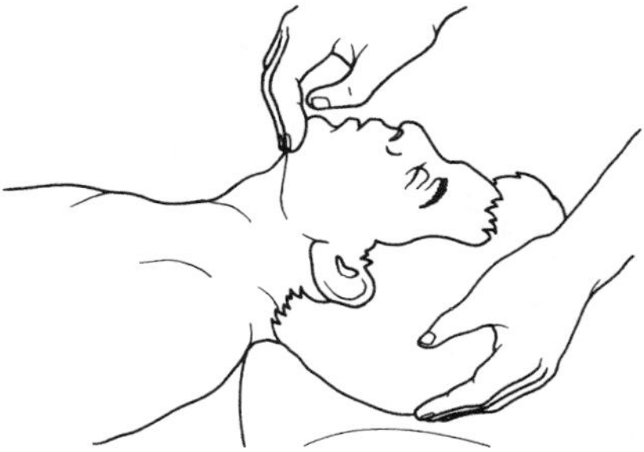

Fig. 8.3 Manual airway manoeuvres 1: Chin lift. The airway should be opened by chin lift and head tilt in the absence of trauma. Two fingers placed on the jaw prominence and lifting slightly, extend the neck into the '*sniffing the morning air position*'. In infants, neck extension should be avoided. The child's face should remain parallel to the surface on which they are lying. The soft tissues of the neck are easily compressed risking airway obstruction. Blind finger sweeps should be avoided because of the risk of forcing a foreign body further into the airway. (Reprinted with permission from Greaves I *et al.* (1995) *Handbook of immediate care*. Balliere Tindall).

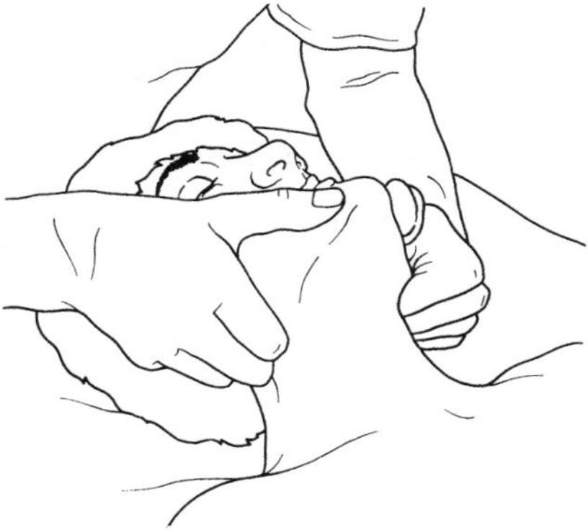

Fig. 8.4 Manual airway manoeuvres 2: Jaw thrust. If cervical spine trauma is suspected (based on mechanism of injury, pain in the neck, or neurological signs and symptoms), a jaw thrust manoeuvre should be undertaken. Two fingers are placed behind the angle of both sides of the jaw, gently pulling the jaw forward without tilting the head. Manual inline stabilization should be maintained and an appropriate cervical collar applied. In non-co-operative patients, reassurance, particularly from parents and friends, may facilitate treatment. In the combative child, the best approach is to attempt to maintain manual inline stabilization. (Reprinted with permission from Greaves I *et al.* (1995) *Handbook of immediate care*. Balliere Tindall).

Breathing

- Ensure adequate oxygenation by using a trauma mask (a face mask with a non-rebreathe valve and an oxygen reservoir) to which oxygen, distributed at 15 litres per minute, is attached.
- COPD is not a problem in children and, therefore, there is no concern about giving high-flow oxygen.
- If the child remains hypoxic despite supplementary oxygen, consider bag-valve-mask assisted ventilation.
- Avoid over-ventilation as this will precipitate gastric distention and a high risk of regurgitation.

Circulation

- High-flow oxygen should be administered to all patients with significant blood loss.
- Vascular access should be achieved by inserting the largest possible cannula into the biggest available vein. Intraosseous access should be the access of choice in the collapsed and/or hypovolaemic younger child, although it is effective in all age groups.
- Transfer to hospital should not be delayed pending vascular access which should be undertaken en route.
- At the time of vascular access, blood should be taken for glucose estimation.
- The initial fluid bolus for a shocked child is 20ml per kg of warmed crystalloid. When using the intraosseous route, it is necessary to use a syringe and 3-way tap to achieve adequate infusion.

Disability

- The management of disability relates to effective ABC management and the determination of a blood glucose level to exclude hypoglycaemia.
- Inadequate airway management (hypoxia), ineffective ventilation, and circulatory compromise (hypovolaemia) all contribute to significant secondary brain injury.

Environment

- Children are prone to hypothermia in view of their relatively large exposed body surface area (head in small babies) and their inability to maintain homeostasis.
- Excessive cooling of burns in children invariably causes hypothermia.
- The child knocked down in the street should be covered appropriately to preserve body temperature.
- Conversely, the febrile child should have unnecessary clothes removed and should not be kept in an over-warm environment.

Paediatric emergencies

Respiratory emergencies

These are common, and whilst many produce mild symptoms, they can be life-threatening. Children differ from adults in their ability to compensate for respiratory compromise by virtue of their different anatomy and physiology. Anatomical and physiological variations in infants and small children include:

- Obligatory nasal breathing (in children younger than 6 months)
- A short neck with a large head
- An anterior larynx (the airway and breathing can be easily affected by neck position and external pressure)
- A large tongue (many children have large tonsils)
- A smaller diameter airway which requires a lesser degree of swelling to cause obstruction
- A trachea narrowest at the cricoid ring
- Mainly diaphragmatic breathing
- A more compliant chest wall (retraction may compromise effective respiration)
- Loose primary dentition (age dependant).

Diagnostic respiratory noises include

- Stridor—of sudden onset in an otherwise unfit child is suggestive of an acute foreign body infection; in an unwell child who appears toxic and is drooling it suggests epiglotitis
- Harsh barking cough—is suggestive of viral croup
- Snoring noises—suggest upper airway obstruction (for example, from the tongue) in the unconscious child
- Bubbly noises—suggest excessive secretions and an inability to clear the airway.

Croup—laryngotracheobronchitis

Clinical features

- Viral illness, more common in autumn and spring
- Initial history of cold, snuffles, mild pyrexia, and malaise
- Followed by typical harsh barking cough
- Inspiratory stridor
- Signs of respiratory distress including increased respiratory rate, use of accessory muscles, nasal flaring, and wall recession **mandate** urgent hospital referral.

Treatment

- The key to successful management is to aim for as little interference as possible, combined with regular monitoring
- Nebulized 1:1000 adrenaline in severe cases
- Nebulized budesonide (2mg, for example as Pulmicort Respules®) or oral dexamethasone (0.15mg/kg) may modify the illness within 45 minutes
- Mild cases can be managed at home; severe respiratory distress will require hospital admission

- Rarely, intubation may be necessary, but in the child who is becoming exhausted, this can usually wait for formal induction of anaesthesia in hospital.

Note

The use of a nebulizer may worsen a child's distress rather than improve it (especially in small children) and should be considered carefully if the child is stable and hospital transfer likely to be brief.

If it is not possible to distinguish between croup and epiglottitis, admission is MANDATORY

Epiglottitis

Clinical features

- Incidence is decreasing due to the use of haemophilus influenza B (HIB) vaccination
- Generally occurs in older children
- Characterized by fever, stridor, (and if severe) drooling, and later, an extended neck and an altered level of consciousness
- Usually no prodromal illness
- Child appears pyrexial and toxic.

Treatment

- Do not examine or disturb the child
- Keep the child comfortable, nursed on the parent's knee
- Accompany the child to hospital
- Collapse is usually due to airway obstruction in which case needle cricothyroidotomy is effective in achieving an airway as an emergency pending a definitive airway in hospital
- Treatment involves appropriate antibiotic therapy (usually a 3rd generation cephalosporin).

Table 8.1 Distinguishing croup and epiglottitis

	Croup	Epiglottitis
Typical age	<3 years	2–8 years
Cause	Viral (many different)	Bacterial (*H Influenza*)
Onset	Slow	Rapid
Prodrome	Usual	Unusual
Toxicity	Apyrexial	Pyrexia (often >39°C)
Feeding	Good	Poor
Cough	Barking, harsh	None
Secretions	Can swallow	Drooling

Bronchiolitis

Clinical features

- Commonly caused by the respiratory syncytial virus
- Occurs in children < 1year old
- Premature and chronically unwell particularly at risk
- Coryza precedes:
  - Cough
  - Increased respiratory rate
  - Wheeze
  - Intercostal recession
  - Widespread crepitations
  - Hyperinflation of the chest
  - Mild pyrexia
  - Cyanosis if severe.

Treatment

- Appropriate positioning, sitting up—for small children this can be achieved using a child safety seat
- Nebulized ipratropium bromide 125μg will reduce secretions
- Antibiotics of no proven value
- If severe respiratory distress, administer oxygen and transport to hospital.

Asthma

Clinical features

- Common medical emergency in childhood
- Common association with atopy and wheeze in infancy
- Diagnostic feature is expiratory stridor
- May be classified as mild, moderate, severe, or life-threatening
- Severity determined by clinical features, peak expiratory flow rate (PEFR) (children over 5), and pulse oximetry.

Clinical classification

Mild asthma

- Minimal signs
- Wheeze detected on auscultation only
- Dry cough at night or after exercise is common
- Heart rate and respiratory rate normal
- PEFR greater than 75% of best or predicted value
- Oxygen saturation above 95%.

Moderate asthma

- Audible wheeze
- PEFR 50–75% of best or predicted
- Mild increase in heart and respiratory rate
- Mild degree of intercostal recession and use of accessory muscles
- Oxygen saturation above 90%
- *May* have difficulty in completing long sentences.

Severe asthma

- Inability to talk or feed
- Respiratory rate greater than 50 breaths per minute (2–10 years)
- Intercostal and sternal recession/use of accessory muscles
- Heart rate greater than 140 beats per minute
- Oxygen saturation less than 90%
- PEFR 33–50% of best or predicted.

Life-threatening asthma

As for severe but with sinister additional signs including:

- Exhaustion
- Silent chest
- Depressed conscious level
- Central cyanosis and bradycardia precede cardiorespiratory arrest
- Oxygen saturation < 85%
- PEFR <33% predicted.

Management

Treatment should follow a stepped plan depending on the severity of the symptoms.

Mild asthma

- Usually managed in the community
- Under parental guidance, 2 puffs from a metered dose inhaler delivering a beta 2 agonist, using a spacer if required
- Repeat beta 2 agonist if no response after 30mins
- If symptoms remain, refer to hospital.

Note

Oral steroids (prednisolone 2mg per kg to a maximum of 40mg) can be considered if there is no response to 24 hours of regular (4–6hrly) inhaled bronchodilator therapy.

Moderate asthma

- Children will be mildly hypoxic and should be given high-flow oxygen pending other treatment
- Beta 2 agonist should be given through a nebulizer driven by oxygen
- Oral steroids should be prescribed in all patients with moderate asthma (prednisolone 2mg per kg to a maximum of 40mg)
- If no improvement after 30 minutes, repeat beta 2 agonist and transport to hospital
- If transport is delayed, repeat beta 2 agonist on a regular basis.

Severe asthma

- Requires urgent management and hospital transfer
- Hypoxia should be treated with high-flow oxygen
- Salbutamol 2.5mg (<5years) or 5mg (>5 years), nebulized (driven by 100% oxygen), repeated as required
- Oral steroids (prednisolone 2mg per kg to a maximum of 40mg)
- If vomiting (or child unable to take tablets), prescribe intravenous hydrocortisone (2mg per kg)
- Nebulized ipratropium bromide (250–500µg) should be added after the beta 2 agonist (child under 5: 125–250µg; 6–12 years: 250µg)
- Monitor carefully and frequently during transport to hospital.

Note

In view of the potential problems with its use, intravenous aminophylline should only be used in hospital.

Life-threatening asthma

- As for severe asthma

  Also
- Consider
  - Salbutamol 5µg/kg intravenously (if available)
  - Bag-valve-mask assisted ventilation
  - Advanced airway measures
- Transport urgently to hospital requesting appropriate medical personnel to be present on arrival.

High pressures risk the development of a pneumothorax or regurgitation due to gastric dilatation.

Always consider pneumothorax or tension pneumothorax in acute deterioration of asthma.

Pneumonia

The range of causative organisms is wider in children than in adults. In the newborn, common organisms include *E coli* (and other gram negatives), haemolytic streptococci, and *Chlamydia trachomatis*. Causes in infancy include viruses (most commonly, respiratory syncytial virus—RSV), Pneumoccocus, haemophilus, and, more rarely, *Staphyloccocus aureus*. Older children are more likely to be infected with bacteria including those listed above and *Mycoplasma pneumonia*.

- Typically presents with pyrexia, cough (usually dry initially, then productive), and general malaise
- Similar physical signs to pneumonia in adults including:
  - Tachycardia
  - Tachypnoea
  - Dullness to percussion
  - Crepitation.

Signs may be difficult to elicit, especially in younger children, and a chest X-ray may be needed to localize pathology. Other symptoms which may occur in children include:

- Neck stiffness
- Abdominal pain.

Patents with significant respiratory distress require hospital referral, otherwise administer a cephalosporin, penicillin, amoxycillin, or erythromycin. If there is any doubt about the diagnosis, hospital transfer for investigation is necessary.

Inhaled foreign body

This is a relatively rare condition and the most likely site of impaction is the cricoid ring—the narrowest part of a child's airway. Severe respiratory distress due to complete obstruction occurs, which untreated will progress to coma and death.

Treatment should follow the Resuscitation Council paediatric choking algorithm (see Fig. 8.5).

If conscious: 5 back blows 5 thrusts chest for infant, abdominal for child >1year

- If unsuccessful, alternate back blows and thrusts
- Between steps, the child's mouth should be inspected for a displaced foreign body
- If unsuccessful, undertake a needle cricothyroidotomy.

If unconscious: attempt 5 rescue breaths

- Then start CPR (do not assess circulation)
- Between steps, the child's mouth should be inspected for a displaced foreign body
- If unsuccessful, undertake a needle cricothyroidotomy.

> The Heimlich manoeuvre should not be undertaken in children under 1 year old due to the risk of abdominal injury

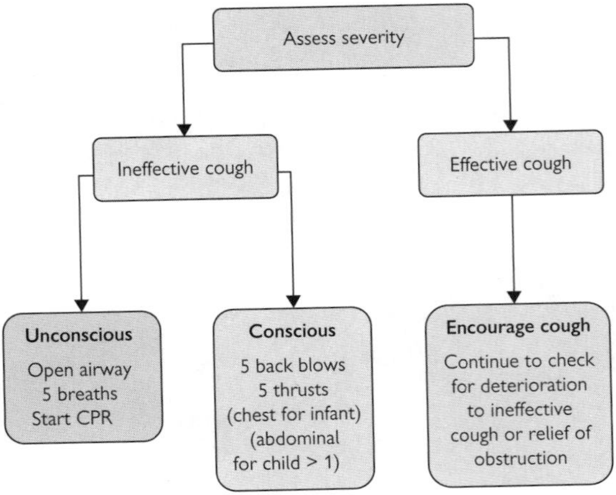

Fig. 8.5 Paediatric choking algorithm. Reprinted with permission from the Resuscitation Council (UK) (2005) *Resuscitation guidelines*.

Convulsions

Causes include:

- Secondary to a febrile illness or are idiopathic in origin
- Hypoxia
- Hypoglycaemia
- Poisoning
- Intracranial infection or tumours
- Failure to take or absorb medication in known epileptics.

Febrile convulsions commonly occur between the ages of 6 months and 6 years and are normally of a short duration and stop spontaneously. However, they cause intense distress to parents (particularly the first time).

The majority of fits are grand mal seizures, although focal or unilateral fits can occur. Status epilepticus occurs when a fit has continued for 30 minutes or fits occur so frequently that the patient does not recover between them. Deaths occur due to hypoxia, airway obstruction, and aspiration of vomit.

Treatment

Whatever the cause of the seizure, the treatment in the pre-hospital care situation follows the ABC system:

- Ensure the safety of the patient
- Establish a patent protected airway
- Do not place anything in the mouth or between the teeth if the jaw is clenched
- Administer high-flow oxygen, 10–15 litres per minute using a non re-breathe mask and a reservoir bag
- In the event of the child not breathing, commence bag-valve-mask ventilation
- In the case of fitting associated with a febrile illness, intravenous access is not usually necessary providing the fit has stopped; remove excess clothing to cool the child
- In children who continue fitting, those with repeated fits, and those in status epilepticus:
    - Vascular access should be obtained (intraosseous access may be the route of choice)
    - Intravenous diazemuls 0.2mg/kg should be given followed by a saline flush
    - If intravenous access cannot be obtained, rectal diazepam should be given (5mg for children less than 5 years of age, 10mg in children more than 5 years of age)
- Blood sugar estimation should be undertaken and appropriate treatment given if indicated
- In all cases, except where the child is a known epileptic and their parents or carers are experienced in post-ictal care, the child should be transported to hospital.

Children with febrile convulsions should be transferred to hospital for investigation of the cause of the fever. Pyrexia may be treated with rectal paracetamol (see p.357 for doses).

Metabolic emergencies

In children, the common metabolic emergencies invariably relate to the diagnosis and treatment of diabetes. However, in the child less than 6 months of age, in-born errors of metabolism can present with fitting and unconsciousness.

Hypoglycaemia

Most cases of hypoglycaemia are due to excessive insulin administration which is normally accidental (but occasionally deliberate, especially in adolescents). The diagnosis should be made by the use of a BM Stix®.

Treatment

- Mild/moderate hypoglycaemia (bizarre behaviour or mild confusion): oral glucose or hypostop
- More severe cases (unable to protect their own airway, reduced conscious level or unconscious): 2.5ml per kg of 10% dextrose intravenously over 5–10 minutes *or* intramuscular glucagon 500μg under 8 years (or under 25kg), 1mg over 8 years (or over 25kg).

Hyperglycaemia

This is most commonly associated with ketoacidosis. This may be the first presentation of diabetes and there may be a history of thirst, polydipsia, polyuria, and general malaise. Associated symptoms include nausea, vomiting, and dehydration. Pre-hospital treatment will depend on the patient's clinical state. Depending on the time to hospital, rehydration may be commenced with normal saline, 20ml per kg given over 1 hour. Following consultation with the receiving hospital, intramuscular insulin may be given at rate of 0.05 units per kg.

The unconscious child

Common causes of coma include:
- Hypoxia
- Hypoglycaemia/hyperglycaemia
- Post-ictal state
- Drugs/poisoning
- Alcohol
- Trauma
- Raised intracranial pressure including meningitis encephalitis, and blocked shunts in children with hydrocephalus
- Sepsis (including meningococcal).

In all cases, assessment and treatment should follow the ABC system.

Airway
- Consider airway adjuncts or endotracheal intubation if necessary.

Breathing
- Administer high-flow oxygen 10–15 litres per minute with a non re-breathe mask and reservoir bag
- Consider 2-person bag-valve-mask assisted ventilation.

Circulation
- Assess and treat shock as necessary.

Disability
- **D**on't **E**ver **F**orget **G**lucose
- If blood sugar is less than 4mmol/litre, give glucose 10%, 2.5ml per kg intravenously
- Assess pupils, look at focal signs; pinpoint pupils suggest opiate ingestion
- Consider and treat opiate overdose with naloxone, where appropriate.

Exposure

Look for evidence of a non-blanching rash suggestive of meningococcal septicaemia. If present or suspected, give benzylpenicillin (under 1, 300mg; 1–9 years, 600mg; 10 years and over, adult dose).

Babies are sometimes described as being 'floppy' or children, inattentive or listless. These are significant observations and, particularly in the case of the floppy child, indicate serious illness.

Common causes of loss of consciousness in children

- Epilepsy/convulsions
- Hypoglycaemia
- Hypoxia (organ failure or any cause of shock including trauma)
- Hypercapnia
- Hypothermia
- Head injury
- Meningitis/encephalitis
- Metabolic
- Poisoning.

Diarrhoea and vomiting

Gastroenteritis is the leading cause of paediatric illness and death in small babies. Vomiting may be a symptom of gastroenteritis or of other conditions including pyloric stenosis (males approximately 6 weeks old), intussusception, intestinal obstruction, urinary tract infections, meningitis, and febrile illnesses.

Diarrhoea is usually infective, though occasionally can be due to food intolerance. Children frequently present dehydrated.

Treatment depends on the level of dehydration which can be assessed as less than 5% (mild), 5–10% (moderate), and greater than 10% (severe).

Mild dehydration

- Treat with oral rehydration solutions (balanced salt glucose solution)—usually 75ml per kg over 4–6hours
- Consider using Dioralyte™ or other proprietary rehydration solution if available.

Moderate dehydration

- May respond to oral rehydration
- Alternatively, normal saline or Ringers lactate given intravenously at 20ml/kg in addition to normal requirements
- Consider transfer to hospital.

Severe dehydration

- Intravenous or intraosseous therapy
- Normal saline or Ringers lacate 20ml/kg over 30 minutes (1hour in infants)
- Then 70ml/kg over 3 hours (5 hours in infants)
- Transfer urgently to hospital.

Table 8.2 Assessment of dehydration

	Mild	Moderate	Severe
Drinking	Normal	Thirsty	Poorly
Skin pinch	Normal	Slow return	Very slow return
Eyes	Normal	Sunken	Very sunken
Mucous membranes	Normal	Dry	Very dry
Level of consciousness	Normal	Irritable	Lethargic/coma

Meningitis

Meningitis is fortunately relatively rare. The mode of presentation varies based on the patient's age.

Under 3 years

Diagnosis in this age group requires a high index of suspicion since symptoms may be non-specific, (for example, not feeding and listlessness). Classical signs (neck stiffness, photophobia, headache, and vomiting) are often absent.

Clinical features include:

- Distended fontanelles may be absent if the child is dehydrated
- Pyrexia (however, the child may be afebrile)
- Nausea
- Poor feeding
- Listlessness, drowsiness, or irritability
- Convulsions
- Apnoeic or cyanotic attacks
- Nausea and vomiting.

Older children

The older the child, the more likely they will present with clinical features similar to adults including:

- Neck stiffness
- Headaches
- Photophobia
- Vomiting
- Pyrexia
- Rash (indicative of septicaemia).

Meningococcal septicaemia

Meningococcal septicaemia may present without signs and symptoms of meningitis. Similarly, meningococcal meningitis may present without evidence of septicaemia. The classical features of meningococcal septicaemia include:

- Non-blanching petechial rash
- The child may be unwell out of all proportion to the physical signs
  Pre-hospital treatment follows the ABC system:
- High-flow oxygen 10–15 litres per minute using a non-rebreathe mask and a reservoir bag
- Ventilatory support, if required
- Intravenous access (peripheral vain or intraosseous)
- Benzylpenicillin
  - 1200mg over 10 years of age
  - 600mg between 1 and 9 years of age
  - 300mg in children less than 1 year of age
- Consider intravenous fluid replacement 20ml/kg normal saline of ringer lactate given over 20–30minutes but DO NOT delay transfer
- Transfer urgently to hospital
- A cephalosporin is usually given in hospital.

Erythromycin is appropriate in penicillin allergy. In established meningococcal septicaemia, ensure that the patient is genuinely penicillin allergic. If not, give penicillin. If genuine allergy is present, transfer immediately to hospital for alternative therapy if this is not immediately available.

Poisoning

Poisoning may be wilful or accidental. Young children may ingest anything they can get into their mouths and adolescents with psychological problems may take deliberate and potentially serious overdoses. The possibility of poisoning should be considered in any child with unexplained illness.

Management

- Identify the poison if possible; send samples to A&E for identification—do not send vomit samples
- Consider specific antidote if available—see p.406
- Do not induce vomiting; do not give charcoal
- Monitor ABC depending on clinical picture
- Transfer to hospital for assessment and monitoring.

Paediatric life support

Pathogenesis of cardiac arrest in children

Children seldom suffer primary cardiac arrest which is commonly secondary to airway and breathing problems producing hypoxia, acidosis, and terminal bradycardia. Cardiac arrest, therefore, has a very poor outcome. However, sudden infant death syndrome (SIDS) and trauma are responsible for most pre-hospital deaths in children. The classical presentation is an unconscious, pulseless, apnoeic child. Preventative measures include the recognition of the acutely unwell child, prompt intervention, and transfer to hospital.

Paediatric respiratory arrest is an infrequent pre-hospital occurrence making skill retention difficult.

Paediatric resuscitation

Follows the same principles as in adults:

- Establish an open airway
- Achieve effective ventilation of the lungs
- Achieve effective oxygenation of the blood and re-establish the circulation.

Airway management

Simple airway techniques

- Head tilt and chin lift or jaw thrust in trauma
- Use of airway adjuncts
  - Oropharyngeal airways will overcome obstruction caused by the tongue. An airway that is too short will be ineffective and, if too long, may induce vomiting. Insertion should follow the contour of the tongue using a tongue depressor.
  - Nasopharyngeal airway may be used in semi-conscious casualties. Insertion involves lubrication of the tube, and gentle rotatory movements in a direction perpendicular to the face. Care is necessary to avoid trauma to the nares and adenoids.

Oropharyngeal airway

Correct size is measured from the centre of the mouth to the angle of the jaw.

Nasopharyngeal airway

Correct size is measured from the tip of the nose to the tragus.

Notes

Avoid overextension of the neck in infants and small children which will, in itself, cause airway obstruction.

If a nasopharyngeal airway is not available, a shortened encuffed endotracheal tube can be used.

Advanced airway techniques

- The laryngeal mask airway (LMA) may have a role in pre-hospital paediatric resuscitation, although it has not been formally evaluated. It must be remembered that the LMA does not properly protect the airway and that there is a risk of aspiration of stomach contents.
- Tracheal intubation is the gold standard for securing and protecting the airway but requires specific training and skill retention. In selected patients, intubation may be facilitated using rapid sequence induction of anaesthesia.
- Specific equipment suitable for the child's age and size is essential. The internal diameter of the endotracheal tube can be calculated from the formula:

$$\text{Internal diameter} = \frac{\text{age}}{4} + 4$$

Neonates require a 3.0 or 3.5. It is essential to have available the size above and below the predicted size. The appropriate length of the tube is calculated from the formula:

$$\text{Length (cm)} = \frac{\text{age}}{2} + 12$$

Uncut tubes are used to avoid the risk of the tube being too short. Paediatric tubes up to a size of 6mm are uncuffed and these should be used on children up to the age of 8 years to avoid damage to the cricoid ring.

Intubation is achieved by:

- Pre-oxygenating the child
- Applying gentle cricoid pressure to bring the larynx into view
- Inserting the tube 2–4cm below the inlet or, alternatively, until the mark on the tube is at the level of the cords
- Checking tube placement by
  - Auscultation over the chest and stomach
  - Pulse oximetry using a paediatric probe
  - End tidal CO_2 monitoring
- Securing the tube in place (noting its position at the lips).

Attempts at intubation should take less than 30 seconds. If unsuccessful, the child should be re-oxygenated by bag-valve-mask ventilation before the process is repeated.

The current evidence base suggests intubation in pre-hospital care is possible but confirms no added benefit over effective bag-valve-mask ventilation with or without airway adjuncts.

Whilst RSI will secure the airway, the low frequency of performing this skill in children in the pre-hospital scene requires a need of training, competence, and skill retention which is beyond most practitioners. The establishment of trained practitioners to deliver advanced airway care (RSI) should be considered for specific circumstances and remote areas, but the skill, otherwise, is likely to remain the remit of the specialist, usually an anaesthetist.

Needle and surgical cricothyroidotomy

For children less than 12 years old needle cricothyroidotomy should be performed using a 14-gauge or 16-gauge cannulae with a Y connection and an oxygen source delivering 5 to 10 litres per minute. In older children, a surgical cricothyroidotomy may be appropriate using a small vertical skin incision, a horizontal incision through the cricothyroid membrane, and a Spencer Wells or similar instrument to dilate the opening to permit the insertion of a size 6 tracheostomy tube or similar sized cuffed ET tube.

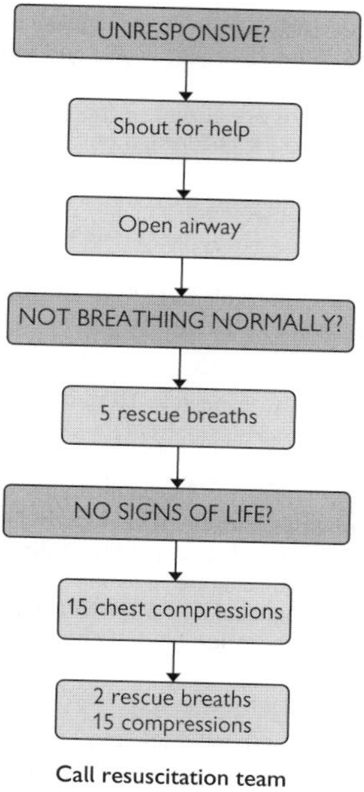

Fig. 8.6 Paediatric basic life support algorithm. (Single rescues CPR is given at 30 compressions to 2 ventilations; dual rescues CPR is given at 15 compressions to 2 ventilations—up to the onset of puberty.) Reprinted with permission from the Resuscitation Council (UK) (2010) *Resuscitation Guidelines*.

Breathing

- If the child is spontaneously breathing, administer oxygen 10–15l/min via a face mask using a non re-breathe valve and an oxygen reservoir bag.
- If spontaneous respirations are absent or inadequate, consider mouth-to-mouth or, in young children, mouth-to-nose rescue breaths or use a pocket mask.
- Ventilation is best achieved using a bag-valve-mask technique with an oxygen reservoir.

Notes

The paediatric and infant reservoir bags have pressure valves at 20cm of H_2O to protect the patient's lungs.

DO NOT overventilate—use enough air to cause modest chest wall rise

Circulation

- Unless there is an obvious peripheral vein, consider intraosseous access 2–3cm below and medial to the tibial tuberosity. The use of a 3-way tap and syringe facilitates infusion.
- The tracheal route can be used if iv an io access is not possible.
- Normal saline is the resuscitation fluid of choice given in a bolus of 20ml per kg.

Notes

Most drugs (except bretyllium) and fluids can be given by the intraosseous route.

Marrow aspirate can be used to determine the haemoglobin, urea, and electrolytes and blood sugar. It can also be used for cross-matching.

For endotracheal use, optimal drug doses are yet to be defined; effectiveness appears to be volume dependant .

After resuscitation from cardiac arrest, fever should be treated aggressively

Otherwise

No attempt should be made to warm the child as a temperature of 32–34 confers survival benefit

Treatment algorithms (non-shockable rhythms)

Asystole

Asystole is the most common rhythm of cardiac arrest in infants and children and is usually secondary to hypoxia. In infants, bradycardia (less than 60bpm) does not produce adequate cardiac output to maintain life and should be treated in the same way as asystole (See algorithm).

- Ensure that the rhythm *is* asystole (check gain and connections)
- If ventilating with bag-mask give 15 chest compressions to 2 ventilations.
- Use a compression rate of 100–120min^{-1}
- Once the child has been intubated and compressions are uninterrupted, use a ventilation rate of approximately 10–12 min^{-1}
- Continue CPR, only pausing briefly every 2 min to check for rhythm change.
- If venuous or intraoesseous (IO) access has been established, give adrenaline 10 mcg kg^{-1} (0.1 ml kg^{-1} of 1 in 10,000 solution).
- If there is no circulatory access, attempt to obtain IO access.
- If circulatory access is not present, and cannot be obtained quickly, but the patient has a tracheal tube in place, consider giving adrenaline 100 mcg kg^{-1} via the tracheal tube. This is the least satisfactory route (see routes of drug administration).
- Give adrenaline 10 mcg kg^{-1} every 3 to 5 min (i.e. every other loop), while continuing to maintain effective chest compression and ventilation without interruption.
- Repeat cycles of CPR

Note

Atropine no longer forms part of the asystole protocol but may be indicated in asystole due to vagal overactivity (for example, following airway manoeuvres). The dose is 20µg/kg (maximum 1mg in children, 2mg in adolescents).

Electromechanical dissociation

The most common cause of an absent pulse with ECG evidence of organized cardiac activity in children is shock.

In all cases of non-VF arrest, treatable causes must be identified:

Four Hs
- Hypoxia
- Hypovolaemia
- Hypothermia
- Hyperkalaemia/hypokalaemia.

Four Ts
- Tension pneumothorax
- Tamponade
- Toxic and thermal
- Thromboembolism.

Electrolyte abnormalities cannot be confirmed pre-hospital, but in patients where this is possible (for example, known calcium channel blockers or renal dialysis patients), treatment with calcium is appropriate.

VF or pulseless VT

VF is less common in children but may occur secondary to electrocution, drug overdose/poisoning (especially tricyclic antidepressants), hypothermia, and heart disease (usually congenital).

- Defibrillate ONCE at 4 joules per kilogram, all further shocks are also at 4 joules per kilogram
- 2 minutes CPR (15:2) without a pulse check
- Repeat defibrillation at 4 joules per kilogram
- Following each shock, without reassessing the rhythm or feeling for a pulse, resume CPR immediately, starting with chest compression
- Give adrenaline 10 mcg kg^{-1} and amiodarone 5 mg kg^{-1} after the 3rd shock, once chest compressions have resumed
- Repeat adrenaline every alternate cycle (ie. every 3–5 min) until ROSC
- Repeat amiodarone 5 mg kg^{-1} one further time, after the 5th shock if still in a shockable rhythm
- Intubate as soon as possible
- Repeat CPR
- Continue giving shocks every 2 min, continuing compressions during charging of the defibrillator and minimising the breaks in chest compression as much as possible
- Higher doses of intravascular adrenaline should not be used routinely in children because this may worsen outcome

In children look for the underlying cause of cardiac arrest—for example, hypothermia, drugs. An AED may be used in children over 8 years, with an electrical output attenuator (50–70J).

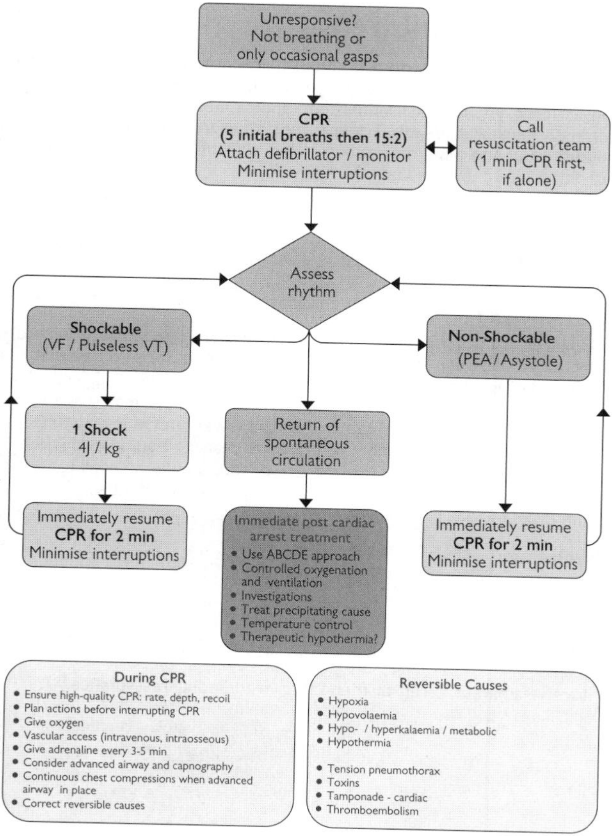

Fig. 8.7 Paediatric advanced life support: cardiac arrest protocol. Reprinted with permission from the Resuscitation Council (UK) (2010) *Resuscitation guidelines*.

Trauma in children

Trauma is the leading cause of death in children over one year of age and 50% of deaths occur immediately or within the first few minutes following the accident. As in adults, untreated hypoxia and hypovolaemia are the common causes of death. Trauma affects children differently, not just physically but also psychologically.

Always look for a child at the scene of a road traffic collision if there is a childseat or toys in the car.
Children can be ejected from the vehicle or be impacted under the seats.

Anatomy and physiology

- Children are smaller than adults, therefore more areas may be injured.
- Increased elasticity of the skeleton leads to a greater risk of internal organ damage in the absence of bony fractures.
- Patterns of injury are different (for example, a bumper may strike a child's abdomen or pelvis, rather than the lower limb as in an adult).
- Appropriate sized equipment is needed to manage trauma in children.
- An aide-mémoire, pocket book, chart, or tape should be used to determine equipment sizes (for example, endotracheal tubes) and drug dosages (see Fig. 8.8).

Psychology

It is important to:

- Be as reassuring as possible
- Adopt a caring attitude
- Explain to the child what you are doing, especially if it is going to be painful
- Involve a parent, carer, or friend to give additional reassurance.

Endotracheal tube

Length (cm)	Internal diameter (mm)
18–21	7.5–8.0
18	7.0
17	6.5
16	6.0
15	5.5
14	5.0
13	4.5
12	4.0
	3.5
10	3.0–3.5

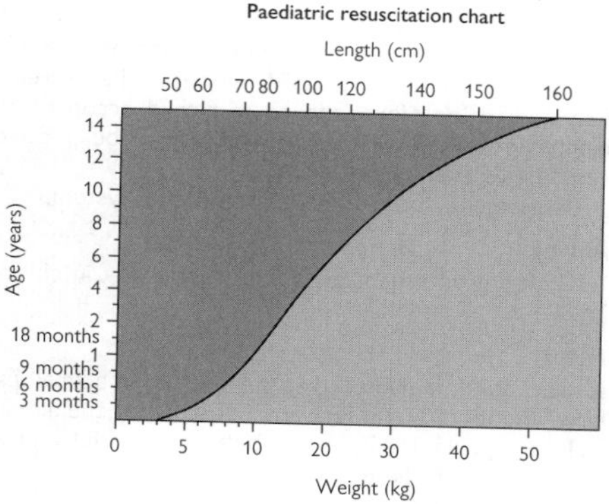

Adrenaline (ml of 1/10000) intravenous or endotracheal		0.5	1	2	3	4	5
Atropine (mg) intravenous or endotracheal		0.1	0.2	0.4	0.6	0.6	0.6
Bicarbonate (ml of 8.4%) intravenous		5	10	20	30	40	50
Calcium chloride (ml of 10%) intravenous		0.5	1	2	3	4	5
Diazepam (mg)	intravenous	1.25	2.5	5	7.5	10	10
	per rectum	2.5	5	10	–	–	–
Glucose (ml of 10%) intravenous		25	50	100	150	200	250
Lignocaine (ml of 1%) intravenous or endotracheal		0.5	1	2	3	4	5
Salbutamol (mg) intravenous		–	2.5	5	5	5	5
Initial DC defibrillation (J)		10	20	40	60	80	100
Initial fluid infusion in hypovolaemic shock (ml)		100	200	400	600	800	1000

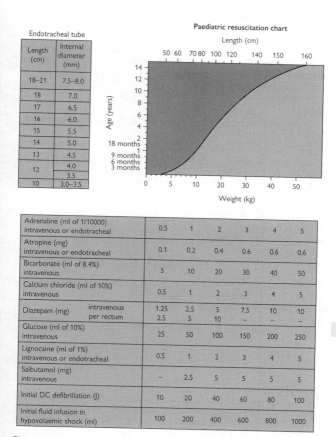

Fig. 8.8 Oakley resuscitation chart. Reproduced with thanks to Peter Oakley.

Scene assessment

Scene safety is the first priority (self, scene, patient). Appropriate personal protective equipment (PPE) is essential. Adequate resources and expertise should be mobilized early. It is vital to read the wreckage carefully and to look for evidence of a child occupant who could have been ejected or hidden within the wreckage or be trapped or hidden by adult casualties. Patient assessment

Assessment always follows the ABCDE system.

Airway

Assessment and management of the airway in children is considered on pp.524–6.

Notes

It must be remembered that the cranium in a small baby is proportionately large and tends to tilt forwards, obstructing the airway.

The important differences between a child and an adult which need consideration include:

- A large cranium
- Compressible soft tissues
- A large tongue
- A more anterior larynx
- A floppy epiglottis.

The airway is narrowest at the cricoid ring.

The size (internal diameter) of the tube is calculated using the formula

$$\text{Internal diameter ETT} = \frac{\text{age}}{4} + 4$$

The length of the tube is calculated using the formula

$$\text{Length of the tube} = \frac{\text{age}}{2} + 12$$

Cervical spine control

The spine should be immobilized based on the mechanism of injury and is mandatory in all unconscious trauma victims. This is in the conventional manner with manual inline stabilization or a semi-rigid collar, side blocks, and tape.

Notes

Adult spinal boards are unsuitable for small children. Consider an alternative, for example, immobilization in a box splint (small baby) or a vacuum splint. A neutral neck position must be maintained. Flexion of the neck risks airway obstruction in small babies.

Collars may be ill-fitting and, if not properly applied, can produce airway compromise due to pressure on soft tissues in the neck. Inline manual stabilization should be considered as an option for providing the safest means of ensuring safe spinal care.

An infant already in a car seat who is at risk of having incurred a spinal injury should be transported to hospital in the seat using a blanket roll and tape to immobilize the cervical spine.

Breathing

Children have pliable ribs and flexible rib cages making fractures rare. Therefore, if rib fractures are clinically present, this implies serious internal damage due to energy dissipation.

Signs of respiratory distress include:

- Increased respiratory rate
- The use of accessory muscles
- Intercostal and subcostal recession
- Grunting respiration
- Head bobbing
- Late features include cyanosis and an altered level of consciousness.

Children with ↑ respiratory distress have both an oxygenation and ventilation problem. Assisted ventilation using a bag-valve-mask system is essential because the depth of inspiration may be insufficient due to the fast rate. (See Fig. 8.1, p.501, for normal respiratory rates in children.)

Immediately life-threatening conditions should be identified and treated :

- **A**irway obstruction
- **T**ension pneumothorax
- **O**pen pneumothorax
- **M**assive haemothorax

Flail chest and cardiac tamponade are extremely rare in children.

Table 8.3 Clinical signs of the four life-threatening conditions

	Position of the trachea in relation to the side of injury	Chest wall movement on the side of injury	Percussion note on the side of injury	Breath sounds on the side of injury
Flail chest	Central	Paradoxical movements	Decreased with pain on palpation	Decreased
Massive haemothorax	Central/away	Normal/ decreased	Decreased	Decreased
Open pneumothorax	Central	Decreased	Increased	Decreased
Tension pneumothorax	Away	Decreased	Increased	Decreased

Management

Flail chest

A rare injury in children because of the pliability of the chest wall. If present, it implies two or more rib fractures, fractured in two or more places. Flail chest is associated with underlying lung contusion. The classical clinical feature is paradoxical breathing. Pre-hospital treatment includes manual splintage and analgesia. Consider assisted ventilation if significant respiratory compromise.

Haemothorax

Clinical features include both hypoxia and hypovolaemia. Management includes intravenous access and judicious fluid replacement. There is usually no indication for inserting a chest drain in the pre-hospital environment; it may worsen an already difficult situation.

Open pneumothorax

Air moves preferentially through the hole in the chest wall if it is greater than ¾ of the transverse diameter of the trachea. The hole should be sealed with an Ascherman chest seal or three-sided dressing and the patient regularly reassessed for developing tension pneumothorax.

Tension pneumothorax

The management is immediate needle thoracocentesis. A chest drain will be required and is usually inserted at a later stage in hospital. Deterioration in a ventilated child may be due to the development of a tension pneumothorax.

Circulation

The essential clinical indicators of the degree of shock include:

- Pulse rate
- Capillary refill time
- Skin colour
- Peripheral temperature
- Respiratory rate
- Mental status.

Systolic blood pressure is maintained until late in hypovolaemic shock and, therefore, hypotension should be regarded as a pre-terminal event.

The degree of volume loss can be determined by collating the physical signs (see Table 8.4).

Shock

Shock is defined as the inadequate delivery of oxygen to the tissues. The classification of shock is the same as in adults. Several types of shock may coexist, for example, septic shock may coexist with hypovolaemia from diarrhoea, distributive shock due to capillary leak, and cardiogenic shock due to toxins.

Children differ from adults in the following way:

- Children with a healthy cardiovascular system compensate very efficiently. Hypotension should be regarded as a pre-terminal event.
- Children vasoconstrict very effectively and can develop a tachycardia in excess of 200bpm before the blood pressure falls.

Children under 2 years of age are unable to compensate effectively for hypovolaemia because they have a fixed cardiacvolume.

Types of shock—see box

Hypotension is a pre-terminal event. In pre-hospital care, it may be difficult to determine. Problems include the range of physiological values based on age, lack of an appropriately sized cuff, and difficulty of measurement in distressed non-co-operative children. Fortunately, the other signs of hypovolaemia will be apparent long before the blood pressure drops. Children rarely show signs of shock until 25% of the circulatory volume is lost.

Causes of shock

Hypovolaemic
- Blood loss
- Heat loss
- Burns
- Diarrhoea
- Diabetic ketoacidosis.

Obstructive
- Cardiac tamponade
- Tension pneumothorax.

Neurogenic
- Spinal cord injury.

Cardiogenic
- Cardiac contusion
- Congenital heart disease
- Myocarditis.

Distributive
- Anaphylaxis
- Capillary leak.

Table 8.4 Physical signs of shock

	Less than 25%	25–40%	>40%
Heart rate	Tachycardia +	Tachycardia ++	Tachycardia +++ or bradycardia
Blood pressure	Normal	Normal or reduced	Falling
Pulse volume	Normal or reduced	Reduced +	Reduced ++
Capillary refill time	Normal or increased	Increased+	Increased ++
Skin	Cool, pale	Cold, mottled	Cold, pale
Respiratory rate	Increased +	Increased ++	Profound respiratory distress
Mental status	Mild aggression	Lethargic	Responds to pain only

Treatment

Shock due to blood loss:

- Arrest external bleeding
- Administer high-flow oxygen
- Splint fractures
- Elevate the legs
- Obtain intravenous or intraosseous access
- Replace fluids at 20ml per kg of warmed normal saline.

Weight can be estimated using the formula:

$$\text{Weight (kg)} = (2 \times \text{age in years}) + 8$$

Avoid Hartmann's solution (contains lactate and potassium) in the treatment of shock in children

Disability

Head injury is the most common cause of death in children. The level of consciousness is assessed using the AVPU system:

A		**A**lert
V		**V**erbally responsive
P	responds to	**P**ain only
U		**U**nresponsive

Pupillary size, reactivity, and equality should be determined. Unilateral pupillary dilatation suggests focal pathology. Bilateral pupillary dilatation may be due to brain injury, hypoxia, or hypovolaemia. Abnormal posture should be noted, for example, decerebrate 'extensor' or decorticate (flexor).

The pre-hospital carer can do nothing about the primary injury. However, preventing secondary brain injury (correcting hypoxia and hypovolaemia) improves outcome and survivability.

High-flow oxygen via a non-rebreathe mask and reservoir bag at 15l/minute should be administered. Inadequate breathing can be supported by BVM ventilation. Judicious fluid replacement should be given to support the circulation but should on no account delay transfer to definitive care.

Exposure and the environment

The child should be exposed, if necessary, to ensure adequate clinical examination after which the patient should be covered and kept warm depending on the time of year and environment.

- Many children become hypothermic because of prolonged exposure to facilitate examination and clinical procedures.
- The ambulance should be kept warm and the doors open for a minimum time to reduce heat loss.
- Pre-hospital fluids, if given, should be warmed.

Secondary survey

This should only be undertaken once the primary survey has been completed and all problems identified have been addressed. For most children, especially those with multiple injuries, this will be undertaken in hospital.

The secondary survey is a head-to-toe examination and may be undertaken in the ambulance en route to hospital—in a warm environment. In practice, the pre-hospital secondary survey should take no more than five minutes.

Important features to note include:

Head

- Scalp for bleeding, lacerations, and boggy swelling
- Ears for evidence of blood/ CSF in the external auditory meatus (suggestive of a middle cranial fossa fracture)
- Nose for blood or CSF loss
- Face for bruising, swelling, wounds, deformity, and dental trauma.

Neck

- For bruising, tenderness, wounds, deformity, and bony tenderness
- Neck veins (distension suggests cardiac tamponade or tension pneumothorax).

Chest

- Chest wall for bruising (including pattern brusing), wounds, swelling, and symmetrical movements, bony tenderness, or fractures
- Percussion for altered resonance.

The abdomen and pelvis

- Abdominal wall for bruising, grazes, swelling, tenderness, guarding, rigidity, and rebound tenderness.

Extremities

Examine for the presence of fractures (indicated by swelling, tenderness, deformity, lack of function, and (rarely) neurovascular deficit). Assess the distal capillary refill which should be the same as a non-injured limb. Compound fractures should be cleaned, dressed, and splinted. Analgesia should be provided if possible. Trained personnel may straighten/reduce fractures.

Monitoring

Careful monitoring should be maintained throughout the child's care and especially during transportation to hospital.

Burns

Minor scalds and burns are relatively common in children. Fortunately, the majority do not represent any significant threat to life. They do, however, cause great distress to the child and its parents.

The relative proportions of different body areas vary with age and an adult burns chart or the 'rule of nines' do not apply. Fig. 8.10 can be used to estimate burns area in children.

The principles of burn management are:

- Stopping the burning process
- Airway assessment and management
- Removal of clothes
- Cooling (the burn, not the child)
- Analgesia.

CHART FOR ESTIMATING SEVERITY OF BURN WOUND

NAME__________WARD________NUMBER______DATE_____
AGE________ADMISSION WEIGHT________

LUND AND BROWDER CHARTS

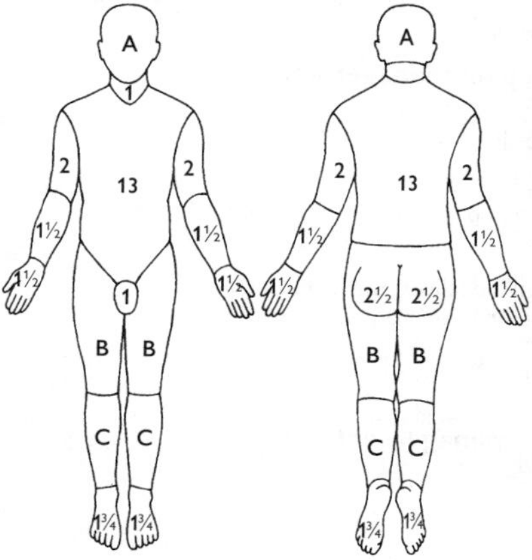

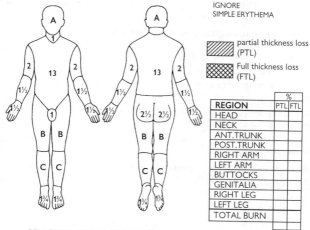

IGNORE
SIMPLE ERYTHEMA

partial thickness loss (PTL)

Full thickness loss (FTL)

REGION	% PTL	% FTL
HEAD		
NECK		
ANT.TRUNK		
POST.TRUNK		
RIGHT ARM		
LEFT ARM		
BUTTOCKS		
GENITALIA		
RIGHT LEG		
LEFT LEG		
TOTAL BURN		

RELATIVE PERCENTAGE OF BODY SURFACE AREA AFFECTED BY GROWTH

AREA	AGE 0	1	5	10	15	ADULT
A=½ OF HEAD	9½	8½	6½	5½	4½	3½
B=½ OF ONE THIGH	2¾	3¼	4	4½	4½	4¾
C=½ OF ONE LEG	2½	2½	2¾	3	3¼	3½

Fig. 8.9 Calculating burns area in children. Reprinted with permission from Greaves I *et al.* (UK) (2005). *Emergency care: a textbook for paramedics*, 2nd edn. W.B. Saunders Co. Ltd.

Analgesia

Children require analgesia just as adults do. In time-critical injury, however, delays on scene to provide analgesia should not occur. The degree of pain may be monitored using a 1–10 pain ladder, but this depends on the child being able to understand what is being asked and to be able to communicate. In young children, pain may be manifested by agitation and crying. Pain management may be achieved using pharmacological and non-pharmacological measures.

Non-pharmacological pain management

Distraction
- Give them something to do.

Reassurance
- Positive reassurance from a parent/carer or friend of the patient.

Environment
- Friendly, sympathetic, and, ideally, single-person contact
- Address the child by their name.

Immobilization
- Use simple splintage.

Pharmacological pain management

Therapeutic options include:

Mild pain
- Oral paracetamol
- Oral ibuprofen.

Moderate pain
- Non-steroidal anti-inflammatory drugs, for example, diclofenac given orally or rectally
- Oral or nasal morphine.

Severe pain
- Intravenous morphine
- Ketamine
- Entonox (can provide short-term effective analgesia but requires patient co-operation for effective administration and is, therefore, unsuitable for young children).

Analgesic doses for children are given opposite.

Local analgesic infiltration may, occasionally, be of value in the management of pain in children.

Paediatric doses

Adrenaline INTRAMUSCULAR for anaphylaxis
- Under 6 years: 150μg, 0.15ml
- 6–12 years: 300μg, 0.3ml
- 12 years and over: 500μg, 0.5ml

Atropine

20μg/kg, maximum 600 μg

Benzyl penicillin
- Under 1: 300mg
- 1–9 years: 600mg
- 10 years and over: adult dose.

Chlorpheniramine
- 1 month–1 year: 250 μg/kg
- 1–12 years: 200 μg/kg

or

- 1–5 years: 2.5–5mg
- 6–12 years: 5mg.

Diazepam
- Rectal—children over 10kg, 500μg/kg, maximum 20mg
- Intravenous
  - Neonate—12 years 300–400 μg/kg
  - 12–18 years 10–20mg

Glucagon
- Under 8 years (or under 25kg): 500μg
- Over 8 years (or over 25kg): 1mg.

Hydrocortisone
- Up to 1 year: 25mg
- 1–5 years: 50mg
- 6–12 years: 100mg.

Ibuprofen
- 3–6 months: 50mg (body weight over 5kg)
- 6 months–1 year: 50mg
- 1–4 years: 100mg
- 4–7 years: 150mg
- 7–10 years: 200mg
- 10–12 years: 300mg.

Ketamine

As adult doses, by weight (See p.331)

Lignocaine

Local anaesthesia, 3mg/kg

Methionine

Child over six: 2.5g initially, followed by 3 further doses of 2.5g every 4 hours

Child under six: 1g initially, followed by 3 further doses of 1g every 4 hours

Midazolam (iv)

- 6 months–5 years: 50–100μg/kg initially
- 6–12 years: 25–50μg/kg, further increments as required.

Morphine

- Up to 1 month: 37.5–75μg/kg
- 1–12 months: 50–100μg/kg
- 1–5 years: 1–2mg
- 6–12 years: 2–5mg.

Naloxone

10μg/kg, subsequent dose of 100μg/kg if no response

Paracetamol

Orally

- 3 months–1 year: 60–120mg
- 1–5 years: 120–250mg
- 6–12 years: 250–500mg.

These doses may be repeated every 4–6 hours, maximum 4 doses in 24 hours

Suppository

- 1–5 years: 125–250mg
- 6–12 years: 250–500mg
- Over 12 years: repeat dosing as above.

Salbutamol

(Over 18 months: 2.5mg as nebulized solution) under 18 months: 1.25–2.5mg as nebulized solution

Consent

Always explain what you are proposing to do to a child. Gillick competent children below the age of 16 are capable of giving informed consent *to treatment;* they *cannot refuse* treatment against the wishes of a parent or guardian until they have reached the age of 18.

Child abuse

Child abuse may be defined as treatment by an adult or another child in a way that is unacceptable in a given culture at a given time. It includes:

- Neglect
- Physical injury
- Sexual abuse
- Emotional neglect.

Factors which alert the practitioner to the risk of child abuse include:

- Delay in seeking medical attention, especially if the injury is serious
- Inconsistent history to account for the injury
- Varying history from witnesses
- Injury pattern is inconsistent with the history
- Injury pattern is inappropriate to the developmental state of the child
- Abnormal parental or carer attitude
- Abnormal child/carer interface
- Unusual patterns of injury, for example, finger marks, burns, and bites.

Under these circumstances, the first priority is to the child, who should be transported to hospital. Concern must be raised with hospital staff and this should be clearly documented.

All health care professionals have a responsibility under the Children's Act 1989 to protect children and should be aware of local procedures for child protection.

Triage

The standard triage sieve used in adult practice presents problems as many children cannot walk. Therefore, triage is a complicated process. Age-specific triage sieves are given on p.604.

Paediatric trauma score

A score of 8 or less on the paediatric trauma score is one way of identifying a time-critical injury for which prompt transfer to a hospital is essential. The mechanism of injury, for example 'run over by a car' also correlates with the severity of injuries.

Table 8.5 Paediatric trauma score

	+2	+1	– 1
Size	>20kg	11–20kg	<10kg
Airway	Normal	Assisted mask	Intubated, cricothyroidotomy, obstruction
Conscious level	Awake	Decreased	Unresponsive
Systolic blood pressure	>90mmHg	51–90mmHg	<50mmHg or only central pulses
Fractures	None	Single closed	Open or multiple
Skin	Normal	Contusion, abrasion, cut less than 7cm, not through fascia	Tissue loss, knife or gun wounds

Chapter 9

The hostile environment

Hypothermia

Body temperature is regulated through the hypothalamus which is activated by changes in blood and skin temperature. The hypothalamus adjusts heat production and loss. Although hypothermia is defined as a core temperature of less than 35°C, medical attention is appropriately directed to any cold patient. It is better to prevent hypothermia than to have to try and treat it.

> Hypothermia is defined as a core temperature of less than 35°C

Mechanisms

The human body loses heat by:
- Radiation: greatest when naked and erect
- Conduction: by contact with another surface such as water or wet clothing
- Evaporation: by insensible moisture loss and sweating, and from the respiratory tract
- Convection: largely dependant on wind velocity, it is increased by limb movement and shivering.

Exacerbating factors

- Air movement ('wind chill')
- Moisture (humidity, rain, or dampness).

Predisposing factors

- Extremes of age
- Poverty
- Inappropriate clothing in a harsh environment
- Nausea and vomiting
- Trauma
- Stress
- Alcohol
- Coincident medical illness (diabetes mellitus, hypothyroidism).

Physiological effects

- Constriction of peripheral vessels (conserves heat but increases the risk of local cold injury)
- Shivering—increases heat production
- Deliberate activity—increases heat production
- Reduced energy reserves—secondary to increased heat production
- Increased oxygen consumption—secondary to increased heat production
- Diuresis—secondary to central redirection of blood.

Increased oxygen consumption secondary to heat generation may lead to hypoxia and is the reason angina is more likely to occur in cold weather. Hypoxia may eventually restrict heat production, leading to loss of shivering. Heat production may also be prevented by exhaustion or starvation as a result of lack of nutrient.

Effects of exposure to cold temperatures

Central nervous system	Impaired co-ordination
	Behavioural changes
	Reduced visual acuity
	Decreased alertness
	Slowed reflexes
	More frequent errors
	Impaired sensory intrepretation
	Hallucinations
Muscular	Shivering
	Increased risk of muscular injury
Cardiovascular	Lowered angina threshold
	Hypertension
Respiratory	Asthma
Peripheral nervous system	Loss of manual dexterity
	Reduced skin sensation

Diagnosis

An approximate indication of likely symptoms and signs as the body temperature falls is given in Table 9.1. It may be difficult to achieve an accurate temperature in the pre-hospital environment and it is essential to stress that the temperature at which any particular clinical feature is seen will vary dramatically from patient to patient. Therefore:

A patient who feels cold should be treated for hypothermia

Management

The key to good management is effective rewarming with prevention of further heat loss.

- Administer high-flow oxygen during rewarming
- Monitor pulse and BP (warming is associated with increasing peripheral blood flow with consequent hypotension if there is trauma)
- Remove and replace cold wet clothing when safe to do so (in a warm place, out of the wind)
- Warm the patient (see below); warm drinks (NO ALCOHOL) may be given if the patient is conscious
- Manage associated injuries—used pre-warmed fluids
- Keep the patient flat whenever possible and remove from the cold environment.

Handle with care: do not precipitate VF!

Table 9.1 The effects of hypothermia

Temperature	Clinical features
37	Normal oral temperature
36	Respiratory rate and pulse increase
35	Shivering maximal
	Slow thinking, dysarthria
34	Patient still capable of functioning; blood pressure normal
33–31	Retrograde amnesia; conscious level clouded; pupils dilated
	BP difficult to measure; shivering largely stopped
30–28	Loss of consciousness; bradycardia; bradypnoea; muscular rigidity; *VF* may supervene secondary to stimulation
27	No voluntary motion
26	Consciousness very rare
25	Spontaneous appearance of VF
24–21	Pulmonary oedema
23	Apnoea
18	Asystole

Spontaneous rewarming

The surface of the victim's head and body are insulated (normally with a space blanket but polythene sheeting is effective) to prevent further heat loss. The hands and feet are kept cool (hands by the patient's side) since warm hands and feet inhibit heat production. Shelter from the wind is a key component of management.

Surface rewarming

- Body-to-body rewarming rarely effective *and may put both the victim and rescuer at further risk.*
- Hot water immersion at 40°C (elbow hot—only for conscious, shivering, uninjured victims). Once warmed, remove from water, lie down and wrap in blankets.

Skin rubbing is contraindicated and hot water bottles are best avoided. Young fit victims may be warmed rapidly. Following admission to hospital, warming can be continued by:

Central rewarming

These procedures can only be carried out after arrival in hospital:

- Airway warming
- Cardiopulmonary bypass
- Haemodialysis
- Peritoneal and pleural irrigation with warmed fluids

Note

Elderly patients with hypothermia should be warmed slowly and carefully. A temperature rise of more than about 0.5° per hour runs the risk of cerebral and pulmonary oedema in these patients. The most appropriate place for ongoing rewarming is an ITU.

Cardiopulmonary resuscitation in hypothermia

- Once commenced, CPR should be continued until the patient recovers, reaches hospital, and is handed over for continued care or the rescuer becomes exhausted.
- Follow the normal cardiorespiratory arrest protocols.
- Defibrillation is usually unsuccessful in the presence of VF if the core temperature is below 30 degrees.
- Adrenaline and other drugs, including amiodarone, should not be used until the temperature is above 30 degrees.
- Always check for hypoglycaemia.

REMEMBER to rule out other treatable causes of cardiac arrest

Cold injury

Frost nip

Is a minor form of frost bite where the skin becomes white and numb. These changes are completely reversible on rewarming, leaving short-term pain and hyperaemia.

Frost bite

- Commonly affects the finger, toes, nose, and ears.
- Is worsened on thawing by reperfusion injury and may produce tissue necrosis.
- Appears white when frozen and becomes blue or purple on thawing and is associated with swelling and severe pain.
- Causes blistering followed by a thick carapace which blackens and eventually separates (some times after several months) leaving healthy tissue underneath. In some cases, auto-amputation of digits occurs.

Management

The key features are:

- Protection from the environment if possible
- No attempt to rewarm until it can be sustained

Active rewarming can be achieved by placing the limb in circulating water at 40°C. This is extremely painful and requires strong analgesia.

Heat-related illness

Temperature regulation

Heat gain results from basal metabolic activity, muscular exertion, heat absorption, and the breakdown of food. Heat is lost through *radiation, evaporation* (of sweat), *convection, conduction,* and *loss of body waste*. The hypothalamus (which responds to core temperature receptors) balances heat production and loss to maintain a body temperature set within precise limits. When core temperature rises above 40°C, enzyme systems begin to break down. Normally, this temperature range is between 36.3 and 37.1°C. In hot weather, there may be a temperature difference of up to 1°C between core and peripheral temperatures.

Adaptation to heat

Acclimatization to heat is largely complete in 7–12 days but may continue for several weeks. Sweating leads to loss of water and sodium. Decreased circulating blood volume results in decreased renal blood flow. As a result of this (and secondary to increased aldosterone secretion), there is reduced secretion of sodium in sweat and urine. This results in re-expansion of the extracellular space. Cutaneous blood flow increases and cardiac output rises to maintain blood pressure despite vasodilatation. Once blood pressure can no longer be maintained, peripheral vasoconstriction occurs which has the adverse effect of preventing heat loss. Other effects of heat include a lower threshold for sweating, anorexia, and loss of interest in activity (both of which result in reduced heat production).

Risk factors

Increased heat production

- Physical activity
- Drugs (cocaine, PCP, ecstasy, amphetamines, LSD, tricyclics)
- Medical conditions such as hyperthyroidism, acute febrile illness.

Reduced heat loss

- Inappropriate clothing
- Alcohol
- Old age
- Poor condition
- Obesity.

Dehydration

- Prolonged exertion
- Diarrhoea and vomiting
- Diabetes
- Mental impairment
- Drugs (diuretics) and alcohol.

Minor heat illness

Oedema

Oedema of the hands, feet, and ankles occurs in the first few days of heat exposure. No specific treatment is required, although elevation and compression stockings are effective. The problem usually resolves spontaneously.

Cramp

Painful muscular contractions, especially of the thighs, calves, upper arms, and abdomen usually occur when large amounts of sweat have been replaced by large volumes of unsalted water. The cramps usually occur during or following exercise. Oral or intravenous administration of salt solution (N saline intravenous) is effective. The condition is more common in unacclimatized individuals.

Tetany

Carpopedal spasm, hyperventilation, and paraesthesiae can be triggered by a change in air temperature. Removal of the patient to a cooler environment and conventional treatment for hyperventilation (see p.138) are effective.

Syncope

Heat syncope results from peripheral venous pooling. It is more common in the unacclimatized and those standing stationary for long periods. Spontaneous recovery occurs once the patient is horizontal.

Exhaustion

Heat exhaustion may be a precursor of sunstroke. By definition, the core (rectal) temperature is less than 40°C (see heat stroke, p.562–3). Gross changes in mental and neurological status do not occur. Symptoms include:

- Weakness
- Tiredness
- Dizziness/lightheadedness
- Headache
- Palpitation
- Nausea and vomiting
- Sweating
- Cramps
- Flushing
- Pilo-erection

It may be extremely difficult to distinguish heatstroke and heat exhaustion. A diagnosis of heat exhaustion is, therefore, no reason for complacency. Heat exhaustion results from the exposure of unacclimatized individuals to a heat load over longer periods (several days) or following short periods of exertion. The elements of treatment are:

- Removal to a cooler place
- Cool oral and/or intravenous fluids
- Fanning and lukewarm water spraying
- Other methods of cooling (see heat stroke p.562–3)
- Admission to hospital for observation

Major heat illness—heat stroke

Heat stroke is the severe end of the heat-related illness spectrum. Its mortality is approximately 10%.

Presentation

The features of heat stroke are those of heat exhaustion, together with a core temperature greater than 40°C and:

- Confusion
- Irritability
- Coma, decerebrate posturing (severe cases)
- Fitting
- Tachycardia, hypotension, and tachypnoea
- Rising core temperature.

Inability to measure core temperature should not prevent the making of a diagnosis of heat stroke.

> The presence of sweating does not exclude heat stroke

Management

The key to management is *rapid* effective cooling. The victim of heat stroke should, therefore, be managed as follows:

- Remove to an area of shade (preferably an air-conditioned room)
- Follow ABC priorities; administer high-flow oxygen
- Gain intravenous access and administer crystalloid 1–2l over the first hour (observe for fluid overload—unlikely in young fit subjects)
- Undress the casualty
- Cool by water spraying and fanning
- Ice blocks (wrapped in cloth) may be placed in the armpits, groin, and neck
- Treat fits with intravenous (or rectal) diazepam (see p.322)
- Transfer urgently to hospital

Complications of heat stroke

Cardiovascular system

- Tachycardia
- ST changes
- Hypotension
- Myocardial infarction.

Respiratory system

- Aspiration
- Hyperventilation syndrome
- ARDS.

Central nervous system

- Cerebral oedema
- Confusion, agitation, delirium
- Convulsions
- Coma
- Hemiplegia
- Ataxia.

Neurological abnormalities may persist following recovery.

Hepatic

- Hepatic complications are not usually encountered in the pre-hospital setting
- Delays in diagnosis and treatment of heat stroke contribute to hepatocellular damage which may progress to hepatic failure.

Renal

- Most commonly seen after exertional heat stroke where dehydration and rhabdomylosis are more common.

Prevention and preparedness

The pre-hospital practitioner may be asked to advise about prevention and preparedness. The risks of heat-related problems can be reduced by:

- Acclimatization
- Maintaining good cardiac fitness
- Adequate hydration
- Wearing appropriate clothes
- Appropriate provision of rest and water breaks
- Identifying susceptible individuals—the elderly, small children
- Awareness of the heat stroke index (see Table 9.2).

Table 9.2 Heat stroke index

Ambient temperature (°C)	Restriction on activity
<24°C	Activities may proceed but remain vigilant for early signs of heat illness
24.0–25.9°C	Rest periods needed
26–29°C	No activity for unacclimatized or at-risk individuals; others need to be carefully monitored
>29°C	No unnecessary activities should take place

Near drowning

It is estimated there are over 500 deaths per annum from drowning in the UK and up to 8–10 times more near drownings, especially in children aged 1–14, adult non-swimmers, and patients with significant co-morbidity. Factors influencing near drowning include:

- Unconsciousness
- Ability to swim
- Exhaustion
- Hypothermia

Unconsciousness may be due to head injury with loss of consciousness (for example, diving into shallow water) or secondary to medical illness (for example, hypoglycaemia, epilepsy, CVA), alcohol, and drugs.

Drowning usually follows a characteristic sequence in which the victim:

- Thrashes about in the water
- Inspires under water
- Ingests water
- Suffers small-volume aspiration and intense bronchospasm

Further attempts to inspire lead to further inhalation/ingestion, unconsciousness, and death.

Exhaustion is commonly associated with long periods of time in the water or occurs acutely in cold water submersion due to onset of hypothermia. So called 'dry drowning', in which no water is found in the lungs, is believed to be a reflex vagal response to sudden immersion. It is critical to appreciate the hydrostatic pressure effect on the body whilst submerged in water which serves to support the circulation.

Hypothermia is common and when the core temperature falls below 35° the victim becomes confused, unco-ordinated, ataxic, and may drown. In children, cold water immersion may provide cerebral protection. There is no significant difference in the pattern of events that occurs between salt water drowning and fresh water drowning and the principles of treatment are the same for both.

Assessment

The assessment priorities are:

- Is the scene safe? Are you safe? Don't become a victim!
- Is the patient breathing? Is the depth of breathing adequate?

Three clinical scenarios result (see below):

1. The patient is conscious and breathing
2. The patient is unconscious, is not breathing, but has a pulse
3. Patient is in full cardiorespiratory arrest

Management

General

Successful treatment and outcome depends on minimizing the 'hypoxic gap'—the time between submersion and relief of airway obstruction.

- The patient should be removed from the water in a horizontal position to avoid catastrophic hypotension and cardiac arrest.
- Vomiting on recovery from near drowning is common and the rescuer should be prepared to turn the patient or use suction as appropriate.
- No attempt should be made to remove water from the lungs other than simple postural drainage of the airway.

> The Victim MUST ALWAYS be removed from the water in a horizontal position

Specific scenarios

The patient is conscious and breathing

- Clear the airway if necessary
- Administer high-flow oxygen (10–15l/min) using a non-rebreathe mask and a reservoir bag
- If breathing is inadequate, consider bag-valve-mask assisted ventilation
- Maintain the patient in a horizontal position
- Consider siting an IVI and give 10ml per kg of isotonic crystalloid depending on the cardiovascular status
- Transport all victims of near drowning to hospital even if they have apparently recovered*.

The patient is unconscious, not breathing, but has a pulse

- Open the airway as a matter or urgency. Most patients have airway obstruction due to water, foreign body, or vomit.
- Consider the possibility of cervical spine injury depending on the mechanism of injury (for example, diving into shallow water). Maintain inline stabilization if required.
- In adults, consider a finger sweep to remove debris. In children, clear the airway if necessary by postural positioning (recovery position) or by elevating the feet and pelvis to allow drainage by gravity.
- When the airway is open, administer high-flow oxygen at 10–15l/min using an non-rebreath mask with a reservoir bag.
- Consider bag-valve-mask assisted ventilation.
- Consider intubation.
- Most patients will vomit on recovery—suction should be available.
- Consider cannulation and IV isotonic fluids 10ml per kg.
- Most near drowning victims are hypothermic; protect from further heat loss.

Steroids and early antibiotics provide no evidence-based clinical benefit.

* Secondary drowning, typified by delayed tachycardia, delayed tachypnoea, cough and frothy sputum, and a risk of developing ARDS occurs in 2–3% of patients in this clinical category.

The patient is in cardiorespiratory arrest
The position may still be retrievable. Important factors influencing outcome include:
- Time spent submerged
- Temperature of the water
- Presenting ECG rhythm

Acute submersion in cold water offers cerebral protection. A two-year-old child has survived 66 minutes' submersion in cold water and made a full recovery.

CPR should follow conventional algorithms. Once started, it should be continued at least until arrival in hospital. Therapeutic and electrical defibrillation is reported to be ineffective in the presence of significant hypothermia. Intravenous access should be obtained and volume resuscitation commenced with warmed isotonic fluid.

Scrupulous airway management is essential:
- Open the airway as a matter or urgency. Most patients have airway obstruction due to water, foreign body, or vomit.
- Consider the possibility of cervical spine injury depending on the mechanism of injury (for example, diving into shallow water). Maintain inline stabilization if required.
- In adults, consider a finger sweep to remove debris. In children, clear the airway, if necessary by postural positioning (recovery position) or by elevating the feet and pelvis to allow drainage by gravity.
- Perform bag-valve-mask assisted ventilation with high-flow oxygen.
- Consider intubation.

Prognosis

Prognosis is excellent in those victims who have not suffered cardiorespiratory arrest. Full recovery, usually without neurological consequences, commonly follows resuscitation of patients who have been unconscious but maintained a pulse. Following cardiorespiratory arrest, the prognosis is not hopeless and full recovery has been recorded, especially in children following cold water submersion.

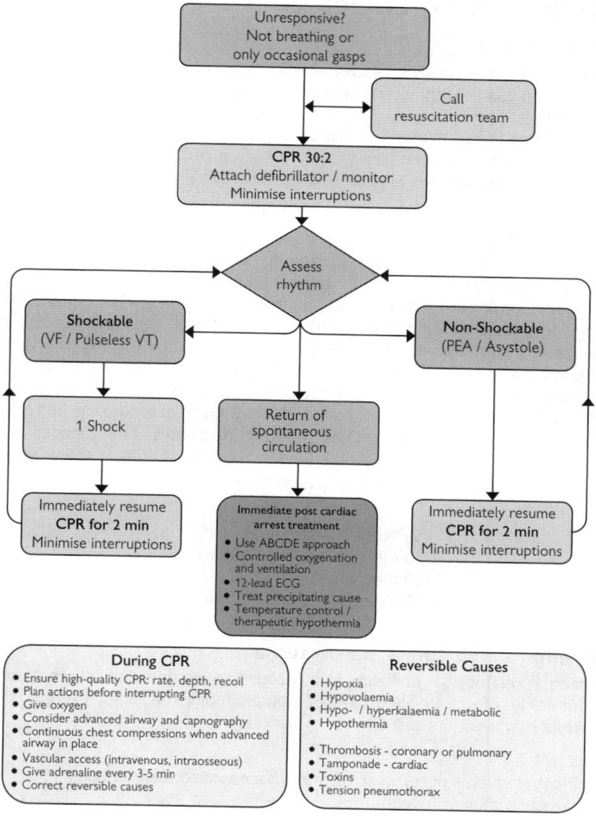

Fig. 9.1 Cardiac arrest algorithm. Reprinted with permission from the Resuscitation Council (UK) (2010), *Resuscitation guidelines.* 1mg adrenaline IV should be given as soon as IV access is obtained and repeated every 3–5 minutes thereafter until return of spontaneous circulation is obtained.

Diving emergencies

Pathophysiology

Atmospheric air consists of oxygen (21%), nitrogen (79%), and carbon dioxide (0.03%). Each exerts a partial pressure in proportion to their percentage concentration. At sea level, this equates to a pressure of 1 atmosphere (KPa). Water is more dense than air. Therefore at a depth of 10m, a diver is subjected to a greater pressure of 2 atmospheres. Boyle's law states that volume (V) is inversely proportional to pressure(P):

$$V \propto 1/P$$

Therefore the volume of a gas will decrease with increasing depth and increase on returning to the surface. In practical terms, at a depth of 10m, the volume of air in the lungs has reduced by a half from that at the surface. Conversely, a diver breathing from a compressed air cylinder will need to exhale during ascent as the volume of air in the lungs doubles in the ascent from 10m depth to the surface.

In addition, because the diver is breathing air at a higher pressure, as per Henry's law, the amount of nitrogen dissolved in blood and tissues increases as the pressure increases. As the diver ascends, the nitrogen will come out of solution as the pressure decreases. The changes that occur are summarized in the box, where it can be seen that the greatest changes occur in the first 10m of descent:

Surface ---------------- 4 litres
10 metres ------------ 2 litres
20 metres ------------1 1/3 litres
30 metres------------- 1 litre

Diving-related illness: barotrauma

Trauma related to pressure can occur on ascent and descent and commonly affects air-filled cavities (for example, the lungs, the gut, the middle ear, facial sinuses, and tooth sockets).

Descent

- Most problems occur near to the surface where the greatest pressure changes occur
- Particularly affects the middle ear, where symptoms of pain can be relieved by swallowing or a valsalva manoeuvre
- May result in tympanic membrane perforation if the diver's eustachian tubes are blocked.

Ascent

- A slow ascent whilst slowly exhaling is essential
- Rapid ascent risks ear perforation, and pulmonary complications (including frothy sputum, cough and pneumothorax, and air embolism, which includes cerebral air embolism resulting in CVA and coronary air embolism which may produce electromechanical dissociation and death).

Diving-related illness: acute decompression illness (ADI)

ADI has previously been divided into:
- mild (cutaneous and limb bends)
- serious (neurological cardiac, respiratory, neurological and gastrointestinal).

Terms such as the bends, hits, and staggers reflect the layman's description of clinical scenarios. On the basis that minor presentations may be followed by more significant problems, all patients with ADI should be referred to a hyperbaric facility.

Symptoms commonly present early after ascent:
- 50% within 10 minutes
- 85% within 1 hour
- A small number present up to 36 hours after ascent

Predisposing factors include:
- Poor physical fitness
- Low water temperature
- Increased physical exertion
- Obesity
- Increasing age
- Injuries
- Dive profile
- Recurrent dives
- Dehydration
- Alcohol.

Pathophysiology

Increased nitrogen is dissolved into blood on descent (Henry's Law) and is variably absorbed depending on blood flow and tissue composition. ADI results from a sudden release of nitrogen when the pressure is reduced on rapid ascent. If the ascent is slow, there is sufficient time for the nitrogen to be excreted by the lungs.

Nitrogen excretion continues for hours after a dive. A reduction in atmospheric pressure such as, for example, during flying, may precipitate ADI. Nitrogen bubbles do not form on the arterial side of the circulation as this blood has just passed through the lungs where pressure equilibrilation has occurred.

Following a rapid, uncontrolled ascent, nitrogen bubbles develop in the venous system. Passage into the arterial circulation is believed to be via a left-to-right shunt through a patent foramen ovale or, more commonly, an A–V shunt in the lung vasculature.

The bubble is eventually resorbed but may produce an acute complement activation, inflammatory response, and tissue damage. Hyperbaric oxygen therapy results in more oxygen in solution which will reach hypoxic areas by diffusion through the tissues. During repressurization in a hyperbaric chamber, the bubble reduces in size.

The chokes

Nitrogen bubbles forming in the pulmonary capillary bed produce decreased perfusion and pulmonary oedema. This can progress to ARDS.

The staggers

Nitrogen bubbles in the spinal vasculature result in neurological signs and may cause permanent disability (spinal bends).

The creeps

Blockage of capillaries in the skin results in an itchy sensation.

Clinical features of acute decompression illness

Generalized
- General lethargy, weakness
- Apathy

Cerebral
- Multi-focal vascular lesions
- Presentations may be similar to CVA (e.g. loss of motor function, sensation)
- May present with headaches and confusion

Cerebellar
- Unsteadiness
- Loss of co-ordination
- Dysarthria and/or nystagmus

Spinal
- Tingling
- Numbness
- Occasionally paralysis
- Spinal pain
- Girdle pain

Musculoskeletal
- May be single joint
- Often a numb feeling progressing to constant pain

The ear
- Vertigo
- Hearing deficit

Peripheral nerves
- Numbness
- Tingling
- Occasional motor weakness

Skin
- Pruritis
- Rash

Management

- ABCDE approach
  - High concentration oxygen via mask with a non-rebreathe valve and reservoir bag to relieve hypoxia and enhance nitrogen offloading
  - Use water for ET tube cuff if intubation necessary
  - Consider possibility of pneumothorax if ventilation becomes difficult or signs suggest the diagnosis
  - Consider intravenous crystalloid
- Analgesia is contraindicated as it will mask developing physical signs
- Nitrous oxide is absolutely contraindicated because of its rapid diffusion potential, therefore increasing the size of nitrogen bubbles
- Benzodiazepine iv for fits
- Transfer to suitable hyperbaric unit
- Most divers have a 'buddy'—check the buddy for symptoms of ADI.

ADI is unlikely to be seen in an isolated organ and should always be regarded as a multi-system problem

Electrocution injury

Types of incident

Industrial/occupational

Often affecting workers on power lines and those in industry using electrical tools and machinery.

Domestic

Due to failure to earth appliances or using electrical equipment near water.

20% of electrocutions occur in children—commonly toddlers playing with electrical appliances and adolescents during acts of bravado.

Lightening

- 75–85% occur in men
- 30% involve people working out of doors
- 25% involve recreational activities

Railway incidents

Electrical injuries involving railways are relatively common and many are suicide attempts. The common electrical systems in the UK are:

- 25,000 volt overhead AC lines
- 750 volt DC third rail system
- 630 volt DC fourth rail system (used by the London Underground)

> Always ensure the electrical system is turned off. Be aware that overhead lines are often disabled by bird strikes and routinely turned back on after 20 minutes.

Electrophysiology

An electric current is a motion of electrical charge where the electrical driving force is known as the voltage and the magnitude of electric current is measured in amperes.

Current flow is dependent on the voltage and the resistance of the tissues (for example, the skin, nerve, and muscle) through which it is passing and is governed by Ohm's law where:

$$I\ (current) = \frac{V(voltage)}{R(resistance)}$$

Current flows preferentially through tissues of least resistance (for example, nerve tissue) and this, therefore, significantly influences the patterns of injury seen. Skin resistance depends on the skin's thickness and its moisture, which is why hands are commonly affected. The amount of damaging themal energy depends on:

- The resistance of the tissue
- The duration of contact
- The square of the current

Current, therefore, is the most critical factor.

Direct current (DC) implies unidirectional current flow (for example, a battery) whereas an alternating current (AC) refers to a changing flow. The latter forms the basis of the UK domestic supply (240V AC current).

Alternating current is much more damaging and, on contact, may produce tetanic skeletal muscle contractions preventing release of any electrical wires. Direct current may produce a violent contraction but tends to throw the victim away from the source.

Lightening

Lightening strike may produce 20–200 million volts with a current of 50,000 amps. However, its duration is usually less than 0.2 seconds. The current pathway defines the injury pattern and, in the case of lightening strikes, the duration is insufficient to break the skin and reaches the earth by a 'flashover' effect, risking cardiac arrest. The flashover phenomenon may result in widespread skin burns. In other patients, respiratory arrest is common. Usually, those who do not suffer a cardiac arrest have an excellent prognosis.

Patterns of injury

Skin

Electrothermal burns result from current flow through the skin generating heat. Electrical burns commonly have points of entry and exit. AC burns tend to be associated with more tissue damage than DC burns.

Nervous system

Damage to the nervous system occurs in 70% of all electrical shock victims. This is because of the conduction potential of nervous tissue. Transient unconsciousness may result. Persistent alteration in conscious level suggests cerebral injury. Similarly, in very severe injury, the spinal cord and peripheral nerves may be damaged with paralysis.

Cardiorespiratory

Cardiac arrest is the principle cause of death following electrical injury. AC currents tend to produce VF and DC high voltage is associated with asystole. Other manifestations include cardiac dysrhythmias including sinus tachycardia, atrial fibrillation, ventricular ectopics, and complete heart block.

Respiratory arrest may occur due to a paralysing effect following prolonged tetanic muscle contractions, therefore risking secondary hypoxic arrest. Cardiac output frequently returns spontaneously but respiratory arrest may persist. Early basic life support is frequently life-saving.

Vascular

May follow deep cutaneous burns, usually with high voltages (1000V).

Limbs and joints

Thermoelectric injury to muscle may produce muscle necrosis, compartment syndrome, rhabdomyolysis leading to renal failure, hyperkalaemia, and the risk of cardiac arrest.

Management

- Ensure that the current is switched off
- Do not approach until it is safe to do so
- A non-conductor such as a wooden pole can be used to move the victim or the electrical source
- In case of electric pylons, be wary of electrical reconnection—unless informed, the electricity board will reconnect the supply after 20 minutes presuming it to be a bird strike
- Assess cardiorespiratory status and commence BLS if indicated
- Excellent recovery has been documented from resuscitation of seemingly dead victims
- Initiate ALS if indicated
- Consider cannulation and fluid replacement—major electrical burns require aggressive volume resuscitation. Lightening strike victims usually have limited burns and do not require fluid resuscitation.
- In lightening strike, seek cover as soon as practical/possible

Consider the risk of secondary traumatic injury if the patient has been thrown to the ground at the time of electrocution.

Chapter 10

Major incident management and triage

Major incident management

Definitions

In health service terms, a *major incident* is defined as:

'Any incident where the location, number, severity or type of live casualties requires extraordinary resources'.

Major incidents may be classified in three ways

- Natural or manmade
- Simple or compound
- Compensated or uncompensated.

The distinction between natural disasters (Tsunami, earthquake, flood, or forest fire) and manmade is self-explanatory. The most common causes of manmade disaster are industrial incidents, mass gathering incidents (such as football stadium disasters), transport incidents, and terrorism.

Simple and compound incidents

In a *simple* incident, the location's infrastructure remains intact and effective: communications are possible and the sick can be treated. When an incident is *compound*, roads, electricity supply, railways, health services, and communications are disrupted.

Compensated and uncompensated

A *compensated* incident is one which can be dealt with by mobilizing extra resources (for example, a major fire in a hotel or cinema). An *uncompensated* incident cannot be managed even when all available resources have been mobilized. Typical examples include natural disasters such as earthquakes and hurricanes.

Disasters and catastrophes

The terms 'disaster' and 'catastrophe' are usually used to refer to uncompensated major incidents (generally natural disasters).

Table 10.1 Major incidents

Date	Place	Incident	Dead	Injured
Natural incidents				
1931	China, Huang He River	Flood	3.7 million	Not known
1970	Peru, Yungay	Landslide	17,500	Not known
1995	Japan, Kobe	Earthquake	5502	Not known
2004	Pacific rim	Tsunami	>250,000	Not known
2005	Pakistan	Earthquake	200,000	Not known
Manmade incidents				
1977	Tenerife	Air crash	583	Not known
1985	UK, Bradford	Stadium fire	55	200
1985	Belgium, Brussels	Crowd crush	41	437
1987	Belgium, Zeebrugge	Ferry capsize	137	402
1988	UK, Lockerbie	Air crash	270	–
1989	UK, Sheffield	Crowd crush	96	200
1995	Japan, Tokyo	Gas attack	12	5000
1998	Omagh	Car bomb	29	200
2005	London	Bombs	52	700

The phases of a major incident

A major incident has three phases:

- Preparation
- Response
- Recovery.

Preparation

The three components of preparation are:

- Planning
- Equipment
- Training.

Major incident planning

Any site where there is a risk of a major incident (for example, chemical plant, major sporting venue, or travel interchange) must have a major incident plan which is regularly updated and regularly practised.

Any agency which will have to respond to a major incident must have a service plan (once again, regularly updated and practised) which can be adapted for an individual incident whether it occurs at a high risk site (such as a chemical plant fire) or is random and unpredictable (for example, an intercity train crash).

All hospitals must have a major incident plan and any health care professional who will be called upon to respond must know his own role and how that role integrates into the overall response.

All major incident plans must be multi-agency, reflecting the skills and responsibilities of all those bodies which will be involved if an incident does happen. In order to facilitate this, many agencies (and all official bodies) now use *MIMMS—Major Incident Medical Management and Support* as their template for a major incident response.

Equipment

Adequate equipment must be available and easily accessible. This will include personal protective equipment, medical equipment, communications, and specialist equipment such as triage cards and major incident commanders' bags.

MIMMS—Major Incident Medical Management and Support

The co-ordinated response to a medical incident is taught on the MIMMS course. This is a three-day course for health care professionals which covers the organization of the response to a major incident, communications, equipment, and triage. Members of the other emergency services and the armed forces also attend. The course concludes with formal major incident exercises at chosen locations such as sports grounds or industrial sites. The MIMMS course is now accepted internationally.

A one-day course is also available for those who may have to respond to an incident but who will not be called upon to assume a command role. *(For details, see useful contact details p.600.)*

Successful completion of a MIMMS course should be considered essential for anyone who is likely to have to respond to a major incident. Possession of '*Major incident management system*' (Hodgetts and Porter, BMJ Books, 2nd edn., 2002) is recommended. *Major incident management System* is distributed to all MIMMS course candidates.

Major incident response

The response to a major incident is considered under the following headings:

- **C**ommand
- **S**afety
- **C**ommunications
- **A**ssessment
- **T**riage
- **T**reatment
- **T**ransport

Command

Command is a vertical process; control a horizontal one:

```
 C
CONTROL
 M
 M
 A
 N
 D
```

Each emergency service will have a commander at the scene Control is enforced by means of cordons (see p.584).

Safety

Safety of responders and victims alike is a key component of the major incident response. The '1–2–3 of safety' is:

1. SELF
2. SCENE
3. SURVIVORS

- Command
- Safety
- Communications
- Assessment
- Triage
- Treatment
- Transport

Control **S**pells **C**alm **A**nd **T**ime **T**o **T**reat

Communications

Effective communications must be established between incident commanders. Regular face-to-face communication is essential. Other methods include:

- Radios
- Runners
- Whistles
- Hand signals
- Telephones (land lines)
- Mobile phones.

Health service communications are an ambulance service responsibility. Communications will be established from the site to ambulance control.

Radios

Ambulance radio systems are usually VHF, allowing communication at the scene and with ambulance control. A radio net will be established with control and call signs. *Single frequency simplex* allows all users to hear all messages (it is 'open') and offers a broader 'picture' of the incident as it progresses. *Two frequency simplex* means that call signs can only speak to and hear control. Control can hear all stations and can let stations hear each other ('talk through'). Two frequency simplex is the usual ambulance service system.

A protected national frequency for doctors at major incidents is currently being trialled.

Runners

Runners are an effective method of communication, but ideally should carry written rather than verbal messages. They should be instructed to return in order to confirm that a message has been conveyed irrespective of whether there is a reply.

Whistles

Repeated whistle blasts by the fire service indicate an immediate need to evacuate an area.

Hand signals

The military use a range of hand signals. These should not be used by civilians unless they are thoroughly familiar with their use and meaning.

Telephones (land lines)

In prolonged incidents, it is possible to set up land lines at the scene of an incident. These can be provided by commercial companies or by the military.

Mobile phones

Mobile phones are an effective means of communication, but have two major problems. There is no central co-ordination of calls, so that confusion and duplication and overload of the system can occur with the result that no calls can be made. The latter is a particular problem once the media have been notified.

In order to prevent system overload and allow continued access to essential users, the ACCOLC (Access Overload Control) system can be activated. Once ACCOLC has been activated, only mobile phones which have been modified will remain in use. Requests for phones to be ACCOLC modified have to be approved at Cabinet Office level.

Assessment

Assessment of the number, severity, and types of injury is a key component of the major incident response.

Triage

Triage is the prioritizing of patients for treatment or transport according to their severity of injury (p.602).

Treatment

Some treatment will be undertaken at the incident scene, although most will take place after evacuation to hospital. In order to achieve the maximum benefit for the victims, this must be co-ordinated so that each patient is delivered to the appropriate facility having received any necessary treatment before departure. In general, treatment at the scene should be restricted to that necessary to allow the patient to be transported safely and comfortably to hospital and to ensure that evacuation is possible.

Transport

The aim is to transport the 'right patient to the right place at the right time' and by the 'right method'. The transport scheme within the incident scene is shown in Fig. 10.1.

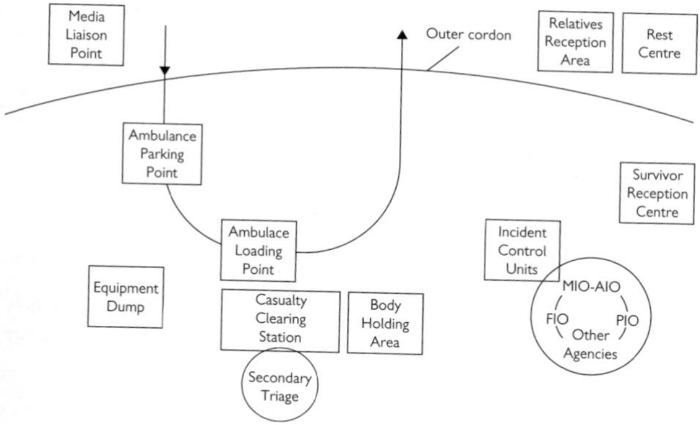

Fig. 10.1 The ambulance circuit.

Decisions regarding patient destinations will be taken under the supervision of the medical commanders. Less injured patients may be transported in patient transport vehicles or in minibuses or taxis. Patients sharing the same vehicle should obviously be going to the same destination. Patients should not be sent to hospitals specializing in a single system if injuries elsewhere have not been excluded. However, patients with a neurosurgical injury should be sent to the local hospital with neurosurgical facilities.

Major incident recovery

Even after the scene of the incident is free of patients, the incident response is likely to continue for some considerable time. Hospitals will have a backlog of surgery to perform, rosters will take time to return to normal, and roads and railways will have to be returned to full function.

Following each incident, all the organizations involved must, separately and together, review their actions. This will highlight areas for improvement and will also identify areas of particular achievement. An immediate operational debrief is usually held to identify key lessons, followed at a later date by a more formal debrief.

Some responders may develop features of an acute stress response, including poor sleep, anxiety, flashbacks, nightmares, poor performance, and inability to concentrate. It is essential that these people are identified and receive the help they need.

Declaring a major incident

A major incident is usually declared by the first representative of the emergency services to reach the scene. The phrase used has been standardized:

'Major incident declared'

Under some circumstances (for example, an aeroplane having difficulty landing), the following may be used:

'Major incident standby'

to warn of a possible imminent incident.

If a warning turns out to be false, or a major incident response is not required, the order is:

'Major incident cancelled'

Methane

The acronym METHANE is used to pass information from the scene to control, but can also be used when passing information between individuals (see box).

M Major incident standby or declared
E Exact location (grid reference if available)
T Type of incident (chemical, terrorist, rail, etc)
H Hazards present and potential
A Access
N Number and severity/type of casualties
E Emergency services present and required

Some emergency services use the mnemonic CHALET:
C Casualties—number, severity, and type
H Hazards present and potential
A Access
L Location
E Emergency services present and required
T Type of incident

The scene of a major incident

Cordons and commands

The inner cordon and bronze area

The *inner cordon* surrounds the actual site of the incident. It contains the wreckage and the hazardous area. The area inside the inner cordon is the *bronze area*. The inner cordon is not always physically marked with tape, but where there is any hazard, access to the bronze area will be strictly regulated with personnel being checked in and out. If the incident has more than one location (for example, wreckage at either end of a railway tunnel), there may be more than one bronze area and more than one inner cordon. In this case, there will also be a command structure for each bronze area (see below).

At terrorist or firearms incidents, the inner cordon is controlled by the police. When there is a fire or chemical hazard, the inner cordon is controlled by the fire service.

The outer cordon and silver area

The outer cordon surrounds the entire incident site, and thus includes the survivor reception centre, casualty clearing station, command post, body holding area, and all the other designated locations which together make up a co-ordinated major incident response. The area between the inner and outer cordons is the *silver area*. There is normally only one silver area (multiple silver areas may be established during the 'sectorization' of a natural disaster effecting a very large area).

Gold command

The gold command is situated away from the scene of the incident at a pre-designated location such as the regional police headquarters.

Command structures and responsibilities

Bronze area

The bronze area is under the authority of the forward commanders, one for each service. A schematic diagram of the bronze command structure is shown in Fig. 10.3.

Silver area

The silver commanders are responsible for the area within the outer cordon. The bronze commanders report to the silver commanders. The command vehicles for the emergency services co-locate to form silver command—the *Joint Emergency Services Control (JESC)*. A schematic diagram of silver command is shown in Fig. 10.4.

Good communication between the silver (or incident) commanders is the key to an effective response. Silver commanders are not tied to the command location but may move around the incident scene gathering information and consulting with other responders. However, they must arrange to meet on a regular basis.

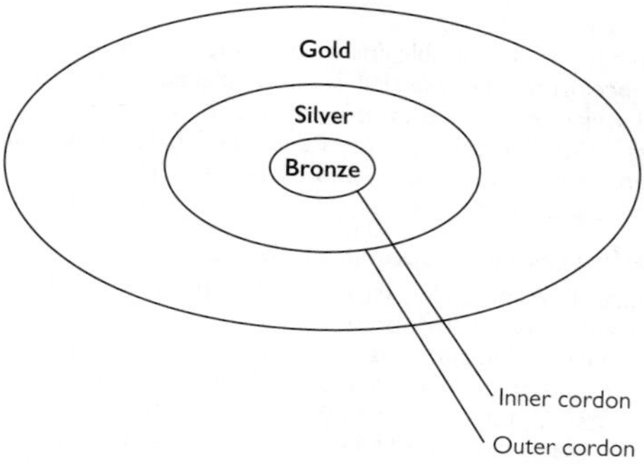

Fig. 10.2 Areas and cordons.

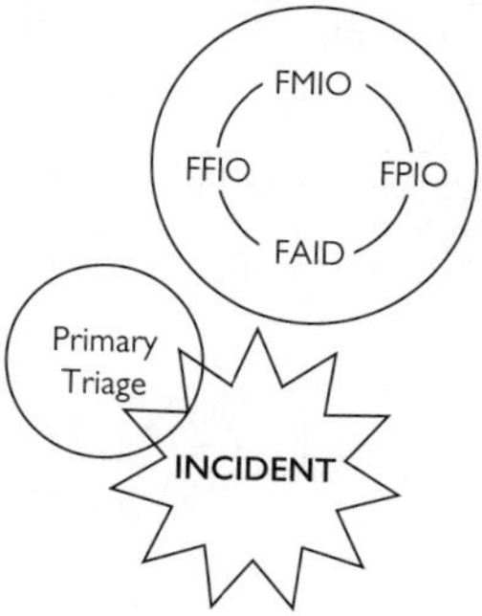

Fig. 10.3 Command in the bronze area (schematic).

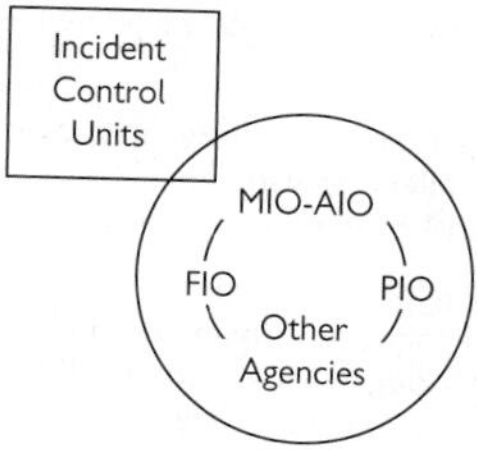

Fig. 10.4 Silver command: the Joint Emergency Services Control—JESC (schematic).

Gold command

Gold command is responsible for multi-agency liaison off site. Requests for assistance from neighbouring services are channelled through gold command which is also responsible for liaison with central government, national agencies (for example, the Radiation Protection Board, Environment Agency, security services), and bodies with multi-area remits such as rail service providers.

The health services response at the scene

The ambulance commander (silver) based at the JESC is responsible for the health services response with the silver medical commander. The ambulance commander is responsible for all ambulance service personnel (including the voluntary aid societies); the medical commander for all doctors and nurses. The ambulance command vehicle is identified by a steady green light. The forward (bronze) commanders report to the silver commanders. The forward control point is within the inner cordon. Primary triage is carried out in the bronze area by the primary triage officer under the authority of the forward medical commander.

A structured response

Casualty clearing station (CCS)

The casualty clearing station is established by the ambulance service for the assessment and treatment of survivors at the scene of the incident. A schematic diagram is shown in Fig. 10.5. Key assets at the casualty clearing station include:

- Safety
- Shelter
- Light
- Heating
- Cooking facilities
- Toilets and washing facilities
- Communications.

Wherever possible, therefore, the CCS should be located in a pre-existing building, although in some circumstances, improvization and the use of temporary shelters may be necessary.

Ambulance parking point

The ambulance parking point is a designated area in which ambulances can wait before being called forward for loading. The ambulance parking point is under the control of the ambulance parking officer.

Ambulance loading point

Ambulances are called forwards (from the ambulance parking point) to the ambulance parking point adjacent to the CCS for loading under the direction of the *ambulance loading officer*.

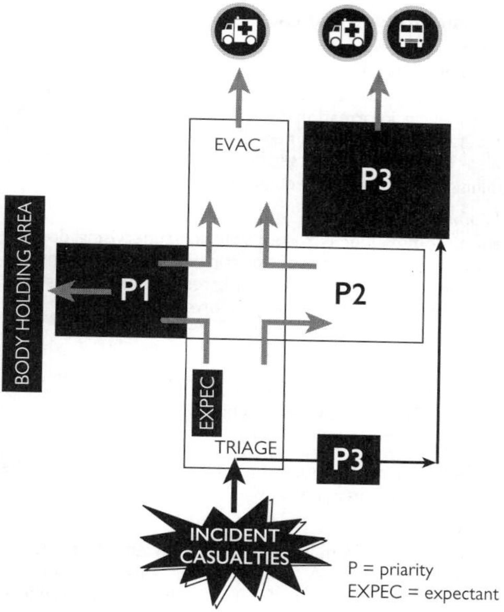

Fig. 10.5 Casualty clearing station (CCS) layout. Reprinted with permission from Hodgetts and Porter (2002). *Major incident management system*, 2nd edn. BMJ Books.

How to recognize incident commanders

Police commander	Blue and white chequer tabard
Fire commander	Red and white chequer tabard
Ambulance commander	Green and white chequer tabard
Medical commander	Text (medical commander) only

Roles and responsibilities—medical

Medical commander

The medical commander (silver) liaises with the other silver commanders and delegates tasks to the available medical and nursing personnel. He is responsible for channelling information to and from local hospitals and for carrying out a full medical assessment of the scene. The medical commander is also tasked with overseeing treatment and secondary triage and determining manpower and equipment requirements.

Forward medical commander

The forward medical commander is responsible for supervising doctors within the bronze area and directing requests for medical equipment and personnel to the medical commander. He is also responsible for ensuring that the medical commander is kept fully informed of developments within the bronze area.

Casualty clearing officer

The casualty clearing officer is responsible for the CCS. The secondary triage officer and the medical teams report to him.

Secondary triage officer

The secondary triage officer carries out triage of patients on arrival at the CCS. He may also assist with treatment of patients within the CCS.

Mobile medical teams

Mobile medical teams sent out from local hospitals may either be used as a team in the bronze area or CCS, or broken up and distributed as appropriate, taking into account the skills of individual team members. A mobile medical team usually contains two nurses and two doctors. Whenever possible, clinicians with no pre-hospital experience or training should NOT be allocated to work in the bronze area. The concept of the mobile medical team is being phased out.

Mobile surgical teams

Life-saving surgical procedures such as amputations are only rarely required due to advances in extrication techniques and pain control. When such a procedure is necessary, a team should be requested from the local hospital to perform it. They should then return to the hospital. The usual composition of a mobile surgical team is a surgeon, an anaesthetist, a scrub nurse, and an operating department assistant (ODA) or anaesthetic nurse.

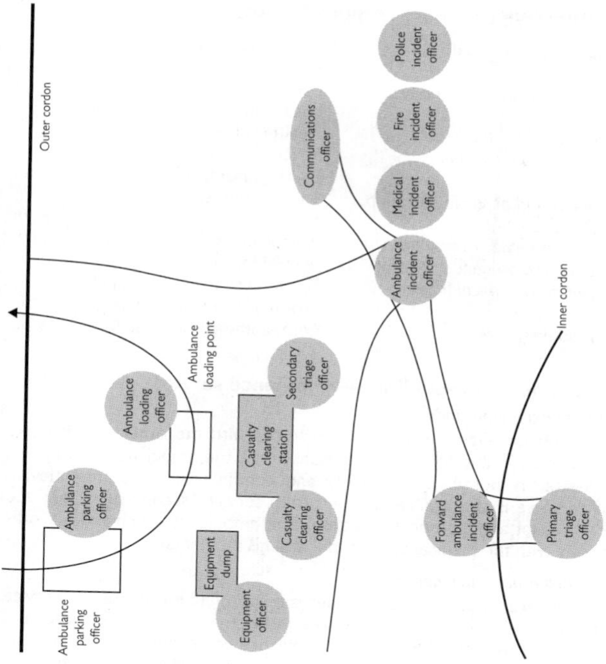

Fig. 10.6 Health services response at the scene of a major incident (schematic). Reprinted with permission from Greaves I *et al.* (2005). *Emergency care—a textbook for paramedics,* 2nd edn. W.B. Saunders Co. Ltd.

Emergency services responsibilities

Care of the injured	Health services Police and fire
Care of uninjured survivors	Police Local authority/social services
Dealing with the dead	Health/police
Evacuation and shelter	Police Local authorities
Social and psychological support	Social services/voluntary aid societies/health
Health service communications	Ambulance service
Explosive ordnance disposal	Armed forces
Fire and chemical hazards	Fire (advice from community health and poisons units)
Field engineering	Local authorities/armed forces

Roles and responsibilities—ambulance service

Ambulance commander

The ambulance commander (silver) liaises with the other commanders and is responsible for task allocation within the ambulance service. He delegates responsibility for safety and communication to the relevant officers. He is responsible for the health services scene assessment and for hospital and transport selection. The ambulance commander works closely with the medical commander and his assistants.

Forward ambulance commander

The forward ambulance commander is responsible for ambulance service personnel in the bronze area. He must ensure effective triage and removal of patients. The forward ambulance commander determines the location of the ambulance parking point with the advice of the police.

Casualty clearing officer

The casualty clearing officer is responsible for the CCS. The secondary triage officer and the medical teams report to him. He must ensure adequate patient documentation and liaise with the doctor in charge of the CCS and the ambulance service regarding patient transfer from the scene.

Ambulance parking officer

Controls the ambulance parking point.

Ambulance loading officer

Controls the ambulance loading point and supervises the loading of ambulances at the CCS.

Ambulance safety officer

The ambulance safety officer is responsible for the safety of all health services personnel within the outer cordon. He must ensure that all personnel are appropriately dressed and advise on the treatment of injured staff. He must also ensure that tired staff are allowed to rest. Liaison with the other emergency services is a key role.

Communications officer

The communications officer co-ordinates all on-site communications between medical and ambulance service staff. He is responsible for the logging of all communications and for ensuring clear and effective communications on-site and with off-site agencies.

Equipment officer

The equipment officer overseas health services equipment requirements at the scene. All requests for equipment must be channelled through the equipment officer if confusion is to be avoided.

Roles of the other emergency services at a major incident

Fire

The roles of the fire service at a major incident are to:

- Establish fire service command and control
- Fight fires
- Save lives
- Prevent escalation of the incident
- Eliminate hazards
- Rescue trapped casualties
- Provide specialist equipment and shelter.

The fire service are responsible for advising on health and safety for all those in the bronze area.

Police

The police will usually take an overall controlling role in land-based major incidents. The roles of the police service at a major incident are to:

- Establish police command and control
- Save lives
- Prevent escalation of the incident
- Supervise evacuation where necessary
- Control traffic
- Maintain appropriate records
- Handle and identify the dead
- Maintain order and protect property
- Carry out any necessary criminal investigation
- Liaise with the media.

Other agencies

The local authority

The roles of the local authority at a major incident include:

- Co-ordination of the response by agencies other than the emergency services (for example, the Environment Agency)
- Provision of heavy machinery
- Provision of manual labour
- Provision of specialist technical advice and assistance
- Provision of environmental health advice and services
- Allowing access to buildings used for shelter of casualties, survivors, and evacuees, temporary mortuaries, and other functions, as required
- Staffing survivor reception centres and other functions (council employees and members of the voluntary services).

In addition, the local authority is charged with co-ordinating disaster planning and training in its area. Each authority has an Emergency Planning Officer (EPO) who works closely with the emergency services and other bodies such as the Environment Agency. The EPO is the point of contact in the event of an incident. A representative is usually sent to silver control for the duration of the incident.

Once the incident is 'over', the local authority will play a major role in reconstruction and the return of 'society' to normal function.

The armed forces

The armed forces provide assistance at major incidents under the *Military Aid to the Civil Powers* (MAC) scheme. The military are usually called in by the local authority. Once assistance has been agreed, the military will appoint a liaison officer who will work closely with the authority.

The armed forces at a major incident can provide:

- Medical, nursing, and technical expertise
- Field medical facilities, tents, and hardstanding
- Ambulances, passenger transport, and other specialist vehicles including helicopters
- Generating equipment
- Communications
- Drinking water
- Field engineering
- Disciplined personnel.

Her Majesty's Coastguard

Her Majesty's Coastguard (part of the Maritime and Coastguard Agency) is charged with co-ordinating the rescue of casualties from off-shore incidents. Specific responsibilities include:

- Identifying the location of the incident
- Alerting nearby vessels
- Establishing communications with the involved vessels and others
- Requesting helicopter support
- Co-ordinating and requesting naval and lifeboat (RNLI) assistance.

The voluntary aid societies

Providers of voluntary aid at major incidents include St John's Ambulance, the British Red Cross, the Women's Royal Voluntary Service, and St Andrew's Ambulance (in Scotland). There are also many smaller specialist bodies, such as BASICS, and appropriately trained individuals. The Samaritans and other organizations provide help to those recovering from the effects of a major incident.

The voluntary services can provide:

- Volunteer medical personnel and skilled assistance
- Trained personnel to run rest and recovery centres and assist with documentation
- Clothing and bedding
- Refreshments to emergency services personnel
- Food, clothing, and shelter to victims of major incidents.

The Faith Communities

The major religious faiths (Christians, Jews, Hindus, Muslims, Sikhs, Buddhists, the Church of Jesus Christ of the Latter Day Saints, and the Chinese Community) have issued detailed guidance regarding specific religious aspects of major incidents (*Guidelines for faith communities when dealing with disasters* available from the Church of England Board for Social Responsibility, Church House, Great Smith St, London SW1P 3NZ).

Other specific responsibilities

Dealing with the dead

Although under certain circumstances, it is permitted for paramedics to *pronounce* death, at a major incident, this role is undertaken by a doctor in the presence of a police officer. However, before this, when triage is being carried out, the triage officer will *label* a patient dead based on the triage algorithm. Pronouncement of death follows. *Certification* of cause of death will only occur following a coroner's inquest. The coroner will issue a death certificate.

Victims who are triaged dead must be clearly labelled as such in order to prevent time wastage in further repeated assessment. Dead bodies should only be moved for two reasons:

- To gain access to living casualties
- To prevent them being destroyed (for example, by fire, chemicals, or crushing).

Bodies that are moved for these reasons and the bodies of those who have died at the CCS should be taken to a *body holding area* which should be close to the CCS but away from public gaze.

Following a major incident, a temporary mortuary will be used to accommodate bodies. In most cases, this will have been identified in advance and included in area major incident plans.

Radio voice procedure

All pre-hospital care practitioners must be familiar with correct radio usage. Nowhere is this more important than during a major incident. The key features of a radio message are:
- Clarity
- Accuracy
- Brevity.

Each message must be clear, unambiguous, and free of unnecessary information. In order to assist with this, speech should be steady, slightly slower than normal, loud enough to be clear without shouting, and at a slightly higher pitch than normal for men (women's voices tend to be clearer over the radio). Certain terms may be used to save time (see box) but unauthorized slang should be avoided. Unusual or difficult words, especially names and addresses, should be spelt using the NATO phonetic alphabet (see box). Numbers should be pronounced as indicated in the box.

Making a call

- Begin a call by stating the *call sign of the number being called*
- Then give your call sign
- Give the message
- Finish with 'over'.

Using 'over' indicates that the recipient of your call can now reply.

Approved radio communications shorthand terms

Go ahead	I am ready to receive your message
Send	I am ready to receive your message
Roger	I understand
OK	I understand
Say again	Repeat *
Acknowledge	Confirm that you have received my message
Send	I am ready to receive your message
Over	Please talk
Spell	Precedes difficult words such as addresses or names (also as 'please spell' when this is requested)
Numbers	Precedes lists of numbers such as telephone numbers
Out	The conversation is finished
Wait	I am unable to speak to you for five seconds (may be repeated once, then wait out)
Wait out	I am unable to reply, I will contact you later
Standby	Be alert, further information to follow

* Say again all after/say again all before.......

The NATO phonetic alphabet

A	Alpha	N	November
B	Bravo	O	Oscar
C	Charlie	P	Papa
D	Delta	Q	Quebec
E	Echo	R	Romeo
F	Foxtrot	S	Sierra
G	Golf	T	Tango
H	Hotel	U	Uniform
I	India	V	Victor
J	Juliet	W	Whisky
K	Kilo	X	X-ray
L	Lima	Y	Yankee
M	Mike	Z	Zulu

Numbers for radio messages

1	Wun	6	Six
2	Too	7	Seven
3	Thuree	8	Ate
4	Fower	9	Niner
5	Fiyiv	0	Zero

Replying to a call

- Begin by giving your call sign.

Ending a call

- Once a message or exchange is complete, the final speaker says '*out*'.
- When speaking to more than one recipient, the phrase '[call sign] *out to you*' can be used to particular recipients, whilst further communication continues with the others.

Corrections

- As soon as you recognize an error, say '*wrong*' and give the correct information.

Repeating

- If a message was unclear and you wish to hear it again, the expression '*say again*' is used. In order to avoid repeating the complete message, the expressions '*say again all after…*', '*say again all before…*', and '*say again all between x and y…*' are used, giving the necessary words from the original message to indicate which sections are to be repeated.

Performing a radio check

- Radio checks can be initiated by control or any call sign
- Begin with the stations being called, then your station, then radio check *('all stations zulu from control, radio check over')*
- Reply with your call sign and OK if reception is clear ('*Zulu 1, OK, over*')
- The initiator ends the radio check with his call sign OK and out ('*Control, OK, out*')
- Other terms are used for unclear transmission:
  Difficult—can be understood but not clear (interference)
  Broken—message only heard intermittently
  Unworkable—occasional words only or continuous interference
  Nothing heard.

Sources of further information

Arrangements for responding to nuclear emergencies. Health and Safety Executive. Available from the Stationery Office

Dealing with disaster, Rev 3rd edn. Brodie Publishing. Available from the Stationery Office (Contains an extensive list of useful website addresses covering all aspects of major incident response.)

Emergency planning in the NHS—health service arrangements for dealing with major incidents. Available from Department of Health Emergency Planning Coordination Unit, Room 603, Richmond House, 79 Whitehall, London SW1A 2NS

Guidelines for faith communities when dealing with disasters. Available from the Church of England Board for Social Responsibility, Church House, Great Smith St, London SW1P 3NZ

Major Incident Medical Management and Support (MIMMS), 2nd edn. Advanced Life Support Group, BMA Publications.

Military aid to the civil community 3rd edn (1989). Available from the Stationery Office

Triage

Introduction

Triage is the sorting of patients, by priority, for treatment or transport. It is a dynamic process. *Primary triage* is carried out in the bronze area, *secondary triage* at the casualty clearing station. Triage may be repeated before evacuation of patients from the site (*triage for transport*).

Triage is the sorting of patients, by priority, for treatment or transport

Triage priorities

Common triage priorities

P	T	Description	Colour
1	1	Immediate	Red
2	2	Urgent	Yellow
3	3	Delayed	Green
1 Hold	4	Expectant	Blue
Dead	Dead	Dead	White or black

In the UK, the T system is conventionally used at a major incident.

Immediate priority

These casualties require immediate life-saving intervention.

Urgent priority

These casualties require significant intervention within 2–4 hours.

Delayed priority

These casualties require intervention, but not within 4 hours.

Expectant priority

Treating these casualties at an early stage in the incident would divert resources from potentially salvageable casualties, with no significant chance of a successful outcome.

The expectant category can be marked by:

- Use of a blue card (not usually available)
- Amending a P3 card with the word expectant
- Turning down the corners of a P3 green card diagonally to expose a red card underneath.

Triage sieve

The triage sieve is a simple reproducible triage method for use as a primary triage tool (see Fig. 10.7).

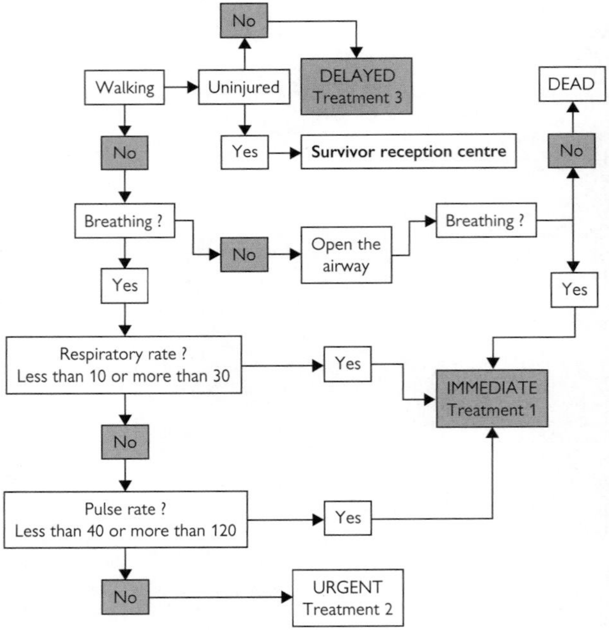

Fig. 10.7 The triage sieve. Reprinted with permission from Greaves I *et al.* (2005) *Emergency care: a textbook for paramedics*, 2nd edn. W.B. Saunders Co. Ltd.

The triage sort

The triage sort is a more complex system designed for use at the casualty clearing station. However, if there are insufficient staff to deal with patients arriving at the CCS, the sieve can be repeated until it becomes possible to carry out the sort. The triage sort uses the triage revised trauma score.

A coded score is derived for each of the three variables (*respiratory rate, systolic BP, and Glasgow Coma Score Scale*). The three coded values are then added together, and the final triage priority is derived as shown in the box.

The triage sort

PHYSIOLOGICAL VARIABLE	VALUE	SCORE
Respiratory rate	10–29	4
	>29	3
	6–9	2
	1–5	1
	0	0
Systolic blood pressure	>90	4
	76–89	3
	50–75	2
	1–49	1
	0	0
Glasgow Coma Scale Score	13–15	4
	9–12	3
	6–8	2
	4–5	1
	3	0
Total score for coding (see box below)		**X**

Coded score	Priority
1–10	T1
11	T2
12	T3
0	Dead

Triage in children

The normal physiological values given in the triage sieve on p.609 do not apply in children and must, therefore, be adapted. Specific triage sieve protocols can be used, based on the child's length (top of head to feet) or weight:

Weight = (2 x age in years) + 8

Alternatively, a *paediatric triage tape* can be used. This is placed alongside the child and the appropriate triage sieve protocol read off the tape according to the child's length.

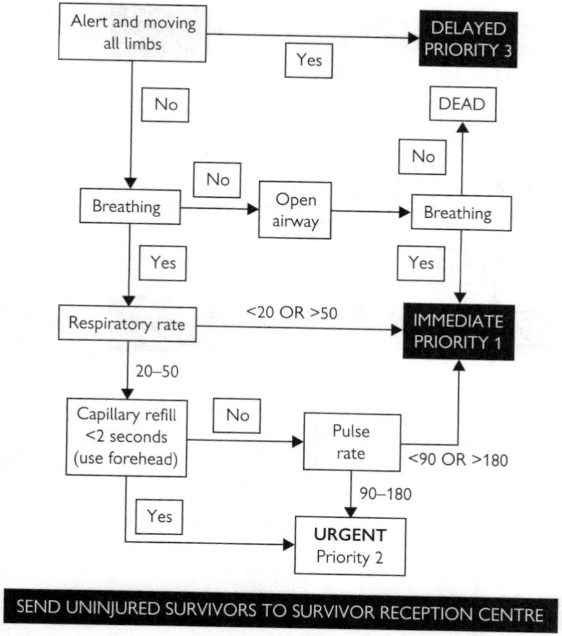

Fig. 10.8 Triage sieve 1: child 50–80cm or 3–10kg. Reprinted with permission from Hodgetts and Porter (2002). *Major incident management system*, 2nd edn. BMJ Books.

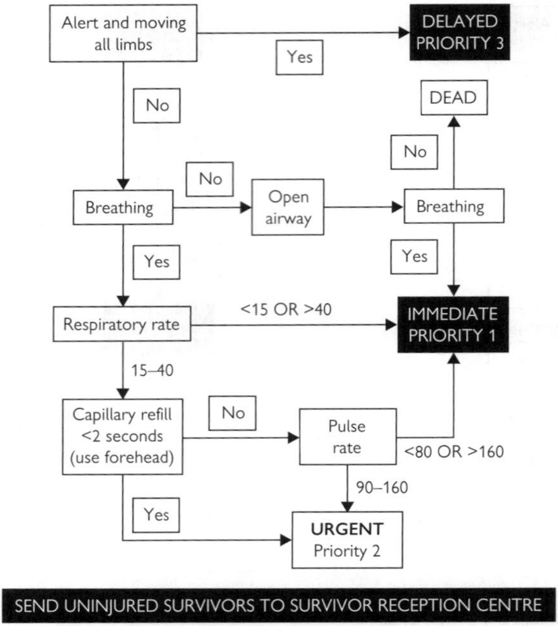

Fig. 10.9 Triage sieve 2: child 80–100cm or 11–18kg. Reprinted with permission from Hodgetts and Porter (2002). *Major incident management system,* 2nd edn. BMJ Books.

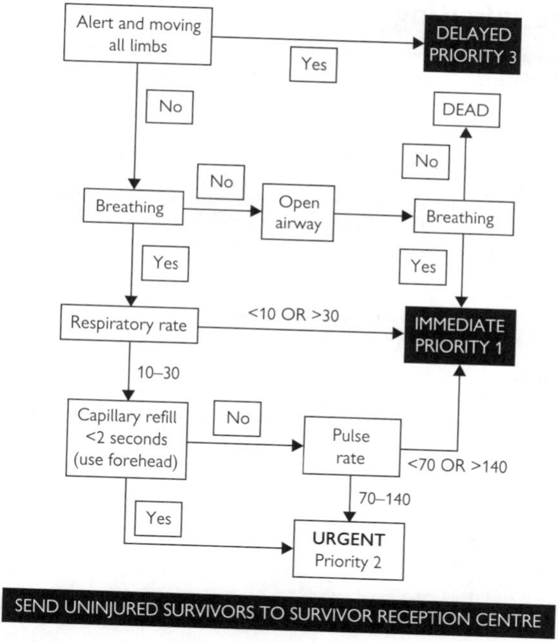

Fig. 10.10 Triage sieve 3: child 100–140cm or 19–32 kg. Reprinted with permission from Hodgetts and Porter (2002). *Major incident management system*, 2nd edn. BMJ Books.

Triage labelling

Because a patient's condition may improve (for example, with treatment) or deteriorate, any effective triage labelling system must allow re-categorization. It is also helpful if clinical notes can be made on the triage card since this will prevent duplication and potential loss of records.

Various triage cards are available, including cruciform cards (*Cambridge Cruciform card* and others), concertina cards (*Smart system*), and multiple single cards. Each of these systems has a different label and colour on a different limb, fold, or sheet of card. Systems which require inappropriate categories to be torn off and discarded are best avoided as any change in the patient's condition requires a replacement card.

Triage is dynamic

Whichever system is chosen, the card should be secured firmly to the patient and protected in a waterproof bag. If no cards are available, the triage category can be marked on the patient's forehead using a waterproof marker.

Trauma scoring

Trauma scores are used to study the outcomes of trauma and trauma care. They are audit and research tools. They cannot be used to predict the outcome for individual patients. In pre-hospital care, the significance of trauma scoring is that it cannot be performed without adequate data. Good record-keeping is a pre-requisite of trauma scoring.

Trauma scoring can be used to identify good quality care (patients who would be expected to die but survived) or to establish the need for improvement (patients who should have survived but died—unexpected deaths.) Trauma scoring is an audit tool as well as a means of determining the effect of financial investment in trauma care.

Physiological scoring systems

Trauma scores can be based on either anatomical data or physiological data, or on both. Anatomical scores use an accurate description of a patient's injuries and do not change. Physiological scores, However, are dynamic—they change as the patient's condition changes. The *Glasgow Coma Scale* is a physiological score. It allows comparison of groups of patient with the same score. The *Revised Trauma Score* (RTS) is probably the most commonly used (see box). This is a coded version of the scoring system used for the triage sort.

Revised Trauma Score

PHYSIOLOGICAL VARIABLE	VALUE	SCORE
Respiratory rate **RRc**	10–29	4
	>29	3
	6–9	2
	1–5	1
	0	0
Systolic blood pressure **SBPc**	≥90	4
	76–89	3
	50–75	2
	1–49	1
	0	0
Glasgow Coma Scale Score **GCSc**	13–15	4
	9–12	3
	6–8	2
	4–5	1
	3	0

Revised trauma score = 0.2908RRc + 0.7326SBPc + 0.9368GCSc

Nearest whole number	Probability of survival (%)
8	99
7	97
6	92
5	81
4	61
3	36
2	17
1	7
0	3

*CRAMS (**C**irculation, **R**espiration, **A**bdomen, **M**otor, and **S**peech)* is an alternative physiological scoring system which has been used in the past to attempt to differentiate major and minor trauma. The available evidence would suggest that it is not sufficiently reliable to be used as a clinical tool for this purpose (see box).

CRAMS Scoring system

Component	**Score**
Circulation (A)	
Normal capillary refill and systolic BP >100mmHg	2
Prolonged capillary refill and systolic BP >85–100mmHg	1
No capillary refill	0
Respiration (B)	
Normal	2
Abnormal	1
Absent	0
Abdomen (C)	
Abdomen and thorax not tender	2
Abdomen and thorax tender	1
Abdomen rigid or flail chest, penetrating wound to abdomen or thorax	0
Motor (D)	
Normal	2
Responds only to pain	1
No response or decerebrate	0
Speech (E)	
Normal	2
Confused	1
No intelligible words	0

Total CRAMS score = A + B + C + D + E

Score ≤ 8 major trauma   Score ≥ 9 minor trauma

The *Paediatric Trauma Score* (PTs) is essentially a physiological score, but includes some simple anatomical components (see box). The PTS is used as a triage tool in the USA where trauma of different severities is taken to hospitals offering different levels of care. It is not widely used in the UK.

Paediatric Trauma Score

	+2	+1	−1
Weight (kg)	>20	10–20	<10
Airway	Normal	Simple adjunct	ET/surgical
Systolic BP (mmHg)	>90	50–90	<50
Conscious level	Alert	Decreased/history of consciousness	loss of Coma
Open wounds	None	Minor	Major/penetrating
Fractures	None	Minor	Open/multiple

Total score range: −6 to 12

Anatomical scoring systems

Anatomical scoring systems are based on a definitive assessment of the patient's injuries: they are static. The most common systems are the *Abbreviated Injury Scale* (*AIS*) and the *Injury Severity Score* (*ISS*). The AIS divides injuries into six body regions and scores injuries from 1 to 6 with increasing severity (injuries scoring 6 are almost invariably fatal). Scores for individual injuries are derived from a list including more than 1200 injuries.

The ISS is based on the AIS. The AIS is recorded for the most severe injury in the three most severely injured AIS regions. These scores are squared and then added together. The maximum score with any chance of survival is 75 ($5^2 + 5^2 + 5^2$). An AIS code of 6 in any region is automatically given an ISS of 75 and implies a fatal outcome. An ISS of 16 or more implies major trauma.

Combined physiological and anatomical scoring systems

The most commonly used scoring system for research purposes is the TRISS (**TR**auma **S**core-**I**njury **S**everity **S**core) system which combines an anatomical method (ISS) with a physiological system (RTS) where:

$$\text{Probability of survival Ps} = 1/\ 1+e^{-b}$$

$$\text{Where } b = b_0 + b_1(\text{RTS}) + b_2(\text{ISS}) + b_3\ (\text{age coefficient})$$

and b_1–b_3 are coefficients for blunt and penetrating trauma

The only relevance of the TRISS methodology in pre-hospital care is as a reminder that careful and full gathering and recording of clinical information is a key component of optimal patient management.

Chapter 11

Chemical, biological, radiological, and nuclear (CBRN) incidents

Introduction

CBRN incidents may occur as a result of accidental events or specific acts of terrorism. Events such as the Chernobyl nuclear incident in Russia, the Sarin gas release on the underground system in Tokyo, and the anthrax release in the USA highlight the necessity for a structured multiagency and multidisciplinary response of which medical support is an essential component.

Chemical incidents

Chemical incidents may occur as a result of an accident involving hazardous materials (HAZMAT) or a terrorist act. The fundamental differences being that for a HAZMAT emergency, the chemical involved is usually immediately identifiable and, in the case of chemical installations, the site will have been pre-surveyed with the result that there will be a site contingency plan already available. Accidental release may also occur as a result of accidents on industrial or commercial sites, in laboratories, hospitals, academic institutions, materials in transit (road, rail, and sea), domestic or commercial spillage, fire, and explosion.

In contrast, a biological or radiological incident may develop from a seemingly innocuous event with the result that the public are unlikely to be aware, initially, that they have been contaminated. As a result, there may be a delay in recognition of such an incident.

Biological incidents

Biological incidents result from the use of living organisms or inanimate poisonous molecules isolated from them (toxins). These biological agents may take significantly longer to take effect than chemicals, depending on the incubation period and mode of transmission of the agent. Recognition of incidents is usually only possible when suspicious symptom clusters are identified or notification of a release is made.

Radiological and nuclear incidents

A radiological emergency results from the emission of various forms of radiation. Such incidents are usually the result of accidents at locations holding radioactive materials, most obviously power stations but also including schools, hospitals, and industrial plants. Deliberately released radioactive materials are a potential terrorist weapon as a result of the detonation of a so-called 'dirty bomb' or following an attack on a nuclear facility. Nuclear explosions produce direct radiation effects, widespread heat, and blast damage.

Mode of presentation

Chemical and biological incidents may present covertly. The initial presentation may be of a number of unrelated and unexpected patient episodes at which the ambulance service may be the only first responders. The NATO model of 'STEP 123' may be the only indication of a covert attack.

- One casualty: note signs and symptoms (*normal incident*)
- Two casualties: note signs and symptoms – similar signs/ symptoms – unrelated patients (*suspect CBRN incident*)
- Three casualties: note signs and symptoms – similar signs/ symptoms – unrelated patients (*strong suspicion of CBRN incident*)
- More than three unrelated patients: showing same signs and symptoms in the absence of any other explanation indicates the presence of an external agent (*CBRN incident*).

In the event of a terrorist chemical incident, there is a clear risk of a secondary device or exposure designed specifically to affect or injure members of the emergency services.

Clinicians likely to be involved in CBRN incidents should be familiar with local policy and be aware of relevant major incident practices including, where appropriate, the use of PPE.

Chemical incidents

A chemical incident may be defined as: *'an event leading to acute exposure of one or more individuals to a non radioactive substance resulting in illness or a potentially toxic threat to health'*. Occasionally, illness may be related to chronic chemical exposure, for example, carbon monoxide in a room with ineffective ventilation.

The management of a chemical incident can be divided into two components:

- Organizational
  - Personal safety
  - Protective clothing
  - Decontamination.
- Clinical
  - Substance identification
  - Decontamination
  - Triage
  - Immediate treatment.

Scene safety

Scene safety is of paramount importance during a chemical incident. It is essential to ensure that it is safe to approach an incident where secondary contamination of responders and emergency personnel is a significant risk. The overall control at the scene is the responsibility of the police. The fire service are responsible for containing any hazard and making the scene safe. Therefore, only when permission has been given should medical personnel approach the scene. A rendezvous point (RVP) will often be used.

The scene is divided into a hot zone, where normally only the fire service will be present; a warm zone, where basic assessment and decontamination may take place involving the fire service and trained health service personnel wearing PPE; and the cold zone, which represents an area where it is no longer necessary to wear special PPE and where more detailed patient assessment and triage can take place. The hot zone is separated from the warm zone by the inner police cordon. The police outer cordon defines the external boundary of the cold zone.

Information gathering

At the scene of a chemical incident it is essential to identify and gain information about the chemical involved including its toxicity and any necessary immediate counter measures. At industrial installations, statutory regulations should ensure that, in the event of a spillage, all aspects of scene management are part of a pre-planned emergency procedure.

In the event of a road transport accident involving chemical vehicles, information regarding the nature of the chemical and its handling should be available from the statutory information plate displayed on the container. For railway incidents, this information may not always be immediately available.

Advisory systems include the HAZCHEM Action Code System, the Kemler Plate, and Transport Emergency (TREM) Cards.

The HAZCHEM warning plate

This is a series of code numbers and letters displayed on a vehicle carrying hazardous substances which provides information about personal protection and the fire fighting methods necessary in the event of a chemical spillage. In addition, it advises whether or not the chemicals can be washed into the normal drainage systems or whether they should be contained. Within a diamond warning sign, the United Nations number for the chemical carried is displayed as well as a contact telephone number of the manufacturer.

The Kemler Plate

The Kemler/ADR system is the European road transport equivalent for hazardous road markings. The plate is in two parts, the upper displays the Kemler code for the substance carried and the lower, the United Nations substance number. The upper numbers contain essential information in relation to the properties of the load. The first digit represents the primary hazard and subsequent two digits, the secondary hazards. If the same number is repeated, this represents an intensified hazard and, for substances which should not be brought into contact with water, the numbers are preceded by the letter 'x'.

The Transport Emergency (TREM) Cards

These are A4 size cards kept in the cab of vehicles carrying dangerous chemicals. Each card provides details of the load, protective clothing requirements, and the action necessary in the event of spillage or a fire. It also contains some information related to first aid for contaminated victims.

Chemdata

All fire service vehicles in the United Kingdom have access to a CHEMDATA system via a computer. This provides accurate information at the scene of an incident including details of PPE and further action in the event of a fire or spillage.

Chemical incidents may be complex events and require multiagency support (for example, the Meteorological Office to give advice on wind direction in the event of a gas leak or the Environment Agency for advice regarding water contamination). The Health Protection Agency (*www.hpa.org.uk*) is available 24hrs a day for support and advice on such issues as:

- PPE
- Decontamination and evacuation
- Toxicological and epidemiological impact on public health
- Antidotes and medical treatment
- Public health impact of industrial sites
- Health effects from chemicals in the environment.

(a)

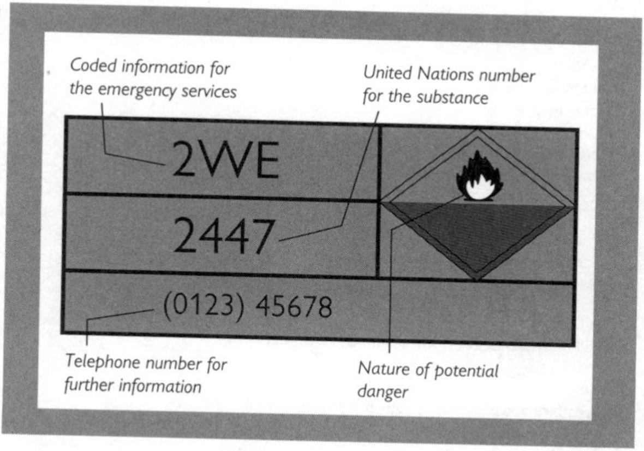

(b) **Hazchem Scale**

FOR FIRE OR SPILLAGE

Hazchem	
UN No	

Issue No 1

1 JETS

2 FOG

3 FOAM

4 DRY AGENT

P	V	FULL	DILUTE
R		FULL	DILUTE
S	V	BA	DILUTE
S (white on black)	V	BA for FIRE only	DILUTE
T		BA	DILUTE
T (white on black)		BA for FIRE only	DILUTE
W	V	FULL	CONTAIN
X		FULL	CONTAIN
Y	V	BA	CONTAIN
Y (white on black)	V	BA for FIRE only	CONTAIN
Z		BA	CONTAIN
Z (white on black)		BA for FIRE only	CONTAIN
E	CONSIDER EVACUATION		

Fig. 11.1 The HAZCHEM Action Code System: (a) the HAZCHEM hazard warning plate; (b) the HAZCHEM code system aide memoire card (front); (c) back.

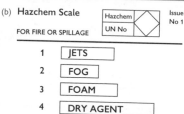

(c) **Notes for Guidance**

FOG
In the absence of fog equipment a fine spray may be used.

DRY AGENT
Water must not be allowed to come into contact with the substance at risk.

V
Can be violently or even explosively reactive.

FULL
Full body protective clothing with BA.

BA
Breathing apparatus plus protective gloves.

DILUTE
May be washed to drain with large quantities of water.

CONTAIN
Prevent, by any means available, spillage from entering drains or water course.

Fig. 11.1 *Contd.*

In particular, advice is available to the medical profession on the best way to manage patients who have been exposed to poisons. This is given through the National Poisons Information Services (NPIS) which are based in Oxfordshire, Birmingham, Cardiff, Newcastle, and London.

Clinical management

Key management tasks in relation to the medical support provided at an incident:

- Establish details of the exact location, type of incident, and hazards (preferably before approaching the incident).
- Approach from upwind and from a safe distance.
- Remain at a rendezvous point (if given) and advance to the scene only when instructed that it is safe to do so.
- Report to the ambulance incident command centre (if already set up) on arrival or the individual acting as the ambulance commander.
- Only wear PPE if you have been trained to do so.
- Establish the casualty clearing station at a safe distance upwind and uphill from the incident.
- Be mindful of the risk of the spread of contamination throughout all the stages of casualty contact.

- Be aware that the risks are dynamic (for example, that the wind may change); it is essential to be in contact with the ambulance incident officer to minimize risk.
- Do not allow clinical care to take place in the hot zone.
- Establish resuscitation based on triage assessment where necessary during decontamination in the warm zone.
- Consider the possibility of secondary trauma as well as chemical contamination.

DO NOT approach an incident unless you are SURE it is safe to do so.

Triage

There are three main categories of clinically contaminated patients:
- *P1*—resuscitation required during decontamination in a stretcher facility.
- *P2*—treatment may be delayed until after decontamination in a stretcher facility.
- *P3*—minor injuries; patients may walk unaided to a decontamination facility.

Following decontamination, normal triage priorities can be used (see p.602).

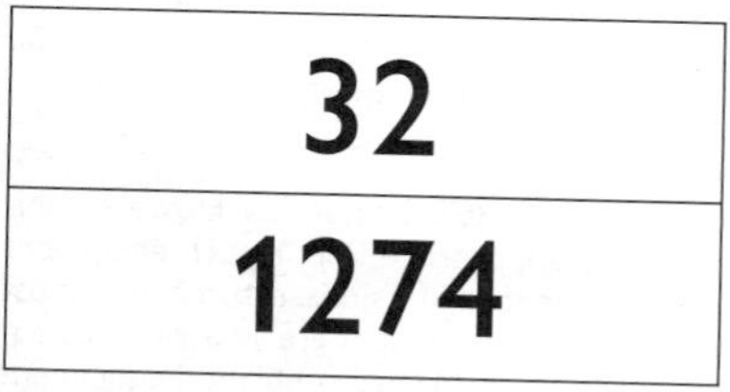

Fig. 11.2 The Kemler hazard warning plate.

Decontamination

Decontamination should ideally take place as near to the source of the chemical exposure as possible, providing that the patient and the scene are safe. At the scene of an incident, decontamination will take place in the warm zone by personnel familiar with the appropriate PPE. It is essential that they have been trained and have experience of working within this environment. Decontamination of casualties is now officially an ambulance service responsibility, although both the fire service and ambulance service are likely to be involved in any significant incident.

Patients may present to emergency departments, risking the spread of contamination. For this reason, selected emergency department personnel are trained in decontamination techniques.

A&E departments must always be warned of the impending arrival of contaminated or potentially contaminated patients.

On arrival at hospital with contaminated patients, instructions from A&E staff MUST be followed. DO NOT enter the department until instructed to do so.

Decontamination is achieved by removing decontaminated clothing and washing the patient thoroughly with water. Under certain circumstances detergent is added. Clothing should be bagged securely for disposal or retained if necessary for forensic purposes. If indicated, emergency life-saving procedures may be undertaken before or during decontamination in the warm zone. Hypothermia is a significant risk from the decontamination process. Appropriate clothing is provided post decontamination.

Resuscitation

Resuscitation should follow the normal ABCDE priorities. However, this may need to be undertaken wearing appropriate PPE. If such equipment is not available, or staff are not experienced in its use, resuscitation must not be attempted. It must be remembered that there is a risk of contamination via the skin or mucosal surfaces. Manual ventilation equipment should be fitted with absorbent canisters if they are to be used in a toxic environment. Should it be necessary to use a defibrillator, both the patient's chest and the emergency responder should be as dry as possible to avoid electrical injury. Expert advice should be sought prior to delivering defibrillation in an explosive or combustible environment.

In the event of a toxicological emergency either contact the National Poisons Advisory Service on 0870 600 6266 or use TOXBASE on *www.hpa.org.uk/chemicals/toxbase.htm*

Note:
Prior registration is necessary before toxbase can be used.

Treatment

It is essential to move the patient as soon as possible from any ongoing exposure to the chemical or toxin. Removal of contaminated clothing constitutes 70% of the decontamination process. Attention to any abnormalities found in the primary survey, the correction of hypoglycaemia if present, and the management of any associated medical conditions constitute the basis for treatment. From the point of view of the chemical exposure, treatment is usually supportive, initially. Intervention (based on expert advice from the HPA or the NPIS) using drugs or specific chemical antidotes may be possible from dedicated pods which will be transported to the scene by the ambulance service.

Transfer

It is important to ensure that vehicles transporting casualties to hospital do not enter a contaminated area. In addition, those vehicles transferring patients who have been contaminated will require equipment and vehicular decontamination afterwards. It is essential to avoid secondary contamination.

Documentation

Contemporary documentation is desirable, though difficult at a chemical incident because of the use of PPE. When and where possible, documentation must be undertaken but should not risk secondary contamination. The first opportunity for formal documentation may be when the patient has been decontaminated and reaches the cold zone.

Debrief

In common with all major incidents, there should be a 'hot debrief' when the incident ends which should identify problems for future consideration as well as allaying concerns with regard to the risks to health care workers.

A planned emergency services/interagency debriefing will permit more attention to detail and allow established plans to be modified.

Individual chemicals

Carbon monoxide—see p.421
Chlorine—see p.423
CS gas and related agents—see p.425
Cyanide—see p.426
Organophosphate insecticides—see p.442
Paraquat—see p.444

Biological incidents

A biological agent (BA) is a micro-organism or a toxin derived from it which causes disease in man. The toxin may be derived from living plants, animals, or micro-organisms. Some toxins are produced or altered by chemical means. Toxins are unable to reproduce themselves and are normally of a simpler biochemical composition than a biological agent.

Historically, biological incidents may be natural or intentional. Intentionally, biological agents have been used in warfare, including World War Two, during the Iran/Iraq conflict, and, more recently, the postal delivery of anthrax spores in the United States in 2001.

Features of biological weapons

- Have the potential to effect large numbers of people
- Have the potential for widespread geographical exposure
- Often have a simple means of distribution
- Are initially untraceable
- Are difficult to detect and difficult to effectively protect against.

Characteristics of biological agents

Pathogenicity

This is the capability of the biological agent to cause disease.

Infectivity

This is the amount of agent required to cause disease.

Pathogens with high infectivity produce disease with a smaller number of organisms compared to those of low infectivity which require larger numbers. Infectivity does not determine the speed of onset or the severity of the illness.

Virulence

This reflects the relative severity of diseases produced by biological agents which can vary between different organisms and strains of the same organism.

Toxicity

Toxicity reflects the relative severity of the illness produced by the toxin. It is dose dependant.

Incubation period

Providing there are sufficient number of micro-organisms to initiate infection, the infectious agent then multiplies to produce disease. The time between exposure and the appearance of symptoms is the incubation period.

In the case of toxins, sufficient quantities must penetrate the body to produce intoxication. The time between exposure and clinical features is known as the *latent period*.

Biological threats

Bacteria	Viruses	Toxins
***Class A agents** (most dangerous due to easy dissemination, high mortality)*		
Bacteria	**Viruses**	**Toxins**
Smallpox	Ebola*	Botulinum
Anthrax	Marburg*	Some mycotoxins
Plague	Arena viruses	
Botulism	Lassa fever	
Tularaemia	Junin and related viruses*	
	Dengue	
***Class B agents** (moderate ease of dissemination, moderate mortality and morbidity)*		
Bacteria	**Viruses**	**Toxins**
Q fever	Venezuelan EE**	Ricin
Brucellosis	Eastern EE**	Epsilon toxin§
Glanders, melioidosis	Western EE**	*Staph. Enterotoxin B*
Salmonella (WC)	Other alphaviruses	
Shigella dysenteria (WC)		
E.coli O157:H7 (WC)		
Cryptosporidium parvum (WC)		
***Class C agents** (low to moderate threat)*		
Multidrug resistant TB		
Nipah virus		
Hantaviruses		
Tickborne haemorrhagic fever encephalitis viruses		
Yellow fever		

*Haemorrhagic fever viruses
**Equine encephalitis
§From *C. perfringens*
WC=potential water contamination agents

Transmissibility

Transmissibility is the potential for a BA to be transmitted from one person to another directly or through a vector. Those agents transmitted easily from one person to another constitute a major concern.

Lethality

The lethality or fatality rate is an expression of the number of deaths in relation to the number of casualties.

Stability

The stability of a BA depends on many factors including temperature, humidity, and exposure to sunlight.

Infectious dose

This is the dose of an organism needed to infect a person. Due to individual variation, this is expressed as the median dose given—the dose needed to infect 50% of those exposed.

Lethal dose

This is the dose of a BA needed to cause death.

Classification

An understanding of the characteristics of a BA is essential for identification, prophylaxis, and treatment. BAs used as weapons can be grouped into:

- Bacteria
- Viruses
- Toxins.

(See box on p.633.)

Dissemination

Dissemination describes the process of dispersal of BAs or toxins. They are most commonly dispersed covertly and by aerosol. Routes of entry are similar to naturally occurring diseases, including percutaneous, inhalation, and ingestion (contamination of food and water).

Recognition

It is quite likely that a biological warfare attack will be covert and late at night or in the early morning to avoid inactivation of an aerosol driven BA by ultraviolet light. Activation within a closed space may have a more profound and obvious effect. It may be difficult to differentiate illness produced by a BA from an endemic disease. Diseases occurring outside their normal geographical location may be more easily identified as suspicious. Alerting features include:

- Large numbers of casualties occurring over a short period of time
- Signs of illness or death in the animal population.

Casualty management

Patients may be a victim of the BA or a traumatic injury. Attempts should be made to minimize cross-contamination without compromising effective clinical care.

ABC management of life-threatening injuries should take priority over decontamination if possible. Clinical care should be delivered by practitioners wearing appropriate PPE.

Treatment should include general supportive measures: maintenance of adequate respiration, intravenous access, and analgesia, as well as the management of any co-existing injuries and pre-morbid conditions. Antibiotic therapy, antiviral therapy, and antitoxin therapy should be given as appropriate. Attempts should be made to separate contaminated victims from non-affected patients.

Medical personnel should be familiar with the local response plan for handling biological emergencies.

All suspected biological agent cases should be evacuated to a specialist centre wherever possible.

Anthrax

Causative organism

Bacillus anthracis

Incubation period

1 to 6 days; may be longer

Symptoms

- Fever, non-productive cough, malaise, fatigue, chest discomfort, sore throat
- May be followed by a brief period of improvement
- Followed by sudden deterioration with severe respiratory distress, sweating, stridor, cyanosis, and shock
- Death 24 to 36 hours after onset of severe symptoms.

Signs

- Pleural effusion, chest wall oedema, meningitis (inhalational anthrax)
- Papule lesion, becoming vesicular with a black scab (eschar); local and systemic infection (cutaneous anthrax)
- Tonsillar ulceration (oropharyngeal anthrax).

Immediate management

- Wear appropriate standard PPE (if there is a risk of anthrax spore contamination, breathing apparatus will be required)
- Decontaminate patient with copious soap and water
- Triple bag and seal patient's clothing
- Transfer urgently to hospital—warn them in advance; DO NOT enter the hospital until advised to do so
- Ensure appropriate decontamination (hypochlorite is appropriate)
- If confident about diagnosis or clinically concerned, give intravenous benzyl penicillin
- Seek advice.

Note

Inhalational anthrax is not infectious; skin lesions and spore-contaminated clothing are.

Nuclear and radiological incidents

Nuclear incidents (i.e. detonations or releases of radioactive material) are, fortunately, much rarer than radiation incidents (release of ionizing radiation).

Radioactive materials occur widely—for example, in industry, medicine, and waste from the nuclear power industry. Associated with these activities is the frequent movement of radioactive materials on road and rail systems.

The Health Protection Agency provides advice and support in the event of a radiation incident through the National Radiological Protection Board (NRPB) who in turn advise both the government and the local emergency centres involved with the incident. This involves specifying and providing guidance on emergency reference levels (ERLs) including ERLs requiring urgent evacuation, shelter, and administration of stable iodine as well as advice on the control of food and drinking water. In addition, the NRPB provides information on recovery methods post incident.

Where the potential for an incident exists, there are statutory obligations to ensure suitable contingency plans to protect workers and the public. In the event of an unforeseen incident, the NAIR arrangements can be implemented. NAIR may provide assistance to local emergency plans and are activated by the police when they feel that there is a need for radiological assistance. Other emergency services, (for example, the fire service, British Transport Police, and the airport and docks police) may also initiate NAIR assistance.

> The NRPB co-ordinates the NAIR arrangements.

Monitoring

NAIR provides prompt assistance to the police and emergency services where no radiation expert is available. Assistance is provided in two stages.

- Stage 1: a radiation expert, with the aid of simple monitoring equipment, can determine whether a hazard exists and can advise the police accordingly. If required, the police can obtain stage 2 assistance.
- Stage 2: comprises more sophisticated resources and a team, usually provided by a major nuclear establishment and consisting of up to four persons who can respond urgently with monitoring, decontamination equipment, and special clothing.

In addition, the NRPB will collate and interpret data from other agencies involved.

Action to be taken in the event of an apparent radioactivity emergency:

- Police will determine whether a pre-existing plan exists. In the event of there being no plan, NAIR assistance will be obtained.
- Stage 1 respondent will determine whether a stage 2 response is required immediately.
- A major spillage will require a stage 2 response immediately.

- NAIR will contact the nearest NAIR respondent who in turn will contact the person dealing with the incident directly.
- NAIR respondent will provide technical advice and assistance to manage the incident.
- NAIR respondent will liaise with the relevant environmental agency to assist.

Press

The NRPB will provide effective communication for the media to ensure consistent advice and information. All of these activities are co-ordinated at its Chilton Emergency Centre.

Types of radiation

For the purpose of this chapter, radiation means ionizing radiation – the form of electromagnetic radiation that produces charged particles (ions) in material with which it interacts. In human cells this may cause short- and long-term damage. Substances which give off radiation are said to be radioactive. This definition excludes microwaves, ultraviolet, infrared radiation, and radio waves. Most day-to-day incidents involve low-dose exposure which constitutes a very small risk to attending medical personnel.

The types of radiation relevant to pre-hospital care are:

Alpha radiation

Small positively charged particles which:
- Travel a short distance in air
- Are easily stopped by paper, clothing, or a dressing
- Can penetrate superficial layers of the skin without causing any harm
- Can be detrimental on inhalation or ingestion.

Examples of alpha emitters are uranium, radon, and plutonium.

Beta radiation

Small negatively charged particles which:
- Travel a few centimetres in air
- Are stopped by heavier clothing and aluminium
- Can damage the skin, producing radiation burns
- Produce most damage when in direct contact with the skin.

Examples of beta emitters include iodine and tritium.

Gamma radiation, X-rays, and neutrons

- All travel great distances
- Produce damage some distance from the source
- Pass through the body causing damage or energy disposition.

Examples of these emitters include caesium and cobalt.

Risk of exposure

Exposure to ionized radiation may effect a part of the body, (for example, producing radiation burns to the skin) or the whole body (producing systemic effects—radiation syndrome). Most commonly, the exposure is going to be of a low dose and the patient is likely to be asymptomatic. If symptoms are present, the implication is of a more significant exposure. Emergency services personnel are at risk due to the spread of low-dose particles as a result of contamination in dust, aerosols, or liquid. The greater risk, therefore, is from gamma rays, X-rays, and neutrons which travel greater distances.

Simple measures will reduce the risk to emergency personnel. Rescue personnel should consider three scenarios which pose a risk:

- Exposure to gamma rays or X-rays from a source near to the patient
- Transfer of contamination from the patient's skin, hair, and clothes
- The inhalation or ingestion of contamination during patient contact.

Type of accident

- Over-exposure to penetrating radiation—this may follow over-exposure to X-rays or gamma rays (for example, incidents involving industrial radiographic sources). These patients are not radioactive and pose no threat to the rescuer.
- External contamination – this may follow release of radioactive material. The patient and their clothes may be contaminated and may present a risk to the carer.
- Internal contamination – exposure due to ingestion, inhalation, or absorption (for example, a casualty exposed to a fire involving radioactive substances).
- Contaminated wounds – an open wound may become contaminated by radiation if there has been a radiation leak at the time of the injury.

Irradiated patients pose no threat to the rescuer

Dealing with a nuclear incident

To reduce the risk external penetrating radiation and of contamination it is important to:

- Assess the risk from all hazards
- Park the ambulance upwind from the accident site
- Undertake an ABC assessment and immediate treatment assuming contamination and taking appropriate precautions
- Keep the on-scene time to a minimum
- Move the patient 10 metres from the source, if there is a risk of continued radiation exposure.
- Consider establishing a 'shield' in cases of entrapment.

Protection

Simple precautions, similar to those used in the case of a chemical incident, will reduce the risk of contamination:

- Assume contamination is present if handling a patient at an incident involving radioactivity.

- Wear a simple face mask with eye protection, gloves, an appropriate disposable impregnable gown, and overshoes or washable boots to avoid contamination of the face and hands.
- Keep activities within the area of the incident to a minimum to reduce airborne contamination.
- Cover open wounds to prevent contamination and reduce the risk from contaminated blood.
- Remove the patient's external clothing and place in an appropriate sealable plastic bag. It is estimated that up to 90% of contamination will be removed with the patient's clothes.
- Wrap the patient in a blanket or contamination control envelope.
- Do not drink, eat, or smoke until checked for contamination.

Clinical assessment and management

It is likely, at an incident, that there will be no overt signs and symptoms resulting from over-exposure to penetrating radiation. In the event of explosions, other traumatic injuries are likely to be apparent.

Early symptoms of significant exposure include:

- Nausea and vomiting
- Erythema on exposed skin.

Features of life-threatening exposure may not be apparent for days or weeks. From the patient's perspective, providing the carer is wearing appropriate PPE, attention should be given to life-threatening emergencies, following the ABCD priorities, prior to patient decontamination.

The doctor should be familiar with the ambulance service policy for handling a radiological/radioactive emergency and should comply with agreed policy and protocols.

Clinical assessment and management

Chapter 12

Emergency obstetrics and gynaecology

Anatomy and physiology of pregnancy

An understanding of the anatomical and physiological changes are essential to the correct management of the pregnant patient and of labour.

Airway

Anatomical and physiological changes affecting the airway and its management include:

- Facial and neck swelling (increased fat deposition) leading to difficulty fitting a cervical collar
- Airway swelling due to oedema leading to difficulty with intubation
- Breast engorgement (may make intubation more difficult)
- Increased risk of gastro-oesophageal reflux
  - Altered gastro-oesophageal junction
  - Relaxation of upper oesophageal sphincter
  - Increased gastric acid secretion
  - Delayed gastric emptying.

  leading to a potential for airway compromise

In addition, pregnant patients can be expected to have a full dentition.

Breathing

Management of breathing during pregnancy is complicated by the following factors:

- Alteration in chest shape (lower ribs flare outwards and diaphragm rises)
- Splintage of the diaphragm and chest by the expanding uterus
- Change from predominantly diaphragmatic to a thoracic movement respiratory pattern
- Ventilation/perfusion mismatch
- Increased tidal volume (+20% at 12 weeks; +40% by 40 weeks)
- Increased minute volume (+50% at term) mainly due to increased tidal volume
- Relative hyperventilation.

It should be remembered that many women are mildly breathless in the later stages of prtegnancy.

Note: FEV_1 and PEFR are unchanged during pregnancy; vital capacity remains effectively unaltered.

Circulation

The circulatory changes during pregnancy include:

- Increased cardiac output (+40% by the end of the second trimester)—both stroke volume and heart rate increase
- Heart enlarges due to muscular hypertrophy, moves upwards and anteriorly, and rotates, resulting in large Q waves and T wave inversion in lead III. A left ventricular strain pattern with inverted T waves in $V_2$and V_3 occurs.
- 3rd heart sound and ejection systolic murmur may be heard
- Plasma volume increases by 50% (hormonally induced peripheral vasodilatation, increased vascular bed-fetus and placenta)
- Relative anaemia (red cell mass only increases by 20–30%)

- Slight reduction in systolic blood pressure; more marked reduction in diastolic pressure
- Vena caval compression by the gravid uterus reduces venous return by up to 40%
- signs of haemorrhage may only occur when 35% of blood volume has already been lost.

Management of vena caval compression

Vena caval compression in the supine position by the gravid uterus reduces venous return by up to 40%. Persisting caval compression may lead to hypotension, reduced cerebral perfusion, and inadequate perfusion of the uterus and placenta. In order to avoid this, the mother should be treated in a position which relieves caval compression. This can be achieved by:

- Holding the uterus to the left, by hand
- Placing a sandbag or pillow (or similar) under the right buttock
- Nursing the patient on a long spine board tilted approximately 30° to the left
- log rolling the patient to the left and then gently rolling them back to rest on the rescuers' knees (the human wedge, see Fig. 12.1).

The safest method, if there is any possibility of a spinal injury in a traumatized patient, is to use a long spine board.

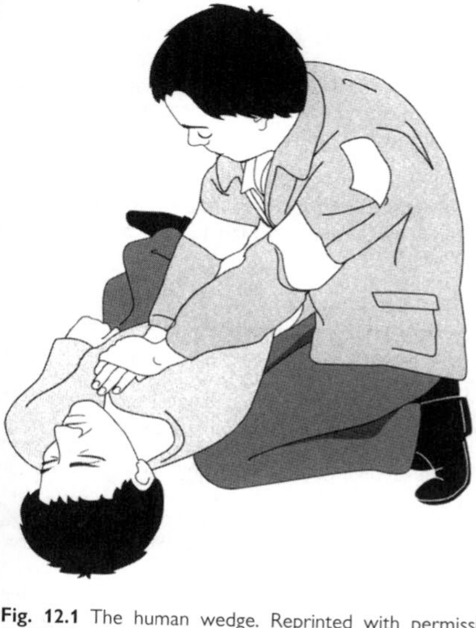

Fig. 12.1 The human wedge. Reprinted with permission from Greaves I *et al.* (2005). *Emergency care: a textbook for paramedics*, 2nd edn. W.B. Saunders Co. Ltd.

The pregnant patient

The approach to the management of the severely ill or injured pregnant patient is essentially the same as that to a non-injured patient, bearing in mind:

- That there are two patients to worry about—mother and fetus
- That maternal anatomy and physiology is different in pregnancy
- That most pre-hospital care practitioners have very little experience in this field.

It is all the more important, therefore, that a structured logical approach is used.

Taking a history

When the patient's condition and time constraints permit, in addition to the patient's history of presenting complaint and past medical history, the following additional features should be established by careful questioning:

- Last menstrual period (LMP)
- Normal period length and regularity
- Gestation in weeks
- Contraceptive usage (use of the IUCD is associated with an increased risk of ectopic pregnancy)
- Previous obstetric history including: miscarriage, premature onset of labour, pregnancy related complications, ectopic pregnancy, previous abdominal/pelvic surgery, assisted conception
- Previous pregnancy and birth history including number and type of deliveries
- Other gynaecological pathology such as fibroids, ovarian cysts, sexually transmitted infections.

The patient's maternity record card, if available, will provide additional important information such as blood pressure recordings and ultrasound scan results.

Examination

The obstetric examination should be limited to that which is necessary in order to carry out immediate treatment and plan further management. Features to note include:

- Assessment of fundal height—is the height 'right for dates'?
- *Inspection* of the perineum for blood loss.

There are three possible indications for pre-hospital vaginal examination:

- For removal of a retained tampon in toxic shock syndrome
- For removal of products of conception from the cervical canal in uterine haemorrhage
- Inspection of open or closed os in miscarriage.

In many cases, it will be more appropriate to wait unit arrival in hospital before an assessment of the os is carried out.

Effective auscultation of the foetal heart is usually difficult in the pre-hospital environment and rarely provides information of immediate benefit. It is usually best delayed until after arrival in hospital.

A full cardiorespiratory assessment is mandatory, but should not delay urgent transfer to hospital when this is indicated by the history or initial examination findings.

Shock in pregnancy

Clinically apparent shock in a pregnant patient is a life-threatening emergency. The pregnant patient may compensate for shock for some time due to an increased blood cell volume and red cell mass as well as restriction of blood flow to the placenta, with obvious consequences for the fetus. Once decompensation occurs, it is likely to be rapid and difficult or impossible to reverse.

General approach

The general approach to the pregnant patient is based on effective resuscitation using ABC principles (bearing in mind the anatomical and physiological changes in pregnancy) combined with rapid evacuation to hospital where appropriate.

Airway

- Ensure that the airway is patent and protected—remember the increased risk of aspiration.

Breathing

- Administer high-flow oxygen (15l/min by non-rebreathing bag) at the earliest opportunity.

Circulation

- Displace the fundus off the inferior vena cava (see above)
- Do not delay transfer to hospital whilst trying to obtain intravenous access.

Ectopic pregnancy

Ectopic pregnancy is defined as any pregnancy occurring outside the uterus. The vast majority are tubal although ovarian, abdominal, and cervical ectopic pregnancies may also occur. The incidence has been variously estimated to be between 1 in 100 and 1 in 400 pregnancies.

Risk factors

- None in 50% of cases
- Previous ectopic pregnancy
- Previous abdominal or pelvic surgery
- Pelvic inflammatory disease; endometriosis
- Assisted conception.

Presenting features

- May be absent
- Amenorrhoea usually between 5 and 10 weeks, but not always present
- Lower abdominal pain
- Vaginal bleeding
- Peritonism and shoulder tip pain (minority of cases only)
- Shock and collapse.

Immediate management

The key to the successful management of ectopic pregnancy is to suspect the diagnosis.

- Ensure a patent airway (effective suction must be available in case of vomiting)
- Administer high-flow oxygen (15l/min via a non-rebreathing mask)
- Transfer urgently to hospital; warn A&E department
- Gain intravenous access and commence resuscitation (if required)—DO NOT delay transfer
- Maintain a systolic BP of 90mmHg (presence of a radial pulse)
- Monitor pulse, BP, respiratory rate, ECG, and pulse oximetry
- Administer analgesia.

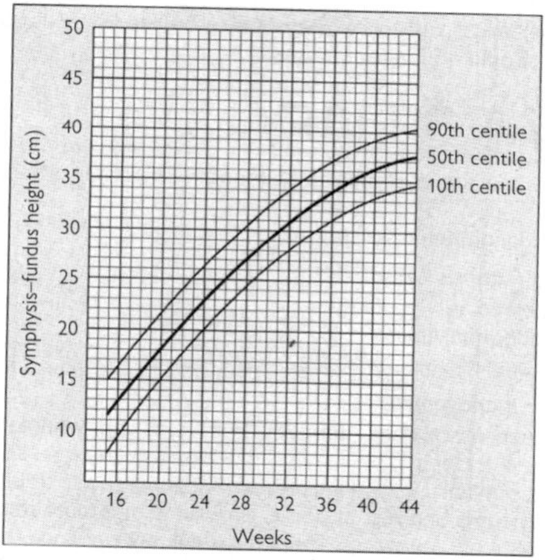

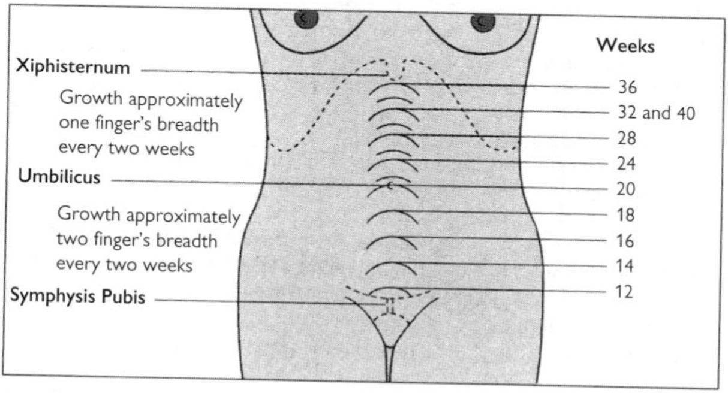

Fig. 12.2 Fundal height and gestation. Reprinted with permission from Greaves I *et al.* (2005). *Emergency care: a textbook for paramedics*, 2nd edn. W.B. Saunders Co. Ltd.

Miscarriage

Miscarriage is loss of a pregnancy before 24 weeks' gestation. The term 'abortion' should no longer be used.

Risk factors

- Smoking
- Alcohol
- Diabetes mellitus, systemic and connective tissue disorders
- Fibroids
- Cervical incompetence.

Presenting features

- Vaginal bleeding
- Lower abdominal pain
- 'Tissue' passed per vaginam.

Immediate management

In threatened miscarriage, the cervical os is closed, whereas in inevitable miscarriage it is open.

- If the os remains closed (*threatened miscarriage*), the traditional management is bed rest at home, avoidance of intercourse, and appropriate GP follow-up. There is little if any evidence that bed rest or avoiding sex effects the outcome of the pregnancy.
- In *incomplete miscarriage*, there is no possibility of successful continuation of the placenta. Persistence of products of conception within the cervical canal may be associated with continuing haemorrhage.
    - Assess ABC, administer high-flow oxygen, gain iv access
    - Administer fluids to maintain a systolic BP of 90mmHg (presence of a radial pulse)
    - Document vital signs
    - Transfer immediately to hospital; warn obstetric team of arrival
    - If there is continuing bleeding, remove retained products from the cervical canal followed by administration of syntocinon
    - Maintain patient nil by mouth
- In *complete miscarriage*, no immediate action is necessary, although appropriate support and counselling will be required.
- If there is significant haemorrhage, immediate transfer to hospital is appropriate. Transfer should not be delayed whilst a line is inserted. This can be done in transit if necessary. Give syntocinon 10 units.

Septic abortion

This condition is fortunately much rarer than when 'back street' abortions were more common. The patient is usually systemically unwell with fever, rigors, sweating, nausea, and headache. There is an offensive vaginal discharge and abdominal tenderness. Shock may occur. The patient must be transferred immediately to hospital. Intravenous access can be obtained in transit or whilst waiting for an ambulance. Intravenous fluids can be administered to maintain a palpable radial pulse or systolic BP of 90mmHg. Scrupulous attention to ABC and administration of high-flow oxygen is essential.

The following patients may require anti-D prophylaxis, depending on their rhesus status:

- Spontaneous miscarriage
- Threatened miscarriage
- Abdominal trauma.

Toxic shock syndrome

An aggressive staphylococcal infection caused by organisms introduced into the vagina on a tampon. It most commonly occurs on the 2nd to 4th day of menstruation. The condition is fortunately rare.

Presenting features

- Fever
- Circulatory collapse
- Diarrhoea
- Macular rash
- Purulent vaginal discharge.

Immediate management

- Immediate transfer to hospital
- Oxygen 15l/min via non-rebreathing mask
- Commence resuscitation as appropriate—DO NOT delay transfer.

Remove tampon if possible

Antepartum haemorrhage

Whatever the cause of antepartum haemorrhage (placenta praevia and placental abruption are the most common), the possibility of massive blood loss cannot be excluded. In all cases, therefore, the patient should be transferred to hospital for assessment. In cases of obvious severe bleeding, transfer urgently to A&E; in apparently minor bleeding, transfer to the local obstetric unit is usually appropriate. By definition, antepartum haemorrhage occurs after 24 weeks' gestation.

Placenta praevia

Placenta praevia occurs when the placenta implants wholly or partly across the cervical os (see Fig. 12.3). With the advent of routine ultrasound scanning, most cases are identified before symptoms occur. Incidence increases with maternal age and a history of previous caesarian sections.

Presenting features

- Painless bright red vaginal bleeding after 24 weeks' gestation—may vary from spotting to life-threatening haemorrhage
- Uterus usually relaxed and non-tender
- Usually painless unless labour has begun.

Immediate management

- Urgent transfer to hospital
- Maintain a patent protected airway
- Administer high-flow oxygen 15l/min via non-rebreathing mask
- Commence resuscitation but do not delay transfer; administer fluids to maintain a systolic BP of 90mmHg (presence of a palpable radial pulse)
- Transport the patient in the left lateral position
- Do not perform a vaginal examination as it may precipitate torrential bleeding
- Maintain nil by mouth.

Vaginal examination is ABSOLUTELY CONTRAINDICATED

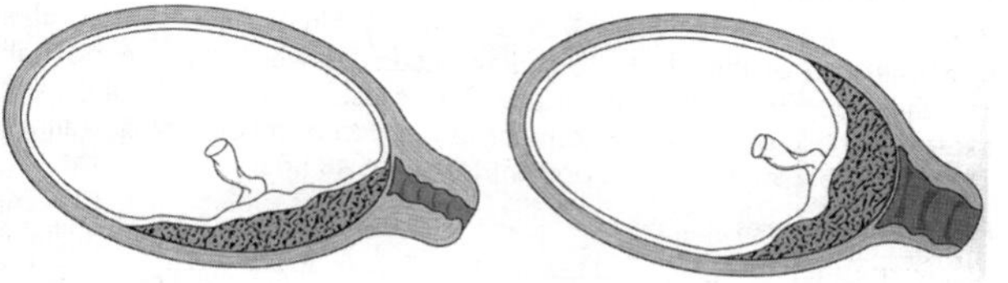

Fig. 12.3 Placenta praevia. Reprinted with permission from Greaves I *et al.* (2005). *Emergency care: a textbook for paramedics*, 2nd edn. W.B. Saunders Co. Ltd.

Placental abruption

Placental abruption occurs when a normally sited placenta separates from the wall of the uterus. Bleeding occurs between the uterine wall and the separated placental surface. The cause is not usually apparent except in those patients in whom abruption occurs secondary to trauma. Traumatic abruption may not present for up to 48 hours after trauma.

Presenting features

- Lower abdominal pain
- Vaginal haemorrhage—may be concealed or revealed (see Fig. 12.4)
- Uterine tender and hard
- Maternal shock (may be disproportionate to observed blood loss)
- Premature labour
- Reduced or absent foetal movements (ask the mother) or heart sounds
- Increased fundal height (compared to dates).

Immediate management

- Vaginal examination is contraindicated although inspection may aid the diagnosis by demonstrating bleeding
- The fundal height should be marked on the abdominal wall
- Transfer urgently to hospital
- Administer high-flow oxygen 15l/min via a non-rebreathing mask
- Gain intravenous access and resuscitate as necessary but DO NOT delay transfer
- Maintain nil by mouth.

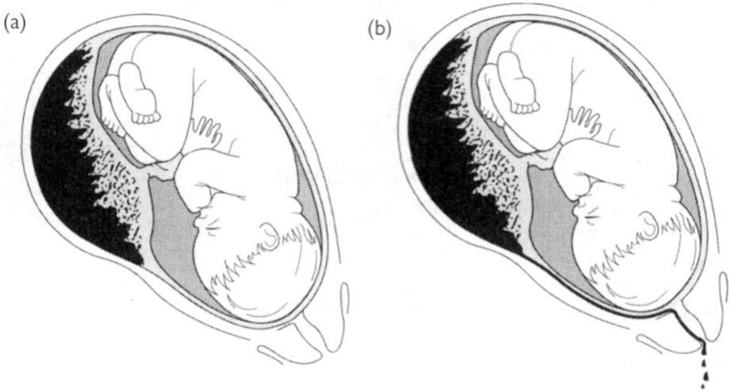

Fig. 12.4 Placental abruption: (a) concealed (b) revealed. Reprinted with permission from Greaves I *et al.* (2005). *Emergency care: a textbook for paramedics*, 2nd edn. W.B. Saunders Co. Ltd.

Hypertensive disorders: eclampsia and pre-eclampsia

Risk factors

- Primagravida
- Age <20 or >35
- Previous history of eclampsia, migraine, Reynaud's disease, hypertension, or renal disease
- Positive family history
- Multiple pregnancy.

Presenting features: pre-eclampsia

- Over 20 weeks' gestation
- Diastolic BP 100 or rapidly rising, BP >140/90 or +30/+15 from booking
- Proteinuria
- Excessive/sudden weight gain
- Upper abdominal pain
- Headache
- Visual disturbance
- Hyperreflexia, clonus.

Eclampsia is the development of fits following a prodromal period of the above symptoms.

Immediate management

Pre-eclampsia

Always recheck an elevated blood pressure

- If BP moderately elevated but otherwise asymptomatic, arrange for further check by GP (or consider hospital referral if no other means of monitoring)
- If symptoms are present, refer to hospital irrespective of degree of hypertension
- If diastolic BP >100mmHg or has risen by >20mmHg, or systolic by >30mmHg since booking, transfer to hospital for assessment.

Eclampsia

- Manage in left lateral position
- Establish and maintain a patent airway, administer high-flow oxygen 15l/min via a non-rebreathing mask
- To control the fitting:
  - Give magnesium 4g intravenous over 10–15 minutes OR
  - Diazemuls 5–10mg intravenous, with further smaller aliquots as required
- Transfer urgently to hospital with minimum stimulation
- Support respiration if necessary.

Other problems during pregnancy

Appendicitis

Occurs in 1 in 1000 pregnancies. Accurate diagnosis of appendicitis is more difficult in pregnancy since the location of the appendix may change. The perforation rate and mortality are both, therefore, significantly higher. In addition, nausea, vomiting, and anorexia may be dismissed as symptoms of pregnancy. Any suspicion of this diagnosis mandates urgent hospital assessment.

Asthma

Asthma often, but by no means invariably, improves during pregnancy. Conventional treatment protocols should be followed.

Fibroids

Fibroids increase in size in pregnancy and torsion or red degeneration may occur. These present (usually after 20 weeks) with abdominal pain and tenderness, vomiting (not always present), and fever. Treatment is with rest and analgesia and symptoms usually settle within seven days. In view of the potential for confusion with an acute abdomen, referral for assessment is appropriate.

DVT and pulmonary embolism

Both these conditions are more common in pregnancy and a high index of suspicion should be maintained. Presenting features include shortness of breath, haemoptysis, pleuritic chest pain, cyanosis, tachycardia, and collapse. Resuscitation should be commenced with urgent transfer to hospital which should not be delayed.

Pyelonephritis

Pyelonephritis is common in the second trimester and presents with fever, vomiting, and loin pain. In severe cases, admission may be necessary.

Preterm labour

Preterm labour is defined as labour before 37 weeks' gestation. Possible features include:

- Reduced or absent contraction pain
- More rapid progression to delivery
- Increased risk of malpresentation
- Early rupture of membranes
- Risk of cord prolapse.

Imminent labour should be managed in situ (with assistance from a midwife if possible, in time). Management is as for normal full term delivery. If delivery is not imminent, transfer to an obstetric unit is appropriate.

Once the baby is born, the priority is to prevent heat loss by wrapping. Immediate transfer is appropriate. A baby which is significantly smaller than would be expected by dates should raise the possibility of twins.

Trauma in pregnancy

A knowledge of the anatomical and physiological changes in pregnancy is essential for the optimal management of these patients. The most common lifethreatening conditions are traumatic placental abruption, uterine rupture, and pelvic fracture. These conditions are, fortunately, rare. However, ALL PREGNANT women should be reviewed in hospital after any significant trauma.

Patient management

Primary survey

The principles of the primary survey are exactly the same in the pregnant as the non-pregnant patient.

- A vaginal examination should NEVER be performed following trauma in pregnancy as it may precipitate torrential vaginal bleeding.
- In the second and third trimesters, the patient should be managed in the left lateral position.
- In the presence of significant trauma, fluids should be administered with less caution than in the non-pregnant patient.

Secondary survey

The secondary survey should be performed after arrival in hospital. An assessment of fundal height may be performed.

Traumatic placental abruption

Presenting features

- History of trauma
- Lower abdominal pain
- Vaginal haemorrhage — may be concealed or revealed (see Fig. 12.4)
- Uterine tenderness
- Maternal shock (may be disproportionate to observed blood loss)
- Premature labour
- Reduced or absent foetal movements (ask the mother)
- Increased fundal height (very difficult to assess pre-hospital).

The presence of a tense hard uterus with contractions and continuous pain suggests the presence of a major abruption and a very poor foetal outcome.

Placental abruption may follow minor as well as major trauma

Immediate management

- Follow ABCDE primary survey protocol as for any injured patient
- Manage the patient in the left lateral position
- Administer fluids to maintain a radial pulse but do not delay transfer
- Treat other *immediately life-threatening* injuries
- Transfer urgently to hospital
- Mark the fundal height on the abdominal wall.

Traumatic uterine rupture

Traumatic uterine rupture is, fortunately, very rare.

Presenting features

- More easily palpable fetus in a severely shocked mother
- Vaginal bleeding (not always present)
- Abdominal pain (not always present).

Immediate management

- Follow ABCDE primary survey protocol as for any injured patient
- Manage the patient in the left lateral position
- Administer fluids to maintain a radial pulse but do not delay transfer
- Treat other *immediately life-threatening* injuries
- Transfer urgently to hospital.

Blunt trauma

Engorgement of pelvic venous plexuses during pregnancy significantly increases the risk of catastrophic haemorrhage following blunt trauma. Urgent transfer to hospital of any patient who has suffered significant trauma is, therefore, essential. Conventional protocols should be followed with the patient in the left lateral position. Intravenous access should be started en route or at the scene, if this will not delay evacuation.

Penetrating trauma

The gravid uterus provides some degree of protection to the mother, at the expense of the fetus, in penetrating injury to the abdomen. Conventional management protocols should be followed.

Normal labour

First stage

What happens

- The cervix effaces and then dilates. Once the cervix is dilated to 10cm, the first stage is complete. After 3cm, dilatation usually occurs at approximately 1cm/hr in a primagravida and 2cm/hr in a multigravida.
- There is a 'show' of blood-stained mucus from the cervical canal.
- The amniotic sac bulges through the cervical os and ruptures.
- Contractions begin and increase in frequency from every 20 minutes to every 2 to 3 minutes.
- The foetal head descends into the pelvis.

Management

- Reassure and support mother; tell her that she is in labour
- Determine whether there is time to transfer to a delivery suite or call for expert assistance
- Gather and record information (see box)
- Check the patient's obstetric records
- If a home delivery was planned, a delivery kit may be available
- Ensure that the environment is warm.

If there is no time to transfer the patient

- Perform a vaginal examination
- Record the progress of labour (length and frequency of contractions is measured by abdominal palpation)
- Listen to the foetal heart before, during, and after a contraction (a toilet roll tube is effective as a stethoscope).

Passage of meconium (dark green, sticky material) during labour may be a sign of foetal distress and an indication for transfer to an obstetric unit:

- Administer oxygen to mother
- Turn mother on side
- Transfer.

History

- Expected date of delivery
- Place of booking
- Problems in this or previous pregnancies
- Time labour started.

Examination

- Maternal vital signs
- Fundal height
- Foetal vital signs
- Progress of labour.

(a)

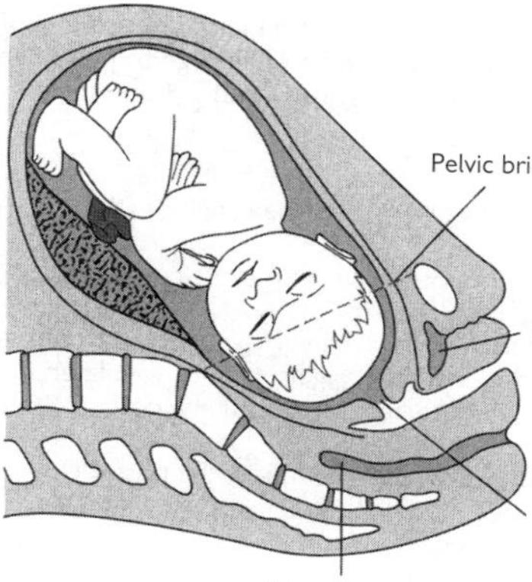

(b)

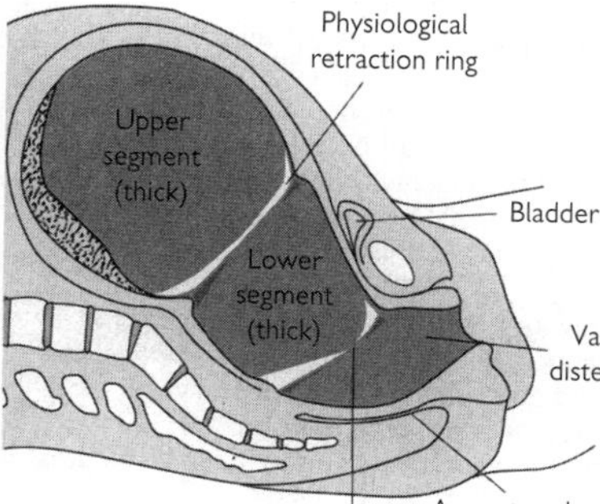

Fig. 12.5 The birth canal: (a) in the early part of the first stage of labour; (b) at the beginning of the second stage of labour. Reprinted with permission from Greaves I *et al.* (2005). *Emergency care: a textbook for paramedics,* 2nd edn. W.B. Saunders Co. Ltd.

Second stage of labour

The second stage of labour is from full dilatation until the delivery of the baby. It is usually marked by the development of an urge to push. Second stage usually lasts 1–3 hours in a primagravida and 1 hour or less in a multigravida.

What happens

- The perineum bulges, the anus dilates, and the baby's head appears at the vulva.
- The baby's head flexes, then rotates, so that the occiput is anterior and the face posterior (see Fig.12.6)
- The occiput delivers first, followed by the vertex, forehead, and face.
- When the head has emerged from the vagina, it turns to a lateral position to allow the shoulders to pass through the widest part of the outlet.
- The anterior shoulder will deliver spontaneously; the posterior shoulder follows.
- The rest of the baby is delivered.

Management

- The perineum may be protected with a pad, but this probably has little effect on the degree of perineal damage.
- The head should be supported once it has delivered.
- Once the head has delivered, the umbilical cord should be checked to ensure that it is not around the baby's neck. If it is, it should be slipped over the head or cut between two clamps.
- Gentle posterior flexion of the head will aid delivery of the anterior shoulder.
- Gentle anterior flexion of the head will aid delivery of the posterior shoulder.
- The baby should be delivered onto the mother's abdomen or onto the bed, dried, and wrapped. Suction of the baby's airway is only rarely needed and should not be carried out routinely. If it is necessary, a double trap device should be used.
- The umbilical cord is cut between two clamps after 2–3 minutes (if not already done).
- Bleeding from a tear is controlled by a sterile dressing and gentle pressure.

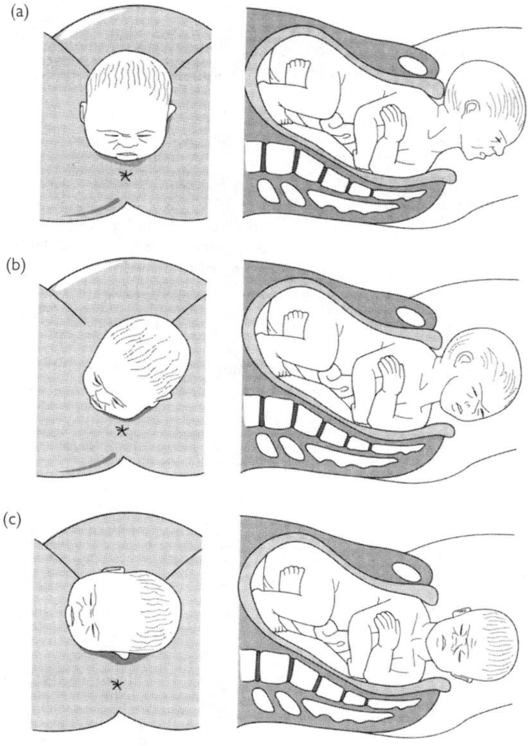

Fig. 12.6 Delivery of the head: (a) delivery; (b) restitution; (c) external rotation. Reprinted with permission from Greaves I *et al.* (2005). *Emergency care: a textbook for paramedics*, 2nd edn. W.B. Saunders Co. Ltd.

The Apgar score

The Apgar score (see Table 12.1) is recorded at 1 and 3 minutes. A score of 7 or above indicates a baby in good condition. If the score is 6 or below:

- Dry the baby with a warm towel
- Administer oxygen.

Provide bag-and-mask ventilation7

Third stage of labour

The third stage of labour is from the delivery of the head to the delivery of the placenta. The separation of the placenta is often indicated by a small rush of dark blood and a lengthening of the cord.

Management

- The placenta will usually deliver itself within 20 minutes. Cord traction is best avoided.
- Delivery of the placenta can be expedited by rubbing up a uterine contraction or by putting the baby to the breast.

Table 12.1 The Agpar score

Sign	**Points**		
	0	**1**	**2**
Colour	Pale	Blue	Pink
Pulse	0	<100	>100
Respiration	None	Irregular	Good
Tone	Limp	Some flexion	Active flexion
Reflex irritability	No response	Limited response	Cry/active movements

Retained placenta

The placenta delivers in 10 minute or less in over 95% of pregnancies. If it has not delivered within 30 minutes, it is unlikely to do so spontaneously.

- Remove the placenta if it is in the vagina
- If the uterus is well contracted, the placenta may be in the cervix and it will probably deliver once the cervix has relaxed
- Try rubbing up a uterine contraction
- Give syntocinon 10 units if not already given
- If no effect, transfer to an obstetric unit for further management.

Avoid excessive cord traction

Postpartum haemorrhage

In the event of a retained placenta and postpartum haemorrhage of more than 500ml:

- Rub up a uterine contraction by abdominal massage
- Put the baby to the breast
- Give syntocinon 10 units im
- Attempt to deliver placenta by controlled cord traction
- Establish access and commence an intravenous infusion
- Administer oxygen 15l/min via a non-rebreathing mask
- Transfer urgently to the nearest obstetric unit
- Obtain intravenous access but do not delay transfer to do so.

Abnormal labour

Prolapsed cord

If the umbilical cord is seen at the vulva, this should be managed as follows:

- Position the mother in the left lateral position and head down (takes pressure of the cord)
- Cover the cord with a large, damp, warm swab
- Transfer to hospital immediately.

DO NOT handle the umbilical cord

Shoulder dystocia

This occurs when the anterior shoulder impacts on the pubic symphysis after delivery of the head, preventing complete delivery of the baby. The following may be helpful:

- Request expert assistance.
- Flex the mother's legs up to her abdomen and try again.
- Roll mother onto her hands and knees and try delivering the posterior shoulder first.
- Deliver the posterior arm. Insert a hand into the vagina anterior to the baby. Ensure that the posterior elbow is flexed in front of the body and pull to deliver the forearm. The anterior shoulder will usually follow.
- Get an assistant to apply suprapubic pressure with the heeal of their hand. Rocking the hand may help.
- If this fails, ensure expert assistance by the quickest possible method. Transfer if necessary.

Malpresentations: breech (see Fig. 12.7)

In multiparous women, the delivery of a breech baby may occur without problems. Otherwise, the only appropriate course of action in non-specialist hands is immediate urgent transfer to the nearest obstetric unit.

Extended breech

This is the most common breech presentation. The buttocks, and often the scrotum and vulva are visible. Meconium may be seen.

Flexed breech

In addition to the above, the soles of the feet may be seen.

Footling breech

A foot or leg (or both feet or legs) emerge first. There is a significant risk of cord prolapse.

Management

- If labour is not well established, transfer urgently to hospital.
- Do not move to hospital if a presenting part is visible unless advised to do so.
- Obtain expert advice from an obstetrician and request midwifery assistance.

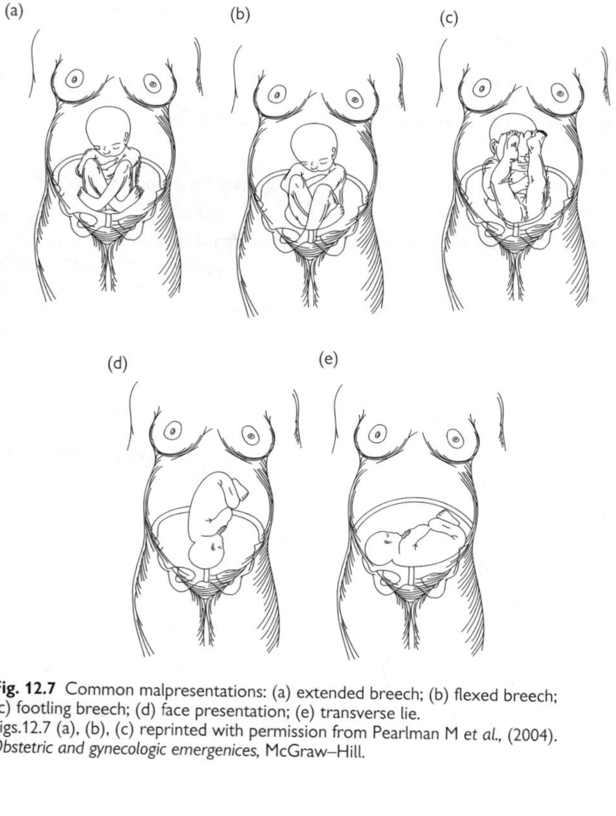

Fig. 12.7 Common malpresentations: (a) extended breech; (b) flexed breech; (c) footling breech; (d) face presentation; (e) transverse lie.
Figs.12.7 (a), (b), (c) reprinted with permission from Pearlman M *et al.*, (2004). *Obstetric and gynecologic emergenices,* McGraw–Hill.

- With the mother in the lithotomy position, once the nape of the neck is visible, lift the baby by the feet to help deliver the head. DO NOT pull. Encourage the mother to push.

If delivery fails to progress after the hips are delivered:

- Seek expert help.
- Confirm that assistance is on its way.
- Put patient on her back with her knees drawn as far upwards and outwards as possible.
- If the baby does not deliver within five contractions, obtain expert obstetric care as rapidly as possible. This may mean moving mother and child to hospital.

Other abnormal presentations/abnormal lie (see Fig. 12.7)

Some *face presentations* may deliver spontaneously, others will require Caesarian section. Brow presentations will normally require a Caesarian section. Vaginal delivery is extremely unlikely in transverse or oblique lies.

Management

- Obtain expert advice
- Ensure expert assistance is en route
- Do not attempt transfer once a presenting part is visible unless instructed to do so
- If delivery fails to proceed, follow the instructions for obstructed breech as above.

Multiple birth

This can usually be managed exactly the same as the delivery of two babies, one after the other. The babies are usually smaller than single babies and often deliver before full term. If the second twin has not appeared within 15 minutes, it is often appropriate to transfer the mother to the nearest obstetric unit for the second delivery.

NEVER give oxytocin or ergometrine until both babies have delivered

Obstructed labour

- Obtain expert advice
- Ensure that expert assistance is on its way
- Do not move the patient unless instructed to do so
- Provide analgesia.

Neonatal resuscitation

The resuscitation algorithm for neonates is shown in Fig. 12.8.

- Suctioning meconium from the nose and mouth before the delivery of the chest is ineffective and not recommended.
- For the first few breaths, the inflation pressure should be maintained for 2–3 seconds in order to assist lung expansion.
- Tracheal adrenaline is not recommended. If there is no alternative, the dose is 100μg/kg.

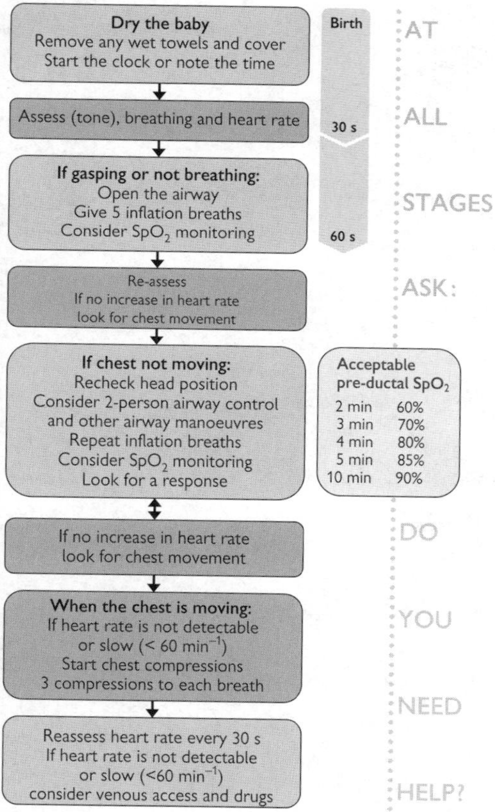

Fig. 12.8 Neonatal resuscitation algorithm. Reprinted with permission from the Resuscitation Council (UK) (2010). *Resuscition Guidelines.*

Chapter 13

Patient rescue and transportation

Immobilization and extrication

Principles of extrication

Management of the airway, breathing, and circulation (ABC) is fundamental in pre-hospital care. In general, with the exception of cervical spine control (**A**irway and cervical spine control) and control of significant external haemorrhage due to limb trauma (assessment of **C**irculation and control of external haemorrhage), fracture management and extrication follows the primary survey unless it is necessary to undertake a snatch rescue.

Entrapments are relatively common in road traffic collisions but may also be seen in industrial accidents, building collapses, and farming incidents.

At the outset, there should be consultation between the senior members of the emergency services on site to determine an extrication plan and whether any additional resources are necessary. An alternative plan should always be available.

Plan A

The likely time for extrication and the time scale that is acceptable, based on clinical need, should be determined. Providing these are acceptable, the best mode of extrication can be determined and a '*controlled extrication*' undertaken.

Plan B

An emergency extrication plan should be agreed in case the patient deteriorates. This may involve compromising some of the routine principles of patient handling, such as spinal immobilization, if there is an overriding clinical need.

Entrapment

Actual entrapment

The patient is physically held in the vehicle or area by the structure impinging on their body (for example, in road traffic collisions or by fallen masonry).

Relative entrapment

The patient is not physically trapped but is unable to extricate themselves as a result of their injuries or the pain associated with them.

Extrication from vehicles

When the scene is safe, the clinician can approach the patient, undertake a primary survey, correct ABC problems where possible, and establish monitoring which should be visible outside the vehicle. With one person in the car supporting the patient's neck (usually from behind), other rescuers should leave the car to allow the fire service to commence the extrication plan. The first priority is to make space within the vehicle and then to facilitate the agreed plan. The procedure can be halted to allow access to the patient for reassessment and interventions as necessary.

Rapid extrication

This commonly involves springing open the door of a vehicle and extrication on a spinal board either by removing the roof or through the rear hatch. Practice is essential in order to understand the principles of extrication and to be a useful member of the rescue team.

Snatch rescue

A snatch rescue is retrieval of a casualty from a difficult environment with minimal stabilization and resuscitation until a place of safety is reached. Examples include impending scene danger, fire, or the removal of a patient in cardiorespiratory arrest to facilitate resuscitation.

Principles of immobilization

The principles of immobilization are straightforward—to maintain casualty safety and comfort and do no harm.

During patient packaging, the patient should be regularly reassessed by repeating the primary survey and, in the case of significant limb trauma, by repeating a neurovascular assessment (sensation, movement, pulses, capillary refill) before and after any limb manipulation.

Reduction and immobilization of fractures is necessary to:

- Prevent further injury
- Provide pain relief
- Reduce blood loss
- Reduce the volume of fat emboli
- Facilitate extrication and rescue.

Prevention of further injury

Appropriate immobilization will reduce the risk of damage to the adjacent skin muscles, nerves, and blood vessels. Where the skin is in jeopardy, for example, in fracture dislocations of the ankle, realignment and reduction may reduce the risk of skin necrosis. Similarly, where there is distal vascular compromise, straightening of the limb will restore circulation in most cases. Protruding bone ends should be returned to a normal anatomical position once major contamination (for example, soil) has been removed.

Pain relief

Fracture immobilization reduces movement at the fracture site, reducing pain from the sensitive periosteum. In addition, painful muscle spasm may be reduced and pressure on adjacent nerves, which may result in pain, relieved.

Reduction of blood loss

The application of a traction splint reduces the potential volume into which bleeding may occur, closes down open venous channels, and restores muscle tension so reducing the overall blood loss.

Reduction of the incidence of fat emboli

Fat embolism occurs as a normal pathological process following major long bone fractures. Whether the patient develops fat embolism syndrome (pulmonary and cerebral manifestations and skin petechiae) depends on the magnitude of embolization and the degree of uncorrected hypoxia and hypovolaemia.

Immobilization of fractures reduces the incidence and magnitude of emboli from fat entering the circulation as a consequence of moving bone ends and open venous channels. Fat emboli can also occur as a result of changes in circulating chylomicrons.

Immobilization principles

- Support to either side of the fracture but avoiding direct pressure over the fracture site.
- Immobilization of the joint above and below the fracture.
- The provision of adequate analgesia (titrated opiates, ketamine, or nerve blocks).
- The reduction of gross contamination in compound factures by irrigation with saline.
- Polaroid photography of the wound at the scene. Further wound inspections are then not necessary in A&E prior to surgical management.
- Dressing of compound wounds with a sterile dressing and pad.
- Splintage.

The features of effective splints are:

- Simplicity
- Ease of use
- Lightness
- Cleanability
- Strength (to avoid damage during use)
- Interchangeability with equipment used in the A&E department.

Methods of immobilization

Cervical spine

Cervical spine immobilization can be achieved by:

- Manual stabilization
- A cervical collar, spinal board, head restraints, and straps.

A cervical collar alone does not provide adequate immobilization.

Manual stabilization

The cervical spine should be protected at the outset based on the mechanism of injury and clinical presentation. As the airway is opened or protected, the cervical spine should be immobilized manually. This can be achieved in road traffic collisions from:

- Behind the patient
- The side of the patient
- In front of the patient.

Immobilization from behind

This is the most frequently used position in road traffic collisions as it facilitates airway management by jaw thrust if required. The neck should be moved to a neutral position. If the patient is conscious, they should be directed to move their neck to achieve this. The patient should stop if they develop severe pain, pins and needles, or weakness. The patient undertaking active movement of the neck will not produce cervical cord compromise. If the patient is unconscious, the rescuer should passively move the neck to the neutral position but stop if resistance is felt and maintain stabilization in that position. Failure to restore a previously normal neck to a neutral position suggests a significant injury. Traction is not applied under any circumstances.

From behind, the rescuer places the hands on either side of the head, ensuring that the ears are not covered. The thumbs should extend upwards behind the posterior aspect of the skull and the little fingers to just under the angle of the jaw (Fig. 13.1a).

Immobilization from the side

This may be the only means of access to the patient initially. One hand supports the patient's head, with the occiput in the palm, and the other supports the jaw between the thumb and index finger. As before, the head is moved to a neutral position. (Fig. 13.1b).

Immobilization from the front

The rescuer's hands are placed over the patient's cheeks with the fingers around the neck and the extended thumbs in front of the ears over the temporomandibular joints. The head is moved to a neutral position (Fig. 13.1c).

In the supine patient, the neck is supported in a similar manner to the technique described for immobilization from behind. It is essential that the rescuer practises these techniques.

Indications for cervical spine immobilization

- Mechanism of injury
- History of unconsciousness in trauma
- Head injury in patients under the influence of alcohol and drugs

- Evidence of injuries above the clavicle
- Spinal tenderness
- Neurological signs/symptoms
- Painful distracting injuries
- Head and neck trauma (even minor) in patients with rheumatoid arthritis and ankylosing spondylitis.

Cervical collars should be correctly sized. Ambulance services currently use either a system of collars which are available in a range of sizes or single collars which are adjustable. The rescuer should be familiar with the sizing technique and adjustment and practiced in collar application.

It is important to note that:

- A collar can only be applied if the neck is in a neutral position.
- The cervical spine cannot be effectively immobilized by a collar alone. A spinal board, head blocks, and straps are also required.
- Ill-fitting collars can be harmful and produce airway compromise.
- Intracranial pressure is elevated by well-fitting collars in the unconscious patient. Once fully immobilized on a spinal board, the collar should be loosened in the unconscious patient.

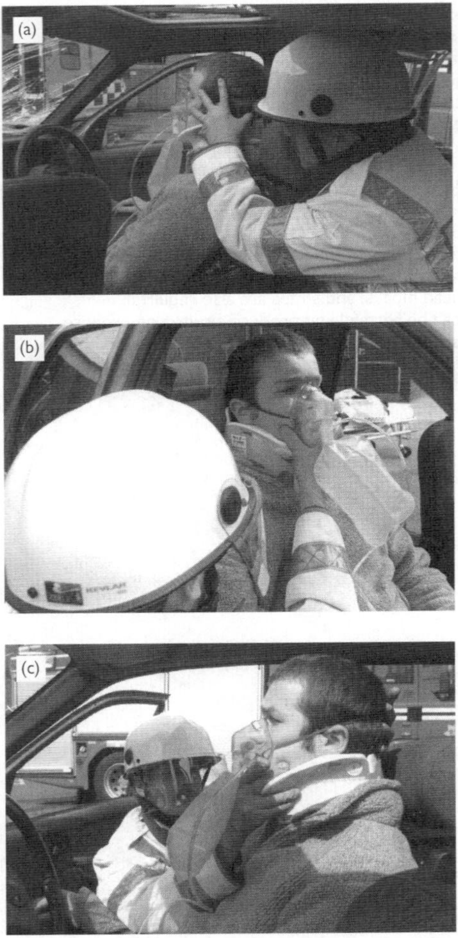

Fig. 13.1 Cervical spine immobilization (a) from behind; (b) from the side; (c) from the front. Reprinted with permission from Greaves I *et al.* (2005). *Emergency care: a textbook for paramedics*, 2nd edn. W.B. Saunders Co. Ltd.

Limb immobilization

Manual methods

Methods of self or buddy help include supporting an injured arm or chest wall at the site of an underlying fracture.

Triangular bandages

The triangular bandage is the mainstay of first aid treatment for upper limb injuries. It can be used in two ways:

- As a broad arm sling
- As a high arm sling.

In the lower limb, a broad or narrow bandage produced by folding a triangular sling two or three times, respectively, can be used to splint the legs together. Triangular bandages can also be used to secure and hold scalp dressings in place.

FRAC Straps™

These are commercially available straps with velcro and have a similar function to the broad and narrow bandages described above. They function to secure one leg to the other, with padding between the legs, or to secure the arm to the chest wall (used in conjunction with a triangular bandage) or to the side of the body.

Neighbour strapping

Neighbour strapping fingers together or one leg to the other provides some degree of support. In the case of femoral fractures, it may permit the patient to be moved to a position where more appropriate splintage can be applied. Strapping the legs together in a patient with a femoral fracture sitting in a car may facilitate extrication prior to the application of a traction splint when the patient is on an ambulance trolley cot.

Inflatable splints

These are clear plastic double-walled splints and require inflation for support. They are used less frequently than before because of the risk of over-inflation and tissue ischaemia. They are also prone to damage and deflation.

Box splints

These consist of three long padded boards and a foot piece. The patient's shoe and sock are normally removed to facilitate neurovascular assessment before the leg is placed in a splint. The foot piece is designed to hold the ankle at right angles. The outer sides of the splint are folded around the leg and secured with velcro straps. Box splints are suitable for immobilizing ankle and tibial fractures and also injuries around the knee. In the upper limb, they can be used to splint forearm and elbow injuries. The splints are available in two sizes.

Mark the location of the dorsalis pedis pulse with a cross to save time finding it next time

Traction splints

Traction splints can be used for closed and open fractures of the shaft of the femur and tibia. Without traction, they can be used to support injuries around the knee. Contraindications to their use include dislocation of the hip, fracture dislocation of the knee, and ankle injuries.

The traction splint is used to secure the leg in an improved and near reduced position. The application of traction involves securing the ankle and applying traction by distracting the device with the proximal end of the splint pressing against the pelvis (separating two fixed points).

The various types of splint include the Donway® splint, Trac3® splint, and the Sager® splint (Fig. 13.2). The attraction of the last is that it can be used to immobilize both legs (bilateral femoral fractures) at the same time.

Before and after application, the rescuer should check the patient's distal neurovascular status. The techniques for application are similar and the rescuer should be familiar with the splint used by their local ambulance service or immediate care scheme and with its application and removal. An exchange splint should be retained in the A&E department.

Before any traction splint is applied, appropriate analgesia should be given and enough assistance must be available. Two people are the minimum required for optimal application of a traction splint. Footwear should be removed and the neurovascular status of the limb must be assessed and recorded.

Donway splint (Fig. 13.2b)

The Donway splint consists of two components which, when fitted together, form a trombone-shaped unit. Only one splint can be applied and only one leg splinted. The Donway splint is bulky and protrudes some distance beyond the patient's foot.

Method of application

1. The ischial ring is placed under the thigh and the strap and buckle loosely fastened across the front of the thigh.
2. The air release valve is depressed to ensure that there is no pressure in the system and the locking screws are unlocked. The footplate is raised and placed under the patient's foot.
3. The splint is attached to the ischial ring; the side arms of the splint are extended like a trombone.
4. The casualty's foot is strapped to the foot plate.
5. The pump is used to increase the pressure within the closed 'U' of the splint which extends, applying traction to the limb. Enough pressure is applied to make the casualty comfortable (approximately 10% of body weight).
6. The supports are positioned under the leg at mid thigh and mid calf and the knee support is secured.

7. The splint stand is lowered and the locking nuts are secured to keep the splint to length.
8. The pressure is released by depressing the air release valve.

Trac 3 splint

The Trac3 and hare splints (see Fig. 13.2a) are effectively the same and share a method of application.

Method of application

1. The splint is adjusted for length against the uninjured leg. The straps are opened and correctly positioned at intervals down the leg. The correct ankle hitch is selected.
2. The hitch is placed under the ankle , the straps are folded across the front of the ankle, and the rings are brought together under the foot.
3. Manual traction is commenced with one hand and the leg supported whilst the splint is put in place. (An effective method is to log roll the patient away from the injured leg, place the splint, and roll the patient back onto the splint). The top padded ring must fit under the ischial tuberosity.
4. The top strap is done up, avoiding the external genitalia.
5. The traction hook is put through the rings and traction taken up (whilst maintaining manual traction).
6. The foot stand is raised and the Velcro straps are positioned and tightened.

The Sager splint (Fig. 13.2c)

The Sager splint is light and can be used to splint one or both femurs. It does not extend significantly beyond the end of the patient's foot. The Sager splint is the authors' splint of choice for pre-hospital use.

Method of application

1. The cushioned 'seat' of the splint is placed between the patient's legs, against the perineum and symphysis pubis. Care should be taken not to trap the external genitalia. The top strap is fastened around the thigh.
2. The splint is extended until the ankle hitch lies at the normal heel position.
3. The ankle harness is applied behind the heel and wrapped around the malleoli and the cushions adjusted to fit the leg.
4. Traction is applied until the patient is comfortable (approximately 10% of body weight).
5. The thigh strap is tightened and lower straps secured.
6. An identical method is used if both legs are being splinted.

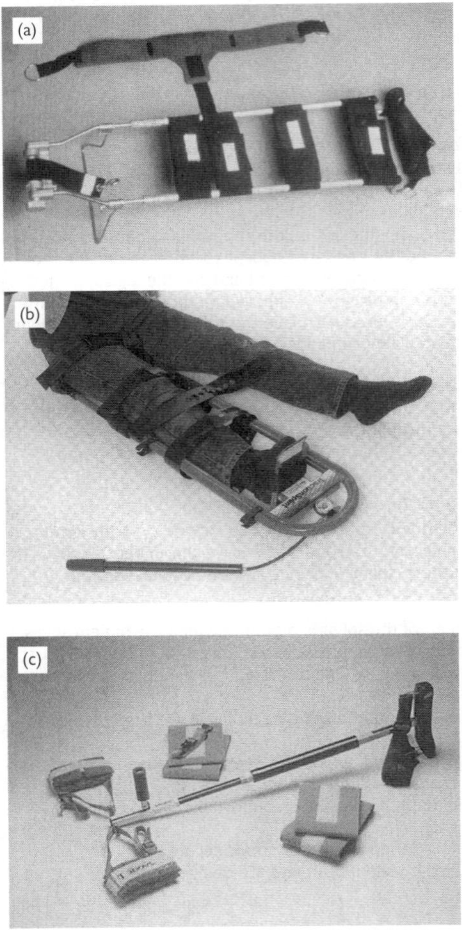

Fig. 13.2 Types of traction splint: (a). Donway; (b). Trac 3; (c). Sager. Figs. 13.2a,b reprinted with permission from Greaves I and Porter K (1997). *Pre-hospital medicine—the principles and practice of immediate care*. Edward Arnold. Fig. 13.2c reprinted with permission from Greaves I *et al.* (2005). *Emergency care: a textbook for paramedics*, 2nd edn. W.B. Saunders Co. Ltd.

Contraindications to traction splintage

- Injuries at the ankle
- Dislocation of the knee
- Fractures around the knee (apply without traction)
- Dislocation of the hip
- Fracture of the pelvis.

Pneumatic antishock garment (PASG)

Also known as the military antishock trouser (MAST) suit, this is an inflatable garment that covers the legs and abdomen and can be inflated to a pressure of 100mmHg. It can be used to:

- Splint fractures of the pelvis and lower limbs
- Facilitate inter-hospital transfer of patients with intra-abdominal bleeding
- Provide some degree of tamponade for patients with ruptured abdominal aortic aneurysms.

It is no longer recommended for use in the treatment of hypovolaemic shock because of the catastrophic deterioration that can occur when the splint is deflated. If it is used to facilitate remote transfer, adequate fluid replacement must proceed at the same time. Specific contraindications for its use include:

- Cardiac failure
- Pulmonary oedema
- Significant chest injuries
- Diaphragmatic rupture
- Advanced pregnancy.

The PASG is difficult and time consuming to apply and its application will delay transfer to hospital. It is therefore contraindicated in all but the most prolonged transfers.

Methods of extrication

Extrication devices

A number of extrication devices are in use in the UK, all of which are fairly similar in design and use. They include the:

- Kendrick extrication device (KED)
- Russell extrication device (RED)
- ED 2000
- Telford extrication device (TED).

These have been introduced to replace the short spinal board. They provide support and stabilization particularly to the upper spine. Whilst maintaining inline manual stabilization and with the patient wearing a cervical collar, the splint is inserted behind the patient by moving the whole patient slightly forward in the sitting position or by retracting the seat. The patient is secured to the device by a series of straps around the trunk and by straps that go around the legs to secure the splint in the groins. Finally, the cervical spine is immobilized using the supporting neck side pieces of the splint. These are secured in place by two velcro straps, one across the forehead, the other across the cervical collar. The splint is provided with lifting handles to facilitate easy and safe movement.

Scoop stretcher

The scoop stretcher provides a means of lifting a patient from a horizontal position onto a trolley cot. It can be split in half longitudinally and is applied from both sides of the patient. It has a supporting head cushion and the bottom part of each component must be extended to fit the patient before application. The two parts of the stretcher are placed one on each side of the patient (ensuring that the narrower foot end is at the patient's feet), then the two components are locked first at the top end and then at the feet. It may be necessary to lift the pelvis slightly to facilitate distal locking of the splint and to ensure that the buttocks are not pinched between the two sides of the stretcher. The patient can be moved in the position they are found, an airway protected position, or supine position. The scoop stretcher can be used as a means of transportation for short journey times or as a means of lifting a patient onto a vacuum mattress or trolley cot.

Spinal boards

Spinal boards are used to facilitate extrication. They provide a stable secure base to which the patient is strapped for full spinal immobilization. Although not designed as a transport device, in UK ambulance practice, spinal boards are commonly used on top of the trolley cot to transfer the patient to hospital. There is a risk of the patient developing pressure sores on the board, especially in those patients with neurological injuries. If the transport time is likely to be more than 20 minutes, consideration should be given to scooping the patient off the spinal board and onto a vacuum mattress.

In hospital, the patient should be removed from the board at the earliest opportunity. In patients with significant trauma, this is normally undertaken at the completion of the primary survey. In non-urgent cases, for example where the board is used as a precautionary measure and where there will be delay in the A&E until the patient is seen by a member of the medical staff, the patient should be log rolled off the board after the first set of stable clinical observations. The patient is then secured on the hospital trolley using sandbags and tape.

Extrication using a long spine board

In road traffic collisions, whilst inline stabilization is maintained and the whole spine supported, the patient can be carefully manoeuvred onto the board in order to carry out a controlled extrication.

The most common approach is to insert the spinal board horizontally through the open door of the vehicle, placing the end of the board on the seat adjacent to the patient's thigh. The patient can then be turned and gently laid backwards onto the board which can then be removed. If the roof has been removed, the board can be inserted behind the patient who can then be laid back against it and moved along the board in a controlled fashion.

If the patient is lying supine, they can be loaded onto the spinal board using a supervised log rolling technique. Alternatively, a scoop stretcher can be used to lift the patient onto the spinal board. All rescuers should be familiar with the technique of log rolling and the use of the scoop stretcher, spinal board, and extrication techniques.

Vacuum splints/mattresses

Vacuum splints/mattresses provide rigid support and can conform to a deformed limb or to the body itself. The splints or mattress consist of a strong, tough, plastic material skin which contains polystyrene beads. Removal of the air from between the beads in the skin makes the splint rigid. The whole body vacuum mattress is a good immobilization device but is unsuitable for lifting.

Vacuum immobilization devices can be used for:

- Limb trauma (upper and lower)
- Spinal injuries
- Inter-hospital transfer of patients with multiple injuries.

Stretchers

The scoop stretcher (described above) is most commonly used and is standard equipment on UK ambulances.

Other forms of stretcher for specific rescue situations are:

- The Neil Robertson stretcher
- The Paraguard stretcher.

The Neil Robertson® stretcher is a canvas stretcher with wooden slats sewn into the canvas and straps to secure the splint in place. The stretcher is then reinforced by poles which have carrying handles. The Paraguard® stretcher is a similar device which is capable of bending around obstacles to facilitate extrication.

Transport in pre-hospital care

Pre-hospital care practitioners are not only responsible for the safe packaging and transport of patients, but must ensure their own arrival at an incident scene in a safe and timely manner.

Medical transport

The immediate care doctor most commonly uses their own private vehicle adapted to the response role:

- A green rotating beacon can be used when proceeding to an emergency/accident (Road Traffic Act 1976). The doctor must be familiar with the legal requirements of this Act.
- In some areas, doctors acting as agents of the ambulance service have special arrangements with the police to use blue flashing lights and audible devices.
- Appropriate car markings approved by the BASICS Equipment Committee are designed for ease of identification of the doctor and for safety.

All doctors who take responsibility for providing a rapid response should undergo specific driver training through the police or ambulance services. BASICS have their own specific driving courses and advanced driving techniques form part of the courses run by the Royal Society for the Prevention of Accidents (RoSPA)

Patient transfer vehicles

Historically, ambulance designs have paralleled those of light chassis vehicles with a coach built body. Gissane and Rothwell from the Birmingham Accident Hospital (UK) were the first to produce a prototype design with the capability to lower the floor of the ambulance to the ground.

A road ambulance may not be the ideal method of transport, particularly for time-critical injuries or illnesses with a long travelling time to hospital. Access may be difficult in rural and remote areas. The use, therefore, of off-road four-wheel drive vehicles or helicopters may be more appropriate.

Mode of transport

The pre-hospital care practitioner should be familiar with:

- The limitations of the vehicle being used
- The effects of the mode of transport on the patient
- The effects of the mode of transport on the medical equipment being used during transit
- The effect of the mode of transport in limiting possible medical interventions
- The importance of correct patient packaging, handling, and loading.

Limitations of the vehicle

UK frontline ambulances conventionally have a single trolley cot which can be secured to the side or centrally, the latter giving increased patient access. Further developments have resulted in the addition of extra equipment and redesign of the cabin layout.

The ergonomics of ambulances are not ideal. Deceleration forces in braking potentially increase intracranial pressure. Ideally, therefore, the patient should be loaded and transported feet first, which is not possible in rear loading vehicles. Vertical forces in passing over road humps and bumps are also a problem and the patient would be best positioned over the area of the wheel base. Most vehicles are designed so that the suspension functions best at 30 miles an hour and there is, therefore, no justification for slow transfer (for example, of spinal injury patients).

Helicopters have their own limitations:

- Limited to flying in daylight hours (civilian helicopters)
- Unable to fly during adverse weather conditions
- Constrained by strict safety regulations governed by the helicopter operator and the Civil Aviation Authority
- Unsuitable for the transfer of certain groups of patients (for example, heavily pregnant females and psychiatrically unstable patients)
- Prone to mechanical problems and require regular servicing.

Effects of the mode of transport on the patient

The problems of deceleration and patient positioning have been previously discussed in relation to land vehicles. Some patients develop motion sickness in transit or become claustrophobic, particularly in smaller helicopters. Fear of flying (or crashing!) may also prevent aeromedical evacuation of some casualties. A prophylactic antiemetic should be given to those patients who admit to travel sickness.

There are potential problems flying patients in non-pressurized aircraft. However, all helicopters in the UK fly at an altitude which will not markedly affect pressure either within air-filled equipment (such as the cuff of an endotracheal tube) or potential sites of injury (pneumothoraces, hollow abdominal viscera). There is no need, therefore, to fill ET tube cuffs with water, although, where relevant, the placement of thoracostomy tubes before take off should be considered since this intervention is likely to be difficult or impossible in flight.

Effects of the mode of transport on the medical equipment being used during transport

Equipment carried on frontline ambulances, including helicopters, is approved by the appropriate authorities for safe patient use during transport. Motion and vibration may effect ECG monitoring which is susceptible to picking up electromagnetic radiation. Pulse oximeters may also be affected by vibration. Although defibrillators are approved for in-flight use, most helicopter services would elect to commence appropriate life support measures in the event of patient collapse and to land the helicopter prior to defibrillation.

In the case of inter-hospital transfer of intensive care unit patients, there may be problems with incompatibility of equipment and the availability of sockets for syringe drivers. It is essential that there is regular liaison between the ambulance service and hospital staff to determine a standard of equipment which will facilitate safe inter-hospital transport.

Effects of the mode of transport in limiting possible medical interventions

A time-critical emergency will dictate on-scene times (in non-entrapment) and also the urgency with which hospital should be reached. When using land-based transportation, a quick ABC assessment and appropriate interventions can be performed, followed by loading onto a spinal board. Monitoring and intravenous access can be established en route to hospital. Liaison between ambulance crew personnel should ensure that the vehicle is going steadily in a straight line when cannulation is attempted. In the event of a cardiorespiratory arrest, the ambulance should stop safely and both crew members should undertake resuscitation.

The relatively confined space of a helicopter and the associated noise makes further assessment (for example, listening to the chest) difficult and puts a reliance on monitoring. The patient should have an adequate ABC assessment and any necessary interventions should be undertaken prior to loading. Intravenous cannulae should be secure. Following packaging it should, however, be possible to make an ABCD reassessment. An in-flight emergency may best be managed by landing the helicopter.

Awareness of importance of correct patient packaging, handling, and loading

Patient handling, loading, and package should be standard practice and compliant with normal manual handling techniques. Patients should be secured on a spinal board, if indicated, and then on to an ambulance trolley cot with access for ABC assessment and monitoring and to any cannulae inserted for administration of drugs and fluids.

Care in transit should include:

- Routine reassessment and monitoring of the patient including a non-invasive blood pressure, pulse rate, respiratory rate, pulse oximetry, and ECG monitoring.
- Completion of appropriate documentation. In the case of seriously injured patients, this is often undertaken after handover of the patient in the emergency department.

Aeromedical evacuation

In many respects, ambulance helicopters are simply ambulances that fly. They do, however, have the ability to fly direct from A to B, therefore reducing transfer time both to the scene and from the scene to the hospital. Air ambulances therefore have a major role in reducing morbidity and mortality in time-critical medical or trauma emergencies (for example, cardiac arrests and major trauma).

Indications for air ambulance use include:
- 999 calls greater than 15 miles or 10 minutes travelling for the nearest land base
- Difficult access to or egress from the scene
- Difficult road terrain including speed bumps. (Particular examples include river banks, large golf courses outside football complexes).
- Weather conditions which allow flying but make land access difficult (flooding, heavy snowfall).

Other potential advantages are:
- Preservation of an essential land-based resource 'freed up' by a helicopter undertaking a long distance transfer
- Provision of a quicker response to rural and remote incidence
- Proven benefit in severe trauma in remote and rural areas
- Transportation of the patient to a hospital that best suits their clinical needs
- Provision of care to lesser emergencies where there are time delays due to difficult access (for example, a patient out in the hills with a fractured ankle)
- Delivery of a doctor or medical team and equipment direct to the scene.

The helicopter is an underused resource for medical emergencies and could assist in achieving compliance with national service frameworks, for example, coronary heart disease. Helicopters do not have an appreciable effect on ORCON performance.

Disadvantages of air ambulances Include:
- Daylight hours' flying only
- Inability to fly in adverse weather conditions
- Requirement for a landing site adjacent to the A & E department
- Need to ensure the patient is appropriately packaged prior to loading
- Limited room for procedures to be undertaken in flight.

Aircrew

London HEMS provides a continuously medically manned service. The Lincolnshire Air Ambulance and the Warwickshire Air Ambulance have doctors as part of the regular air crew. The other services usually have two well trained paramedics as the basis of their response. Aircraft pilots are specifically tasked with the safe flying of the aircraft and are not involved in any medical care.

Regulations

In the UK, the Civil Aviation Authority covers aviation practice and there are clear definitions relating to mission types, crew types, and the use of the aircraft. The providers of a helicopter service must have an Air Operations Certificate (AOC). The Joint Aviation Authority (JAA) has defined two types of crew and two types of mission:
- ***HEMS crew members***—these are normally paramedics or doctors who have been specifically trained and are assigned to the HEMS flight to provide medical assistance to the patient and assist the pilot during a mission with such roles as navigation and air craft radios.

- ***Medical passenger***—a medical person, usually a doctor, nurse, or paramedic who is carried during a HEMS flight and whose role is directly focused on the patient care. No specific training is necessary other than pre-flight briefing.
- ***Helicopter air ambulance flight***—is a pre-planned flight requiring medical assistance where immediate transportation is not essential, for example, an inter-hospital transfer between dedicated landing sites.
- ***Helicopter emergency medical service (HEMS) flight***—a flight by helicopter for the purpose of emergency medical assistance where immediate and rapid transportation is essential for medical personnel, supplies, or ill or injured patients.

Safety

Safety regulations apply to the flight crew and emergency service personnel should be briefed on ground safety issues. Important considerations include:

- The danger of walking into the tail rota.
- The dangers of the main rota if the aircraft has landed on uneven ground or the rotas are displaced when it is windy.

As a consequence, a helicopter should never be approached unless the pilot has given a clear signal to do so.

- Only trained air crew should be allowed to move equipment and patients in and out of the aircraft when possible.

At the scene

The pilot has the ultimate decision with regard to the landing site. An ideal landing site, at a minimum, should be twice the diameter of the rotating blades. In the case of the Bolkow 105 or Squirrel helicopter, this is about 25 metres in diameter or approximately half the size of a tennis court. The ground should be firm and flat, free of debris, and away from any power or telephone lines. The site should be kept clear of people at the time of landing and those near by should be instructed to look away as the downdraft close to landing may blow foreign objects into their eyes.

Choice of aircraft

The size of the helicopter and its engine performance will determine restrictions such as the number of crew and the amount of equipment that can be carried. Wind speed, atmospheric pressure, and temperature all affect performance. The weight that can be carried varies from day to day; on very hot summer days, performance is reduced and appropriate measures to lighten the load will be necessary. This may involve reducing the number of people carried, the medical equipment, or fuel.

Aircraft used in the UK

Aerospatiale Dauphin

This has a large cabin and can carry two patients and two medical crew. It can be a single or twin pilot operation. Access to the patient is complete from head to toe.

Aerospatiale Squirrel

This is a smaller aircraft, usually crewed by a pilot and two medical crew. It is normally used to carry a single patient, although a double fit is possible. Access is to one side of the upper body only, making in-flight procedures very difficult.

Bolkow 105

This is a twin engine aircraft with a small interior cabin which limits the number of patients to one and medical crew to two. The second crew member acts as a navigator. Access to the lower half of the patient is limited in flight.

Bolkow 135

Larger than the 105, the 135 has the additional capacity to carry a medical passenger.

Other helicopters

These include the search and rescue helicopters of the Royal Navy and Royal Air Force. The Sea King helicopter is suitable for long-range transfers in difficult conditions and at night. Military helicopters are not subject to CAA rules regarding night flying.

Chapter 14

Sporting events and mass gatherings

Mass gathering medicine

A mass gathering is defined as a collection of 1000 people or more.

Legal requirements

The number and diversity of casualties depends on:

- The nature of the event
- The venue
- The attendees
- The climate.

For example, politically related marches and derby football matches are often associated with hostile crowds and violent situations, often compounded by the effects of alcohol. Peaceful gatherings (for example, summer fetes) may produce few casualties from the event itself but will produce the usual number of day-to-day minor and major emergencies.

Depending on the nature of the event, the incidence of casualties is variably reported to be between 0.11 per thousand to 9.0 per thousand. At pop concerts, 1–2% of the audience will seek medical assistance during the event of which approximately 10% will need treatment on site. Approximately 1% of those needing medical assistance will require referral to hospital. These figures may be significantly altered by adverse weather conditions, poor facilities, and alcohol abuse.

Landmark events in mass gathering medicine in the UK include:

- The Ibrox Park football disaster, 1972
- The Bradford fire, 1985
- The Hillsborough Stadium disaster, 1989.

Following the Wheatley Report into crowd safety after the Ibrox Park incident, *The Guide to Safety at Sports Grounds* (commonly referred to as *The Green Guide*) was produced in 1973 and has subsequently been revised. This was followed shortly afterwards by the *Safety at Sports Grounds Act 1975* stipulating legislation for safety at certain grounds.

Following Lord Justice Taylor's report into the Hillsborough Stadium disaster in 1989, the medical arrangements for football league grounds were reviewed in the Gibson Report and, as a consequence, the concept of crowd doctor was developed and an acceptable level of clinical competence was defined. It is currently recommended that all doctors attend an appropriate pre-hospital care course run by the Football Association in conjunction with the Faculty of Pre-hospital Care of the College of Surgeons of Edinburgh and that all such doctors should be the holder of the Diploma in Immediate Medical Care, again of the Royal College of Surgeons of Edinburgh.

The Gibson Report for football ground events made the following recommendations:

- One first aider per 1000 spectators
- One or more first aid rooms with appropriate equipment
- A doctor should be present if the attendance is about 2000 or more
- One ambulance with a paramedic crew should be present if the crowd is above 5000
- 5000–25,000 attendance—one A&E ambulance (with a paramedic crew) plus one ambulance officer
- 25,000–45,000 attendance—one A&E ambulance (with a paramedic crew) plus one ambulance officer, one major incident equipment vehicle and a paramedic crew, and one control unit
- 45,000 or more attendance—two A&E ambulances (with paramedic crews) plus one ambulance officer, one major incident equipment vehicle and a paramedic crew, and one control unit.

Contingency planning

All stadia should have a contingency plan for emergencies as well as a major incident plan. The suggested recommendations for a contingency plan include the following, which can be adapted to fit most situations:

- Fire
- Bomb threat, suspect package
- Buildings and services
  - Damage to structures
  - Power cut or failure
  - Gas leak or chemical incident
- Safety equipment failure
  - Turnstile counting mechanism
  - Closed circuit television
  - Public address system
  - Electronic information boards
  - Stewards' radio system
  - Internal telephone systems
- Crowd control
  - Surging or crushing
  - Pitch incursion
  - Late arrivals or delayed start
  - Lock outs
  - Disorder inside the ground
  - Large-scale ticket forgery
  - Emergency evacuation
  - Ticketing strategy in the event of an abandoned fixture
  - Features/considerations specific to the location.

Each stadium should have its own major incident plan which has been agreed by all involved in the major incident response including the planning officers, emergency services, and health and safety organizations. It should be noted that a paramedic, for the purpose of mass gathering medicine, is a person who holds a current certificate of proficiency in ambulance paramedic skills as issued by the Institute of Health Care and Development and who has immediate access to appropriate levels of specialist equipment including drug therapy as per their normal practice. In addition, a paramedic crew, as a minimum, consists of a paramedic and IHCD trained technician.

Any practitioner who is involved in providing support at mass gathering events should be familiar with the *Guide to Safety at Sports Grounds* (*Green Guide*) (4th edn, 2003) and the *Event Safety Guide* (1999, reprinted 2002). In addition, the practitioner should be familiar with the major incident plan and, most importantly, take part in regular major incident exercises.

Index

B

D

E

T